STUDIES IN GLOBAL EQUITY

GLOBAL HEALTH CHALLENGES FOR HUMAN SECURITY

STUDIES IN GLOBAL EQUITY

GLOBAL HEALTH CHALLENGES FOR HUMAN SECURITY

EDITED BY

LINCOLN CHEN, JENNIFER LEANING,
AND VASANT NARASIMHAN

PUBLISHED BY
GLOBAL EQUITY INITIATIVE
ASIA CENTER
HARVARD UNIVERSITY

DISTRIBUTED BY HARVARD UNIVERSITY PRESS
CAMBRIDGE, MASSACHUSETTS AND LONDON, ENGLAND 2003

Library of Congress Cataloging-in-Publication Data

Global health challenges for human security / edited by Lincoln Chen, Jennifer Leaning, and Vasant Narasimhan.
   p. ; cm.
Includes bibliographical references and index.
  ISBN 0-674-01453-7 (alk. paper)
  1. World health. 2. Medical policy—International cooperation. 3. Globalization—Health aspects. 4. Epidemics. 5. Poverty. 6. Basic needs.
  [DNLM: 1. World Health. 2. Disease Outbreaks. 3. Health Policy. 4. International Cooperation. 5. Poverty. 6. Security Measures. 7. Violence. WA 530.1 G5625 2003] I. Chen, Lincoln C. II. Leaning, Jennifer. III. Narasimhan, Vasant. IV. Global Equity Initiative. V. Harvard University. Asia Center.
  RA441.G567 2003
  362.1'0422—dc22

                                        2003022886

Executive Editor: Patricia M. Tyler, Newton, MA USA
Design and Production: Digital Design Group, Newton, MA USA
Printed by Webcom Ltd, Toronto, Ontario, Canada
Cover photograph: © Copyright United Nations (Operation Lifeline Sudan) UN/DPI Photo #187725C

TABLE OF CONTENTS

AUTHOR AFFILIATIONS VII

PREFACE XV

INTRODUCTION.. XVII

SECTION I: HISTORY, ETHICS, AND POLICIES

1. A HUMAN SECURITY AGENDA FOR GLOBAL HEALTH 3
   Lincoln Chen and Vasant Narasimhan

2. HUMAN SECURITY AND CONFLICT: A COMPREHENSIVE APPROACH. 13
   Jennifer Leaning, Sam Arie, Gilbert Holleufer, and
   Claude Bruderlein

3. HEALTH AND SECURITY IN HISTORICAL PERSPECTIVE 31
   Simon Szreter

4. BIOETHICS, HUMAN SECURITY, AND GLOBAL HEALTH 53
   Giovanni Berlinguer

5. HEALTH AND SECURITY FOR A GLOBAL CENTURY 67
   Jonas Gahr Støre, Jonathan Welch, and Lincoln Chen

SECTION II: GLOBAL EPIDEMICS

6. HEALTH AND SECURITY: GLOBALIZATION OF INFECTIOUS
   DISEASES 87
   Mary E. Wilson

7. EVOLVING INFECTIOUS DISEASE THREATS TO NATIONAL AND
   GLOBAL SECURITY 105
   David L. Heymann

8. HIV/AIDS: THE SECURITY ISSUE OF A LIFETIME 125
   Alex de Waal

9. AIDS: A THREAT TO HUMAN SECURITY 141
   Olive Shisana, Nompumelelo Zungu-Dirwayi, and
   William Shisana

SECTION III: VIOLENCE AND RISKS

10. VIOLENCE AND HUMAN SECURITY: POLICY LINKAGES 161
    David R. Meddings, Douglas W. Bettcher, and Roya Ghafele

11. GENDER, HEALTH, AND SECURITY 181
    Sonali Johnson and Claudia García-Moreno

12. HEALTH PROBLEMS AS SECURITY RISKS: GLOBAL BURDEN OF
    DISEASE ASSESSMENTS 209
    Kenji Shibuya

SECTION IV: POVERTY AND HEALTH ACTION

13. HUMAN SECURITY AND PRIMARY HEALTH CARE IN ASIA:
    REALITIES AND CHALLENGES 233
    Mely Caballero-Anthony

14. HARNESSING SOCIAL CAPITAL FOR HEALTH, SECURITY, AND
    DEVELOPMENT IN BANGLADESH 257
    Alayne M. Adams and Mushtaque Chowdhury

15. LIVELIHOOD SECURITY THROUGH COMMUNITY-BASED HEALTH
    INSURANCE IN INDIA 277
    Mirai Chatterjee and M. Kent Ranson

INDEX 301

AUTHOR AFFILIATIONS

Alayne M. Adams is Assistant Professor in the Department of Population and Family Health at Columbia University's Mailman School of Public Health. She received her doctorate in Public Health from the London School of Hygiene and Tropical Medicine, and pursued postdoctoral studies as a MacArthur Fellow at Harvard University's Center for Population and Development Studies. Her research interests focus on the social and behavioral aspects of health, including women's social networks, poverty, gender and HIV/AIDS, and community-based approaches to health promotion. In addition to longstanding research activities in Mali, West Africa, Dr. Adams sustains an active collaboration with the Research and Evaluation Division of BRAC, a large NGO in Bangladesh, and with Right to Play, a humanitarian NGO.

Sam Arie contributed to this paper while studying for a master's degree in Public Administration at Harvard's Kennedy School of Government. After graduating, he worked in the World Bank's Poverty Reduction and Economic Management sector, where he contributed to social sector expenditure analysis in Cameroon and Mali, and was responsible for the preparation of a public expenditure review in the Democratic Republic of Congo. He has also worked for the Asian Development Bank in Manila, and currently works for the Boston Consulting Group in London.

Giovanni Berlinguer is a physician and Professor Emeritus at *La Sapienza* University in Rome. He was Professor of Social Medicine from 1969 to 1974, and of Occupational Health from 1974 to 1999. He served as President of the National Bioethics Committee (1999-2001) and as a member of the National Health Council (1994-1997) and the International Bioethics Committee of UNESCO (2001-2003). He was also a member of the Board of the *International Journal of Health Services* and of the Global Equity in Health Initiative (1996-2001), and he delivered the opening conference at the World Congress of Bioethics (Brazil, 2002) on Bioethics, Power, and Injustice. He has published many articles in Italy and in international journals, and 43 books, including his latest, *Bioetica Quotidiana* (Florence, 2000), translated as *Everyday Bioethics: Reflections on Bioethical Choices in Daily Life* (Baywood, 2003).

Douglas W. Bettcher is the Coordinator of the Framework Convention on Tobacco Control team, Tobacco Free Initiative at the World Health Organization in Geneva. He holds a Ph.D. in International Relations from the London School of Economics and Political Science, and a Doctor of Medicine degree from the University of Alberta, Canada. Dr. Bettcher sits on the Editorial Boards of the *Bulletin of the World Health Organization* and *Global Governance*, and is a Vice Chair of the public health interest group of the American Society of International Law. He has written widely on several topics, including globalization and health, foreign policy and health security, international law and public health, tobacco control, and trade and health policy issues.

Claude Bruderlein is the Director of the Program on Humanitarian Policy and Conflict Research at the Harvard School of Public Health. He has been engaged in international humanitarian protection since 1985. He has a law degree from the University of Geneva Law School, with a specialization in international law, and a master's degree in law from the Harvard Law School. In 1996, he joined the United Nations in New York as Special Advisor on Humanitarian Affairs. Mr. Bruderlein has written extensively on the role of nonstate actors in the implementation of humanitarian law and on human security challenges in conflict areas. His research and policy interests include human security, conflict management and prevention strategies, law in transitional societies, and the innovative use of information technology to develop conflict prevention strategies. He teaches at the Harvard Law School and the Harvard School of Public Health.

Mely Caballero-Anthony is Assistant Professor at the Institute of Defence and Strategic Studies (IDSS) in Singapore. Her research interests include regionalism and regional security in the Asia Pacific region, multilateral security cooperation, politics and international relations in ASEAN, conflict prevention and management, and human security. She has been heavily involved in Track II work, having run the Secretariat of the Council for Security Cooperation in the Asia Pacific (CSCAP) from 1997 to 2001, and as a member of the ASEAN Institutes of Strategic and International Studies (ASEAN-ISIS) network.

Mirai Chatterjee is Coordinator of Social Security at the Self-Employed Women's Association (SEWA), a 700,000-strong labor union of workers of the informal economy. Ms. Chatterjee has been with SEWA since 1984 and served as its General Secretary from 1996 to 1999. She earned a master's degree in public health from John's Hopkins University, and currently serves on the board of several India-based organizations, including Friend's of Women's World Banking, affiliated with Women's World Banking of New York and HealthWatch. Ms. Chatterjee is based in Ahmedabad, India, and is the author of several papers and articles on organizing and women's empowerment, health, population, and development issues.

Lincoln Chen is Director of the Global Equity Initiative at Harvard University and a member of the Commission on Human Security. His previous positions include Executive Vice President for Strategy at the Rockefeller Foundation, Taro Takemi Professor of International Health at the Harvard School of Public Health, Director of the Harvard Center for Population and Development Studies, Representative of the Ford Foundation in India, and Scientific Director of the International Center for Diarrheal Disease Research in Bangladesh. Dr. Chen has an M.D. from Harvard Medical School and an MPH from Johns Hopkins University. He has published extensively on world social development, especially in health, population, and food and nutrition, and is a member of the American and World Academies of Arts and Sciences.

Mushtaque Chowdhury, MSc, Ph.D. (London), is Deputy Executive Director of BRAC, one of the largest indigenous NGOs in the world. He has wide research and program interest in health, education, poverty alleviation, and the environment, and has published extensively in journals and books. He maintains professional associations with various national and international initiatives including the Global Alliance for Vaccines and Immunizations, Global Equity Gauge Alliance, and Bangladesh Health Equity Watch. Currently Dr. Chowdhury is a Visiting Professor at Columbia University, on sabbatical from BRAC.

Alex de Waal is a writer and activist who has worked since 1984 on issues of war, famine, human rights, and governance in Africa. He currently serves as Program Director of the Commission for HIV/AIDS and Governance in Africa (CHGA) at the Economic Commission for Africa. Dr. de Waal obtained a DPhil in social anthropology at Oxford University. He is author of numerous articles and eight books, including *Demilitarising the Mind: African Agendas for Peace and Security* (Africa World Press, 2002). Previously he worked for African Rights, InterAfrica Group, and Human Rights Watch, and was Chairman of the Mines Advisory Group.

Claudia García-Moreno is Coordinator, Gender and Coordinator, WHO Multicountry Study on Women's Health and Domestic Violence Against Women, in the Department of Gender and Women's Health, World Health Organization. García-Moreno is a Medical Doctor with a master's degree in community medicine from the London School of Hygiene and Tropical Medicine. She has worked more than fifteen years in public health in Latin America, Africa, and Asia, particularly in primary health care and women's health, including reproductive health. She was Chief of Women's Health in the World Health Organization from 1994 to 1998 and is now responsible for work on gender and on violence against women. She has published extensively on issues relating to gender, women's health, and violence against women.

Roya Ghafele has a background in international affairs and international history. She studied at Johns Hopkins University, the Sorbonne, and Vienna University. Her Ph.D. on *Globalization, Africa, and the WTO* was awarded by the Austrian President. She gained professional experience with McKinsey & Company and UNIDIR. At present she is working with the OECD analyzing levels of market openness in France and Germany.

David L. Heymann is currently Executive Director of the World Health Organization (WHO) Communicable Diseases Cluster. From 1995 to 1998 he was Director of the WHO Program on Emerging and other Communicable Diseases Surveillance and Control; previously he was Chief of Research Activities in the Global Program on AIDS. Dr. Heymann also spent thirteen years working as a medical epidemiologist in sub-Saharan Africa on assignment for the U.S. Centers for Disease Control and Prevention (CDC). In Africa, Dr. Heymann investigated the first outbreaks of Ebola in the 1970s, and in 1995 directed the international response to the Ebola outbreak. Dr. Heymann holds an M.D. from Wake Forest University and a diploma in Tropical Medicine and Hygiene from the London School of Hygiene and Tropical Medicine. He has published 139 scientific articles on infectious diseases in peer-reviewed medical and scientific journals.

Gilbert Holleufer was for 13 years a delegate with the International Committee of the Red Cross (ICRC). In 1999, as a communication advisor at ICRC headquarters, he launched and participated in the implementation of the People on War project, a randomized inquiry in 12 countries that surveyed 12,000 ordinary people exposed to recent wars about their war experience and their opinions on issues such as the rules of war and international intervention. From 2000 to 2001 he was a Visiting Fellow at the Harvard School of Public Health, during which time he conducted an in-depth analysis of the quantitative and focus group data that resulted from the People on War consultation.

Sonali Johnson has a background in Asian History and an MSc in gender and development from the London School of Economics. She has worked in the department of Gender and Women's Health at the World Health Organization for the last two years, and has contributed to several publications on gender and women's health issues. She has also written on the health implications of using skin whitening products in India.

Jennifer Leaning is Professor of International Health at the Harvard School of Public Health, where she directs the Program on Humanitarian Crises and Human Rights, and Assistant Professor of Medicine at Harvard Medical School. She holds academic degrees from the Harvard School of Public Health and the University of Chicago Pritzker School of Medicine, and is board certified in both internal medicine and emergency medicine. Dr. Leaning has written widely on problems of disaster response and human rights. Her research and policy interests include problems of international human rights and humanitarian law, humanitarian crises, and medical ethics in settings of disaster and emergency. She serves on the board of directors of Physicians for Human Rights (where she was a founding board member), Physicians for Social Responsibility, The Humane Society of the United States, and the Massachusetts Bay Chapter of the American Red Cross.

David R. Meddings works in the Department of Injuries and Violence Prevention of the World Health Organization, where he coordinates a multicountry study examining the health impacts of small arms-related violence. He holds Doctor of Medicine and Master's of Health Sciences degrees. His clinical work in humanitarian contexts began in Africa in 1989. In 1990 he began a series of missions in conflict areas with the International Committee of the Red Cross (ICRC), and served as epidemiologist for the ICRC at their Geneva headquarters from 1997 to 2002. He has published in the medical literature on civilian involvement in modern conflicts, the direct and indirect effects of armed violence, and patterns of weapon use and wounding in highly militarized settings.

Vasant Narasimhan is a research fellow at the Global Equity Initiative at Harvard University and a consultant to the Rockefeller Foundation. He most recently served on the transition team of the new Director-General of the World Health Organization as a strategy advisor. He has previously served a number of country health programs, including Botswana's national AIDS treatment program with the Merck-Gates Initiative, the Peruvian Ministry of Health through the PARTNERS tuberculosis program, and multiple African AIDS treatment program sites through the Harvard AIDS Institute. His research experience includes the financing and operations of malaria control, the economics of disease outbreaks, the impact of global human resources for health crises, and child health in India. He is a graduate of Harvard Medical School and the John F. Kennedy School of Government.

M. Kent Ranson is a Lecturer in the Health Policy Unit, London School of Hygiene and Tropical Medicine, and a Research Coordinator, Self-Employed Women's Association Insurance (Vimo SEWA). Dr. Ranson has degrees in clinical medicine (M.D., McMaster University), public health epidemiology and biostatistics (MPD, Harvard University), and health economics and financing (Ph.D., University of London). He is currently heading a three-year research project to assess several interventions aimed at optimizing the equity impact of Vimo SEWA. His other research interests include the cost-effectiveness of public health interventions (anti-tobacco, anti-malaria, and anti-trachoma-blindness) and the identification and measurement of characteristics of health systems that prevent implementation of the most cost-effective interventions.

Kenji Shibuya has doctorates in both medicine and international health economics. He is currently a scientist for the Global Program on Evidence for Health Policy at the World Health Organization, responsible for major causes of disease burden, costs and effectiveness of health interventions through the WHO-CHOICE project, health and human security, and equity.

Olive Shisana holds a doctorate from the Johns Hopkins University School of Public Health. She is Executive Director of a South African national research program on Social Aspects of HIV/AIDS and Health at the Human Sciences Research Council (HSRC), and is the founder of the program. Previously she served as Professor of Health Systems at the National School of Public Health at the Medical University of Southern Africa, and as Executive Director of Family and Community Health at the World Health Organization. She also served as Director General of South Africa's post-apartheid government. She has written on the HIV/AIDS epidemic, policy, and planning in Africa. She was a principal investigator for the Mandela/HSRC study of HIV/AIDS, and for a national survey of HIV prevalence among health workers and patients in South Africa. She is currently principal investigator on a study of the epidemiology and social situation of orphans and vulnerable children in Botswana, South Africa, and Zimbabwe.

William Shisana holds a master's degree in industrial psychology from the University of Baltimore. In South Africa, he was a lecturer at the University of the Western Cape, where he introduced coursework for a master's degree program in industrial psychology. Later, he served as Senior Psychologist for Old Mutual in South Africa, and subsequently as Deputy Director in the Psychology Directorate for the South African Defense Force, focusing on selection and performance management. He has expertise in competency-based selection, managing diversity, performance management, and facilitation, where he addresses issues related to HIV/AIDS in the workplace. He currently serves as an independent consultant in human resource management, and teaches diversity management to graduate students at Israel College.

Jonas Gahr Støre served as Executive Director of the Director General's office during Dr. Gro Harlem Brundtland's first two years in office at the World Health Organization (1998-2000). A political scientist from the Institut d'Etudes Politiques de Paris, Mr. Store served as foreign policy advisor and Head of the International Department of the Prime Minister's Office of Norway from 1989 to 1998. In 2000 he was appointed State Secretary and Chief of Staff of Prime Minister Jens Stoltenberg. He is now chairman of ECON Analysis, a Nordic research and consulting company based in Oslo.

Simon Szreter, Ph.D., is Reader in History and Public Policy at the University of Cambridge, and Fellow of St. John's College, Cambridge. His principal publications have been in demographic history and the history of empirical social science: *Fertility, Class, and Gender in Britain 1860-1940* (Cambridge, 1996), and *Changing Family Size in England and Wales 1891-1911: Place, Class, and Demography* (coauthored, Cambridge, 2001). He is currently coauthoring a book on the history of sexuality in marriage in early 20th century Britain. He has also published a series of articles on economic change, mortality, public health, and social capital. He coedits www.historyandpolicy.org, a recently launched website and joint initiative of Cambridge History Faculty and the Institute of Contemporary British History, London.

Jonathan Welch is a student at the Harvard Medical School and a research fellow at the Global Equity Initiative of Harvard University. Previously, Mr. Welch was a Fulbright Scholar in Peru with Partners In Health and the Peruvian Ministry of Health, assisting in community health projects designed to control and treat multidrug-resistant tuberculosis. He has worked as a Technical Officer at the World Health Organization in the Evidence and Information for Policy cluster, and he participated in the Brookings Institution Summer Institute in Washington, D.C., where he worked on tuberculosis drug procurement and quality assurance in the Office of Health, Infectious Diseases, and Nutrition at the United States Agency for International Development.

Mary E. Wilson is Associate Professor of Medicine at Harvard Medical School. She is board certified in internal medicine and infectious diseases and served as Chief of Infectious Diseases at Mount Auburn Hospital in Cambridge, Massachusetts for more than 20 years. Her main academic interests include tuberculosis, the ecology of infections and emergence of new infections, determinants of infectious disease distribution, travel medicine, and vaccines. She is a fellow in the Infectious Diseases Society of America and the American College of Physicians. She served on the Advisory Committee for Immunization Practices (ACIP) of the Centers for Disease Control from 1988 to 1992. In 2002 she was a fellow at the Center for Advanced Study in the Behavioral Sciences in Stanford, California. She has published widely, serves on several editorial boards, and is author of the book, *A World Guide to Infections: Diseases, Distribution, Diagnosis* (Oxford University Press, 1991).

Nompumelelo Zungu-Dirwayi is a researcher at the Social Aspects of HIV/AIDS and Health program at the Human Sciences Research Council (HSRC). She has a special interest in mental health and the social and behavioral aspects of HIV/AIDS. She recently completed her master's degree in psychology from the University of Cape Town. Previously, she worked for the MRC Research Unit on Anxiety and Stress Disorders. Her work includes the first scientific study published on the mental health impact of testifying in The Truth and Reconciliation Commission of South Africa. She has authored or co-authored several papers on AIDS, and participates in a number of HIV/AIDS research projects at the HSRC.

Preface

The 15 papers in this volume are invited contributions from distinguished leaders in global health. The authors were asked to explore the breadth and depth of the interconnections between health and security. These two goals — security and health — are shared by all societies and have recently resurged in public awareness. The impact of violence associated with war and conflict now reaches into every home. But so too do insecurities generated by epidemics of disease such as HIV/AIDS, tuberculosis, and childhood infections, which create daily insecurities among the poor. How should these long-standing challenges of health and security be viewed in today's context? What are the linkages between human security and global health? And does improved understanding offer some policy guidance for global health action?

The papers in this volume were commissioned by the Harvard Global Equity Initiative, a research unit supporting the work of the international Commission on Human Security. Cochaired by Sadako Ogata, the former UN High Commissioner for Refugees, and Amartya Sen, the Nobel Prize winning economist, the Commission promoted research, consulted widely, and encouraged public dialogue as part of a participatory process in formulating its final report. Global health was one major area of interest to the Commission. After probing the many threats to people around the world, the Commission released its independent report, *Human Security Now,* which presents the Commission's official views. These papers informed those views and are part of the intellectual and public discourse encouraged and facilitated by the Commission. Ultimately, however, these papers are solely the responsibility of the authors and are not the position of the Commission or affiliated institutions.

The intellectual development process on health and security consisted of a regular seminar series sponsored by the Harvard research unit and two workshops. The first workshop to delineate the concept was conducted in cooperation with the World Health Organization's Evidence and Information for Policy Cluster in Montrieux, Switzerland in April 2002. The Global Equity Initiative at Harvard University hosted a second workshop in November 2002. These workshops brought forth helpful suggestions and constructive dialogue, and many of the workshop ideas were incorporated into the final papers assembled for this volume. It should be noted that similar versions of the paper by Lincoln Chen and Vasant Narasimhan and the paper by David Heymann were published in July 2003 in the *Journal of Human Development* (Volume 4, Number 2). These papers were included in that special issue to illustrate health dimensions of 'new insecurities' in our global age. We thank the editors of that journal for their permission to reprint these papers in this volume that is devoted exclusively to global health.

Acknowledged with deep admiration is the leadership provided by the Commission's cochairs. Also appreciated is the support of the ten other Commissioners and the Commission's secretariat based at the United Nations in New York City, especially Viviene Taylor, deputy director, who was the liaison to the Harvard research unit. Thanks are due to the Ministry of Foreign Affairs of the Government of Japan, the UN Human Security Trust Fund, and the United Nations Development Program (UNDP, Human Development Report Office) — all responsible for the financing of these and related studies. The early planning work to launch the Commission was provided by the Japanese Ministry of Foreign Affairs; Keizo Takemi of the Upper House of Parliament; Tadashi Yamamoto, President of the Japan Center for International Exchange; and Peter Geithner, advisor to the Rockefeller Foundation.

Special thanks are due to Patricia Tyler, Executive Editor, for her valued management of the editorial process and meticulous editing of the entire volume. The supportive contributions of Ellen Seidensticker and Jonathan Welch are acknowledged with appreciation. The works presented here would not have been possible without the enormously important work of research fellows and staff at the Harvard Global Equity Initiative — Prea Gulati, Juan Carlos Hincapie, Chris Linnane, Sarah Michael, Paul Segal, and Florence Werthmuller. These professionals made the entire journey pleasurable and intellectually rewarding.

Lincoln Chen
Jennifer Leaning
Vasant Narasimhan

Cambridge, Massachusetts
September 2003

INTRODUCTION

Health and human security are fundamentally valued in all societies, but their connections and interdependencies are not well understood. In this volume, 15 chapters explore the linkages between global health and human security, demonstrating that pursuit of these two social goods can best be accomplished by understanding the richness, complexity, and opportunities presented by the nexus between them. From a policy perspective, these contributions explore a range of innovative strategies to build upon these linkages.

The chapters are organized into four clusters — history, ethics, and policies; global epidemics; violence and risks; and poverty and health action. We begin with an open exploration of the breadth and depth of health and security linkages in history, ethics, and policy. Two health fields closely related to security interests — global epidemics and violence and risks — are then analyzed, seeking to bring more specificity to an understanding of health and security. The final section on poverty and health action recognizes that preventable illness and premature death are among the daily insecurities faced especially by the world's poor, and that innovative health actions exist to protect individuals against ill health and insecurity.

The chapters in this volume underscore three basic aspects of global health and human security. First, recent developments present enormous challenges for human security and global health. With the end of the Cold War, the security landscape is changing rapidly. The traditional approach of national security by military defense seems inadequate and incomplete in an increasingly interconnected and unstable world. Additionally, conflicts are proliferating in the midst of failed states, and new forms of violence, especially terrorist attacks exemplified by September 11th in the United States, are fueling public fears. In global health, millions continue to die from diseases of poverty, despite the accumulation of impressive knowledge and modern technologies. Health inequities are widening. Violence, it all its forms, continues as a pressing public health problem, and the advent of HIV/AIDS has generated an unprecedented global health crisis, especially in sub-Saharan Africa. New germs are emerging and have the potential, as the SARS epidemic demonstrated, to spread rapidly throughout the world, inextricably linking the health and security concerns of all individuals.

Second, the interconnections between health and security are deep, subtle, and long-standing. Today's context of new conflicts, pervasive poverty, and accelerating global flows has brought the health and security fields closer together. Health as a security priority in some cases has been quite direct, as in the deliberate use of germs as a weapon of terror. In other cases, catastrophic health crises, such as the devastation caused by HIV/AIDS, may pose an even greater threat to societal security than conflict. Internal or civil wars directly target civilian populations, causing high morbidity and mortality as well as widespread collapse in the psychosocial dimensions of security, impeding the possibilities of post-conflict reconstruction. In all situations where health of populations is eroding or security is under threat, understanding and integrating the factors that are common to or that link both health and security would improve the search for solutions.

Finally, a human security approach can help identify new strategies for meeting the goals of global health and security. Preventive action and the capacity for rapid and appropriate responses are critical, as are protecting and empowering individuals to pursue their own safety and self-determination. In all cases, strategies for human health and security depend upon individual and collective action — often anticipatory, preventive, and reactive.

The ultimate question in all policies and programs is, "Whose security?" Core to the concepts of human security and health in these chapters is the recognition that these social goods derive from a focus on people and populations, not institutions and governments; that they must be pursued within an ecological and social context; and that strategies in support of them must be viable through time. All of the contributors in this volume share a vision of global health as indivisible from security in an increasingly interdependent world.

History, ethics, and policies

The first section of the volume consists of five chapters that address the historical, ethical, and policy aspects of global health and human security.

The opening chapter by Lincoln Chen and Vasant Narasimhan traces the emergence of the concept of human security, as well as its evolution and usages. Accepting a comprehensive definition parallel to 'sustainable development,' the authors examine the human security dimensions of three major global health fields — infectious disease, poverty-related diseases, and violence and crisis. In these explorations, the authors show how each health area is intertwined with the security of people. The chapter concludes with a discussion of how a human security approach would enrich contemporary global health policies and programs.

Based on field experience and the security literature, Jennifer Leaning, Sam Arie, Gilbert Holleufer, and Claude Bruderlein examine the definition of human security during conflict. They note that attention in conflict situations to the provision of physical goods, while essential, is too restrictive. Individuals trapped in conflict must adapt and mobilize physical, social, and psychological resources for survival and dignity. People in crisis depend powerfully on social relationships and community trust. A richer construct of human security, the authors argue, focuses on 'resilience,' the psychosocial capacity to adapt to and control threatening and rapidly changing conditions. During war, resilience can be either sustained by the international community acting within the realm of international law to protect civilians, or undermined by failures to engage early enough with sufficient effect.

Simon Szreter examines human security from the perspective of European history. He argues that tight linkages between health and security have been prominent for centuries and that their recent separation is unusual. Both health and security in 18th and 19th century Britain were profoundly disrupted by unbridled economic growth and invariably accompanied by the 'four Ds' — disruption, deprivation, disease, and death. The historical record suggests that in those precarious times, three policies were essential for advancing health and security — registration of all people, an active civil society, and universal welfare policies. Today, these basic policies are notably absent in many low-income countries, which are further disadvantaged by extensive histories of imperialism and colonialism. Ultimately, health and security in both low- and high-income countries are linked, and the advancement of human security in low-income countries should be seen as central to the self-interest of the global public.

According to Giovanni Berlinguer, health and security raise historical and ethical challenges that can be further elaborated by bioethics. The author notes the changed security environment provoked by fears generated in the September 11th attacks in the United States, with broad health implications. He argues that health equity is the fundamental value underpinning global health; it is both intrinsically valuable as well as instrumental in achieving human freedom. The globalization of health responses should be based on the value of equity, on the application of knowledge, and on moral indignation over health injustice.

The final chapter in the section, by Jonas Støre, Jonathan Welch, and Lincoln Chen, examines the implications of health and security for global health governance. The authors argue that health risks and the institutional responses to them have increasingly shifted focus from national, to international, to global. The key functions of a 21st century global health infrastructure — knowledge management; laws, regulations, and conventions; health and development; and institutional partnerships — are examined systematically. The authors conclude that political commitment, new financing systems, and the development of a common international health and security ethos will be essential for global health governance.

Global epidemics

Only two decades old, the HIV/AIDS pandemic is perhaps the greatest health disaster in human history, and the recent SARS epidemic has generated enormous fears. These viruses are among more than two dozen new infectious agents that emerged or reemerged in recent years. With their global reach and ability to devastate through epidemics, these infections vividly demonstrate the linkages between health and security. Contemporary contexts have introduced new dynamics in the emergence, transmission, and impact of these infectious agents. The four chapters in this section offer complementary perspectives on global epidemics and human security.

Mary Wilson introduces the subject by reviewing the contemporary factors relevant to the global spread of infectious diseases. Today people and germs are linked by unprecedented global travel and trade. Increased human interactions are compounded by demographic changes in the growth, density, and urbanization of populations. In addition to these risk factors, microbes are demonstrating an impressive ability to develop antibiotic resistance. The author reminds us that humankind and germs are involved in an eternal struggle for ecological supremacy.

Health and security, David Heymann argues, have been profoundly affected by recent events, including bioterrorism with anthrax, HIV/AIDS, and recently SARS, as well as concerns over the proliferation of weapons of mass destruction. The author proposes that a strong global health infrastructure in disease surveillance and control is needed to mount an effective global response to these human security threats. The initiatives of the World Health Organization demonstrate how an integrated and comprehensive system could be developed. One of the major advantages of such a system would be its 'dual use' to detect and respond to naturally occurring infections as well as the intentional misuse of germs as weapons. Recent world experience with the SARS epidemic provides an early and positive indication of the effectiveness of this proposed model.

Alex de Waal argues that assumptions and perceptions of the HIV/AIDS pandemic, especially in sub-Saharan Africa, are based erroneously on either complacency or past experiences. The author notes that the spread of HIV/AIDS in Africa is an unprecedented event in human history; the disease stands to have an extraordinary health impact on adult populations. Truncation of the adult lifespan, he notes, could have profound effects on a wide range of societal functions — demography, fertility, and mortality. Governance will be an especially challenging task in hard-hit societies, where institutional infrastructure has been devastated. Finally, the chapter identifies perhaps the most significant impact of HIV/AIDS:

gravely diminished social reproduction capacity of families and societies across generations.

Olive Shisana, Nompumelelo Zungu-Dirwayi, and William Shisana examine the HIV/AIDS epidemic in southern Africa. They note the dire increase in morbidity and mortality and its consequent impacts on all aspects of society. The underappreciated effects of HIV/AIDS include the concomitant increase in political tensions, slowing or reversal of health and social progress, and economic setbacks. No dimension of societal function and productivity — health, education, or military — is spared from the HIV/AIDS epidemic.

VIOLENCE AND RISKS

Violence in its varied forms is often perceived as the major threat to human security. Traditional security action has focused on the control of violence through national defense and civil policing. It is increasingly recognized, however, that violence manifests itself in collective, interpersonal, and self-inflicted forms, constituting a spectrum of violent actions within social life, rather than distinct phenomena separate from the underlying dynamics of social relations. Violence is associated not only with political conflict but also with local crime, domestic disputes, and psychosocial pathologies, with gender bias strongly driving many forms of violence.

Violence worldwide has been increasingly addressed as a global health problem recently, using traditional public health tools such as epidemiology, the evaluation of interventions, and behavioral modification activities. As a manifestation of behavioral pathologies, violence, like unsafe sex and tobacco use, has important health and security consequences. The three chapters in this section offer a health perspective on violence and the risks it presents to health and human security.

The opening chapter by David R. Meddings, Douglas Bettcher, and Roya Ghafele examines the recent WHO study on global violence — collective, interpersonal, and self-inflicted. The authors present not only a typology of violence but also a summary of the global epidemiological picture. They note that all forms of violence share some common determinants — low economic development, high poverty levels, gross income inequalities, and weak governance. The authors underscore that violence is a core public health problem amenable to the approaches of public health, and that the health and human security framework permits the capture of all forms of violence as threats to human insecurity.

Sonali Johnson and Claudia García-Moreno examine violence through a gender and human security lens. The authors note that 'gender analysis' deals not simply with women but also with the social relations between the sexes, which are deeply embedded in virtually all human health and security interactions. Thus, the chapter reviews literature across a range of security crises — gender and conflict, rape, sexual and domestic violence, the trafficking of women, and gender-based risks associated with HIV/AIDS. Gender-based human security policies must wrestle with false divisions between what traditionally has been considered legitimate terrain — the public sphere and private spheres of life. The human security approach adopts a comprehensive and balanced policy stance toward all threats to human security, public and private.

Kenji Shibuya broadens the reach of health issues that threaten human security by reviewing global data on the burden of disease. Based on WHO estimations on morbidity and mortality in all countries and world regions, he notes the huge diversity in patterns of disease worldwide. Common infectious diseases predominate in low-income countries, whereas chronic cardiovascular, oncological, and mental diseases are important in both high- and low-income countries. Based on the best available epidemiologic knowledge, the chapter undertakes risk assessments, both proximal and distal, of major health threats amenable to behavioral modification. The author concludes that poverty and lack of economic development are powerful contextual determinants for many preventable diseases, and that modification of several major risky behaviors, such as unsafe sex and tobacco use, could generate enormous improvements in health and security. Achieving these gains will depend upon appropriate perception of risks, modification of risky behavior, and the application of cost-effective interventions.

POVERTY AND HEALTH ACTION

Health and human security ultimately depend upon the actions of individuals, families, and nations in diverse communities around the world. While the diverse range of issues they raise is global in scope, the three chapters here concentrate on South and Southeast Asia. The Asian perspectives on health action and human security demonstrate both positive and negative lessons. More importantly, they point to approaches that can be used by new initiatives to engage communities in health and security issues.

The chapter by Mely Caballero-Anthony distills and synthesizes in-depth case studies of health insecurity in several Southeast Asian countries. Her conclusions are unmistakable. Despite the persistence and scale of poverty and preventable diseases, public commitments are weak throughout the region. Primary health care for all remains more rhetorical than a practical reality in the daily lives of the poor. Caballero-Anthony tracks the deficiencies to skewed priorities of political leaders, elite institutions, and weak governance. If these trends are to be reversed, health care must be elevated to a 'security priority,' considered equally with military security expenditures for national defense.

The two chapters from South Asia present a positive picture of poor people and communities organizing to improve their own health and security. The Bangladesh case study by Alayne M. Adams and Mushtaque Chowdhury describes the work of BRAC, one of the world's largest non-governmental organizations (NGOs). BRAC adopts a comprehensive and holistic approach, recognizing that human security is inherently multidimensional. Much of its efforts are devoted to building village-based groups among the poor as well as 'social' or 'relational' capital that enables villagers to advance common security. The authors describe innovative approaches to health and related development challenges, demonstrating that practical and effective protection is feasible when the poor are empowered.

The case from India by Mirai Chatterjee and M. Kent Ranson describes how innovative actions for health and security can emerge when individuals are empowered to establish and pursue their own priorities. The case is based on the experience of the Self-Employed Women's Association (SEWA), a membership organization of women in the informal sector of the economy in Gujarat. As a women's trade union, SEWA's priorities are determined by democratic means. Through such participatory processes, SEWA initiated a community-based health insurance program as a critical strategy for promoting the human security of its members. The authors emphasize that innovative community-based action is feasible when it draws upon the contributions of local members, and its scale and effectiveness is strengthened when health and human security policies are also enacted at the national level.

By focusing on protection and downside risk for disadvantaged populations, human security fundamentally reorients security from an exclusive focus on the nation-state to one that also considers the security of individuals and communities. The contributions to this volume offer an ambitious agenda for future policy, action, and research. As health crises mount, the global community must mobilize to acknowledge that without the protection of health, the security of people will remain in peril. It is clear from the chapters in this volume that the relevance of human security to health is substantial and that the policy implications for international, national, and community actors will be critically important in the years to come.

SECTION I

HISTORY, ETHICS, AND POLICIES

CHAPTER I

A HUMAN SECURITY AGENDA FOR GLOBAL HEALTH[1]

LINCOLN CHEN AND VASANT NARASIMHAN

INTRODUCTION

The concept of 'human security' has emerged slowly but steadily over the 1990s, a development with important implications for health and human development. Human security attempts to broaden security thinking from 'national security' and the military defense of political boundaries to a 'people-centered' approach of anticipating and coping with the multiple threats faced by ordinary people in an increasingly globalizing world. Promulgated by the United Nations (UN) and interested governments, the concept of human security has steadily gained ground, culminating in the establishment of an independent international commission on human security in 2001. Cochaired by former UN High Commissioner for Refugees, Sadako Ogata, and Nobel Prize economist, Amartya Sen, the commission is mandated to clarify the concept of human security for global policy and action (1).

What are the implications of the emerging concept of human security for health and human development? The purpose of this paper is to address this question by analyzing three associated questions. What is human security and in what ways could it be related to global health? Why have some health problems been associated with human security, while others have not? What are some policy and operational implications for health action? These three questions address the basic challenge of understanding what value, if any, the concept of human security brings to global health.

EMERGENCE OF HUMAN SECURITY

Three major trends in the 1990s generated the contextual forces that facilitated the emergence of human security. The most influential was the end of the Cold War, which dramatically changed the world peace and security environment. Rather than a bipolar stalemate imposed by the nuclear arms of two superpowers, new forms of conflict emerged in the post-Cold War decade. These so-called 'new wars' have often taken place within, rather than among, states, sometimes sparked by ethnically based divisions. In these new conflicts, the security of people cannot be protected through reliance on military defense of national borders. As an example, while established conventions on international refugees protect those who flee political oppression across international boundaries, today's conflicts generate large numbers of internally displaced people about whom international covenants are mostly silent.

Second, an improved understanding of socioeconomic development shines light on the neglected everyday insecurities faced by the world's poor and excluded. When given voice to express their views, poor people repeatedly underscore the many insecurities of daily life — economic impoverishment from income insecurity, threats of physical violence, and the devastating impact of catastrophic illness (2, 3). The insecurities of health, interestingly, relate not simply to preventable suffering and avoidable death, but also to the economic erosion of the people's precarious asset base to purchase urgent medical services. These emergencies often trigger a vicious spiral of impoverishment.

Third, the process of globalization — the accelerated transnational flows of goods, services, finance, technology, information, people, and disease — has generated uncertain rapid social changes. In a matter of months, the 1997 Asian financial crisis engulfed a vibrant economic region, impoverishing literally millions of people. The macroeconomic shock exposed long-standing social gaps, including the absence of social safety nets and fragile health services. The past decade also witnessed the accelerated transmission of infectious diseases, such as HIV and dengue fever, fueled by the movement of people and goods (4). Even the September 11 terrorism attack and the subsequent anthrax bioterrorism incident underscored the transnational vulnerability of the rich as well as the poor. All of these factors generated an impetus to reexamine traditional approaches to national security and human development. Human security emerged as a concept that has the potential to link seemingly divergent fields and to capture and address some of the world's most pressing demands.

An early task of the Commission on Human Security was to define just what human security means. The proposed working definition was:

> The objective of human security is to safeguard the vital core of human lives from critical pervasive threats while promoting long-term human flourishing (5).

This definition of human security focuses on protecting people from the downside risks they might face due to particular circumstances. In addition, it attempts to clarify human security by concentrating on the 'vital core' of human lives and 'critical and pervasive threats,' while promoting immediate action without compromising 'long-term flourishing.'

While compelling in terms of explaining and responding to new challenges, human security has also faced criticism. Human security, some argue, is merely 'old wine in new bottles,' combining traditional concerns about 'freedom from fear' and 'freedom from want.' The former addresses political liberties and the latter economic entitlements, roughly parallel to the first and second generation of human rights. Others argue that the concept is 'too idealistic,' and fails to take into account the real-world politics of geopolitical power in a rapidly changing international system. Human security appears to appeal to 'middle powers,' neither the most powerful nor the weakest states.

Perhaps the strongest argument against the concept is its vagueness and breadth. If human security is comprehensive, it may be impossible to prioritize policies and actions. A series of associated terms has developed — people's security, the security of displaced people, livelihood security, environmental security, comprehensive security, and health security. How can all of these insecurities be grouped into a single concept? Which threats should be prioritized? And can any be excluded?

LINKAGES: HEALTH AND SECURITY

Global health has been increasingly drawn into these human security debates. Indeed, some aspects of health are intrinsically linked to security; terms such as 'health security' have become increasingly used. The health field also has produced several major policy papers on health and human security (6). At the simplest level, premature and unnecessary loss of life is perhaps the greatest insecurity of human life. Of the planet's six billion people, about 56 million die annually, many prematurely (7). Depending upon the assumptions employed, about one-third of these deaths may be preventable or curable with existing knowledge, technologies, and resources. The ethos and mission of global health to prevent and treat these unnecessary health insecurities situates health in the mainstream of human security.

Beyond the generalized connection, however, health and human security linkages have emerged in a series of health fields. Throughout the 1990s, three specific linkages emerged: violence and conflict, global infectious diseases, and poverty and inequity. The relationship between these health fields and the working definition of human security is depicted in Figure 1.

VIOLENCE AND CONFLICT

The September 11 attack in the U.S., the war in Afghanistan, and earlier conflicts in Kosovo, Bosnia, and Rwanda — all illustrate the changing nature of warfare in the post-Cold War era. Today, there are about 50

Figure 1.   Human security and its relationships to health. Global health
plays a critical role in preventing and treating unnecessary
health insecurities and unavoidable health crises.

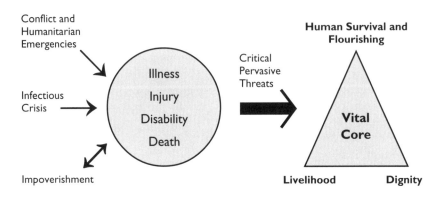

conflicts in the world affecting more than 100 million people (Figure 2).
Many of these conflicts are within rather than among nation-states and
are characterized by the collapse of effective governance reflected by the
loss of centralized authority to control violence (8). Internal divisions
between ethnic or religious communities, fueled by intergroup tensions,
sometimes drive the armed conflict. Civilians are not simply 'collateral
damage': if they are of certain ethnic or religious groups, they may be the
intended target of violence. Such conflicts usually provoke massive flows
of people, both international refugees and internally displaced people;
gross violations of human rights; and, tragically, genocide, including the
use of rape as a weapon of war.

Complex humanitarian emergencies can extend beyond conflict to
natural disasters, as illustrated by the recent volcano eruption on the
Congo-Rwanda border, Hurricane Mitch in Guatemala, the earthquake
in Gujarat, India, and the 1998 floods in Bangladesh. The widespread
devastation caused by these natural disasters demonstrated the vulnerability of increasingly concentrated poor populations in ecologically fragile
environments. These crises are of serious concern for both their scale and
speed of human devastation. In countries with wholly inadequate support
systems, these short-term devastations can rapidly translate into long-term
regional economic and political instability.

Crisis-linked deaths are not all due to wars and disasters. Recent research increasingly recognizes violence in all forms as a major determinant
of population health (9). Deaths due to violence may result from many
causes — war and conflict, local crime, domestic violence, and even self-
inflicted violence. Deaths due to conflict-related violence, interpersonal
violence, and domestic violence are common in all regions of the world,

Figure 2.   War, crisis, and disasters in 2000

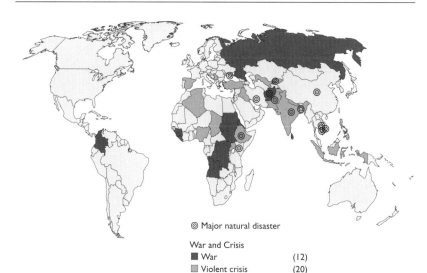

◎ Major natural disaster

War and Crisis
■ War   (12)
▨ Violent crisis   (20)
□ Limited or no violence   (158)

Source: ECHO presentation to UN Agencies in Brussels, 16 June 2001.

rich and poor, although the determinants and levels of violence-related deaths vary greatly among populations.

Health programs in humanitarian crises have been inextricably drawn into these complexities, creating entirely new challenges for global health. Often, conflicts expose the long neglect of basic public health and curative services, where the social trust that underlies health services has eroded. Based on the long tradition of 'medical neutrality' supported by humanitarian covenants and human rights conventions, health interventions have had to adapt and move beyond distinct medical emergencies and a focus on epidemiological intelligence and disease control. Health action has been compelled to cooperate with military, political, and economic activities of the UN, interested governments, and nongovernmental organizations to create the space for effective health action. Indeed, health action sometimes has been used as an effective diplomatic tool for peace negotiations. Ceasefire days have been recognized by combatants, for example, in order to enable health workers to immunize children. Health action has also increasingly diffused to other interventions and actors, including military health and relief efforts.

GLOBAL INFECTIOUS DISEASES

The 1990s marked a major shift in approaches to global infectious diseases. Once considered as either disappearing in rich countries or confined to poverty-linked common childhood infections, infectious diseases have risen markedly on the global agenda. Many factors explain this emergence: the discovery of more than two dozen new viral and bacterial agents, the spread of resistance to common antibiotics, and the devastating impact of new epidemics — cholera in Peru and Latin America, plague in India, Ebola virus in Africa, dengue fever in Asia, West Nile Fever in the southern U.S., and bovine spongiform encephalitis (mad cow disease) and hoof-and-mouth viruses in Europe. The economic and political impact of these epidemics has been massive — cessation of exports, driving away of foreign tourists, and discrediting or paralysis of government. Public visibility accorded to new or resurging infections has been accompanied by growing recognition of 'silent,' 'neglected,' or 'orphaned' diseases like malaria and tuberculosis. Figure 3 shows the global burden of these and other leading infectious diseases.

Two infectious agents have powerfully influenced thinking about the linkage between human security and global health. The anthrax bioterrorism attacks in the U.S. underscored the vulnerability of even the world's richest populations to the use of bacteria and viruses as weapons. Bioterrorism aims both to generate public fear and to increase a society's sense of vulnerability. Although anthrax caused only five direct deaths, the still-unsolved attacks virtually paralyzed some systems of American society, including the postal system and congress. It is reported that, at one time, nearly one-third of workers at the U.S. Centers for Disease Control were assigned to combat the anthrax attack. This attack also generated new fears about other infectious agents, like smallpox, for which the U.S.

Figure 3.   The global burden of infectious disease worldwide

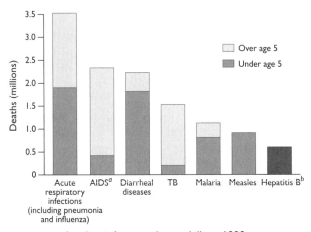

Leading infectious disease killers, 1998

a HIV-positive people who died with TB have been included among AIDS deaths.

b Figure for hepatitis B is for 1997 and is not broken down by age.

Source: WHO; 1998, 1999.

government was compelled to rebuild a national stockpile of nearly discarded vaccines. To the public, the attacks also exposed the ill-preparedness, decay, and underinvestment of the national public health infrastructure. Political leaders were warned and began to recognize that public health protection, like fire and police forces, remains an essential public good that must be provided by government. With public safety from health threats a renewed priority, a countervailing concern has grown over the politicization of public health. Will public health priorities prevail over the political imperatives of 'homeland security'?

Beyond bioterrorism, the major driver linking health and human security has been the global HIV/AIDS pandemic. By the early years of the 21st century, there have been more than 40 million people infected by the HIV virus, more than 20 million cumulative deaths, and more than three million deaths annually. At the turn of the century, the HIV/AIDS pandemic, especially in high-infection regions like sub-Saharan Africa, was finally recognized as perhaps the greatest human security threat of our time or, indeed, in all of human history. The death toll from HIV/AIDS already exceeds that of the plague of Black Death in the 14th century. Two decades after its discovery and global spread, the UN Security Council in 1999 declared HIV/AIDS a threat to national security, especially in heavily infected, economically weak, and politically fragile countries in sub-Saharan Africa. The G8 meetings of heads of state in Okinawa (2000) and in Genoa (2001) similarly accorded high political priority to this health and human security threat. Recently, an entire session of the UN General Assembly was devoted to HIV/AIDS, and a Global Fund for AIDS, Tuberculosis, and Malaria was launched.

POVERTY AND INEQUALITY

Although security is usually equated with physical violence, the insecurities of daily life among ordinary people, especially the poor, gained visibility in the 1990s. The United Nations Development Program Human Development Report in 1994 proposed that human security complemented human development since, without a sense of security, exercising the freedom of choice inherent in human development would not be possible (10). The introduction of the concept coincided with international debates about the alternative social investment opportunities made possible by the freeing-up of post-Cold War military budgets. The relationship between poverty, health, and human security was vividly revisited during the Asian financial crisis when millions of people were suddenly impoverished due to macroeconomic shocks. While human development is a positive concept focusing on equitable growth, little attention had been devoted to protecting people during economic downturns. For many developing societies that have not yet developed social protection systems, economic shocks can suddenly precipitate enormous social hardship among society's most disadvantaged people.

These connections between poverty, health, and insecurity were highlighted by the series of Voices of the Poor studies produced by the World Bank for its *World Development Report 2000*. Because of the vast numbers of the world's poor and the severity of their multiple deprivations, the toll of these insecurities far surpasses the suffering and death due to either conflict or infectious epidemics. Voices of the Poor revealed that the poor feared not only violence from crime (including corrupt local police) and the loss of wages and jobs; severe illness was a source of worries about the economic toll of paying for emergency health care. For the poor with weak asset bases, catastrophic illness among working adults not only deprives the family of daily wages, but also puts enormous pressure on the family's limited assets to purchase requisite health services. Sometimes, such expenditures precipitate a vicious cycle of illness, asset depletion, and impoverishment. The health-associated insecurities of poverty thus are exacerbated by the gross failure of many countries to implement the primary health care movement goal of 'health for all' promised two decades ago.

Recognition of the linkages between health and development has grown on the global political agenda. Four of the eight UN Millennium Development goals focus on health attainment — reductions in infant, child, and maternal mortality, morbidity, and malnutrition. The recent World Health Organization Commission on Macroeconomics argued that, since ill health is a significant impediment to economic development, donor resources supporting health programs in developing countries should be dramatically expanded. The recent Monterrey conference on financing for development stimulated pledges of enhanced foreign aid by most Organization for Economic Cooperation and Development countries. Some hope to witness a doubling of aid volume over the next five years. Even the U.S., the lowest contributor to aid based on per-capita Gross Domestic Product, pledged to increase its foreign aid, conditioned upon certain macro policy changes in recipient countries.

Policy implications

The evolving linkages between security and health are not due to happenstance or coincidence. Rather, they reflect fundamental contextual shifts in our era of globalization, to which the human development field must adapt, respond, and lead. We postulate the following commonalities for why health and human security have become inextricably linked to human security.

First, we believe that new wars, emerging infectious diseases, and the health linkages to poverty reflect either changing vulnerabilities in these globalizing times or improved knowledge and recognition of the everyday insecurities confronted by marginalized peoples. The end of the Cold War, new thinking in international development, and the forces of globalization all have introduced new risks for human security, including health security. These contextual changes also challenged traditional modalities and mechanisms of response to the many insecurities we face. Human security as a policy concept emerged, not out of thin air, but propelled by these new global forces.

Second, human security starts from a people-centered perspective that generates a different set of priorities than does traditional state-centric security. The security needs of internally displaced people, the poor, or those at high risk to infectious diseases cannot be met by traditional approaches to security and development. Military control of national borders can do little to protect people against many new health threats. Traditional development theory focuses on economic growth, treats health as consumption, and views mortality as an averaged, long-term secular process. Yet sickness, as it affects individuals, can be particularly devastating. People fear catastrophic illness and its crippling consequences, and want protection and a sense of confidence about the future. A new people-centered paradigm, with its policy and operational implications, can complement and strengthen state security to protect people in an unstable and interconnected world.

Third, human security helps to capture the depth and extended impact of health crises, which are deep because conflict, epidemics, and catastrophic illness generate profound economic, social, and political disturbances. Social institutions, including governments and health services, are deeply disrupted. Health policy and action, moreover, must cope with emergencies as well as extended crises. Internal conflicts have continued for more than two decades in Afghanistan and Sudan, for example. Often, the health and human insecurity linkages underscore the weakness of baseline primary public health and curative services in most countries, rich as well as poor.

Finally, human security captures the comprehensiveness with which the health sector must face many of these challenges. Health actors can no longer simply act alone without regard for the many other issues and actors involved. That is certainly the case in complex humanitarian emergencies. It is also the case that control of global infections is not possible without surveillance, control, and response linked to international trade, migration, and movements. The September 11 attack reminded the world that people's insecurities are interdependent. Someone else's insecurities may soon spill over to one's own insecurities in an increasingly interconnected world.

These linkages confirm that the concept of human security should be comprehensive, not forced into restrictive or artificial narrowness. While many might prefer to limit the concept, focusing on some insecurities and excluding others, we believe that human security will necessarily remain comprehensive and integrative. Moreover, human security may be defined by the nature of the threat it is intended to respond to, as much as by its people-centered 'value base,' its insights into new strategies, or its capacity to mobilize and energize diverse constituencies. In this respect, human security may follow the path of the Brundtland Commission on Environment and Development. This acclaimed commission of the 1980s coined the term 'sustainable development,' and developed a comprehensive concept that enhanced, rather than diminished, its impact. The concept's value base has helped to augment its usefulness in planning complementary environment and development activities, and in galvanizing diverse stakeholders and constituencies for social action. Human security as a comprehensive concept holds similar potential.

NOTE

[1] This article was originally published under the title, 'Human Security and Global Health,' in the *Journal of Human Development*, Volume 4, Number 2, July 2003, Carfax Publishing, Taylor & Francis, Abington, U.K.

REFERENCES

1.   Sen A. Why Human Security. Presentation at the International Symposium on Human Security, Japan Ministry of Foreign Affairs; 2000 July 28; Tokyo, Japan.

2.   Narayan D, Patel R, Schafft K, Rademacher A, Koch-Schulte S. *Voices of the poor: can anyone hear us?* New York: Oxford University Press for the World Bank; 2000.

3.   Narayan D, Chambers R, Shah MK, Petesch P. *Crying out for change: voices of the poor.* New York: Oxford University Press for the World Bank; 2000.

4.   Chen LC, Berlinguer G. Health equity in a globalizing world. In: Evans T, Whitehead M, Diderichen F, Bhuiya A, Wirth M, editors. *Challenging inequities in health: from ethics to action.* New York: Oxford University Press; 2001.

5.   Alkire S. Conceptual framework for human security; 2002. Available from: URL: http://www.humansecurity-chs.org/doc/index.html, accessed on 2002 Oct 10.

6.   King G, Murray C. Rethinking human security. *Political Science Quarterly* 2002;116(4):585–610.

7.   World Health Organization. *World health report.* Geneva: World Health Organization; 2003.

8.   Leaning J, Briggs SM, Chen LC, editors. *Humanitarian crises: the medical and public health response.* Cambridge (MA): Harvard University Press; 1999.

9.   World Health Organization. *World report on violence and health.* Geneva: World Health Organization; 2002.

10. United Nations Development Program. *Human development report 1994: new dimensions of human security.* New York: Oxford University Press; 1994.

CHAPTER 2

HUMAN SECURITY AND CONFLICT: A COMPREHENSIVE APPROACH

JENNIFER LEANING, SAM ARIE, GILBERT HOLLEUFER, AND CLAUDE BRUDERLEIN

INTRODUCTION: HUMAN SECURITY AND PSYCHOSOCIAL NEEDS

In the last decade of the twentieth century, observers celebrated the declining number of interstate wars just as a proliferation of complicated intrastate disputes, conflicts, and emergencies began to take hold. These situations present a different class of crisis, one where the international community has been unable to recognize, forestall, or even mitigate the effects of a rapid collapse in human security among targeted civilian populations.

In an earlier analysis, we argued that as these crises unfolded, a narrow focus on material resources in strategies of relief and development prevented analysts from identifying the true sources of vulnerability or resilience in a population (1). In this earlier paper we outlined a conceptual approach to human security that paid due attention to the psychological and social bases of community stability, and explored the underlying conditions or factors that support constructive coping mechanisms in the face of threats or hazards.

This approach is briefly summarized here to provide context for the main focus of this chapter: a discussion of the ways in which current conflicts subvert the core basis for human security. The argument, based on empirical observation and analysis of survey data, is that failure to protect combatant and noncombatant populations from the worst excesses of war results in social and psychological distress that can best be expressed in terms of breakdowns in human security. This failure to protect is in the first instance the responsibility of the local warring parties, whose war strategies deliberately target civilian populations and enlist combatants in the commission of atrocity. In a larger sense, however, this failure also arises from inattention and laxity on the part of the international community, whose members have not been asked to understand the impact of such wars over time on the societies and individuals forced to endure them.

CORE COMPONENTS OF HUMAN SECURITY[1]

A core bundle of basic resources — material, psychological, and social — is needed in order for an individual, community, or society to be resilient. The first essential component of human security is basic material and survival inputs: *food, water, shelter,* and *safety.* These core inputs ensure a minimum level of survival, establish a basis for human development efforts, and decrease the potential for conflict.

The second component of human security consists of core attachments to *home, community,* and *the future*[2] (2). Links to these three domains underpin a sense of identity and facilitate participation in society at large, from the small group to the nation-state. These attachments are often undone when populations are uprooted and dislocated, when families are dispersed and communities are destroyed, and when arbitrary violence and discrimination render the future distant and unpredictable. Individuals in these situations turn to other — often less constructive — sources for participation, recognition, and empowerment. When sections of a population identify less readily with the collective enterprise than with these alternative groups — formed around race, religion, geography, or age and characterized by an ideology of resentment and aggression — credible dispute resolution becomes unlikely and the paths to violence and disorder are manifold.

In the earlier paper we developed a working definition of human security, noting the extent to which these core inputs to human security were essential preconditions for the more complex and contingent enterprise of human development.

> "Human security is an underlying condition for sustainable human development. It results from the social, psychological, economic, and political aspects of human life that in times of acute crisis or chronic deprivation protect the survival of individuals, support individual and group capacities to attain minimally adequate standards of living, and promote constructive group attachment and continuity through time."

MEASURING HUMAN SECURITY

Measurement of the first component of human security — the fulfillment of basic needs[3] — requires agreement on what constitutes a minimally acceptable standard of living (with basic survival levels of food, water, and shelter). The issue of safety, however, remains an outstanding but critical aspect for the fulfillment of basic needs, and is a particularly challenging requirement in the context of crisis and conflict. We return to this problem later in the chapter.

The second, psychosocial component of human security requires measuring the relatively intangible domains of home, community, and the future. We proposed using negative measures, or *inverse indicators*, of these three domains to provide greater sensitivity to the presence or absence of human security in a given situation. The three negative measures are: *social dislocation, dynamic inequality between groups*, and *high discount rates*. Different metrics — some already in use in UN indices and others aimed at capturing less concrete aspects of human need — might be used to assess each of these inverse indicators.[4]

Measuring the strength of these three psychosocial domains requires a focus on *dynamic changes* at the local level. Dynamic changes carry the potential to ignite or reignite conflict, and can occur in the social, political, or economic realm. Close attention to these changes will improve the capacity of systems for *threat assessment* and early warning, to anticipate crisis in order to build resilience and mitigate vulnerability. We posited in the earlier paper that use of the human security model would help the international community to identify the sources of crisis at an early stage and to be better equipped to offer support or intervention before conflict arises.

In this chapter we employ the definition of human security in the analysis of what happens to populations exposed to current conflicts, as intentional targets of nonstate actors in regional or civil wars. Two aspects of human security found in the earlier discussion to be important in understanding resilience in the face of threat — capabilities and vulnerabilities — surface here as pivotal concepts.

CAPABILITY AND VULNERABILITY

Human security is a capability-based concept, as approached by Jean Drèze and Amartya Sen. Drèze and Sen insist on the importance of social functioning as well as biological health, and argue that in order to lead a secure life, people rely on appropriate psychological as well as material relationships (4). Focusing on *capacity to function* rather than on the simple provision of goods allows us to recognize that because individuals and local circumstances differ, the inputs required to secure an acceptable standard of human security will also differ. "The focus here is on human life, as it can be led, rather than on commodities as such (4)."

Capacity to function underlies the relationship between coping and vulnerability. Patrick Webb maintains that vulnerability to disaster should not be thought of as an absolute state or condition, but rather as the combined impact of a threat and the possible adaptive reactions it provokes. He suggests that vulnerability can be expressed as the net impact of the hazards one faces offset by the mechanisms one has for coping with them (7). Such coping mechanisms, when constructive, contribute to one's capacity to function, as posited by Drèze and Sen.

Humanitarian protection in war

To assess the valence of human security in the context of war, it is necessary to search for legal regimes, enforcement mechanisms, and coping strategies that combine to protect populations from the harmful effects of conflict. In the paradigm of human security advanced in the previous section, issues of safety, or protection from gross violence, become paramount. As we discuss here and in the next section, however, the prominence of psychosocial factors in creating the reality as well as the perception of safety holds firm.

The traditional legal effort to protect civilians from the harmful effects of war has centered on enhancing the distinction between civilian persons or objects and military targets. This approach was based on two key assumptions: first, that civilian targets were of limited military value and attacking them would provide little military advantage; and second, that parties to a conflict, quite apart from and in addition to their legal or moral obligations, would thus seek to optimize the use of their resources by targeting military assets. International Humanitarian Law (IHL) has built on this basic assumption that rational military preference supports civilian protection.[5] The concept of civilian distinctiveness has been promoted in all international legal treaties relating to the conduct of war. An essential element of this regime of civilian protection in war is the commitment of the parties to the conflict to abide by the laws.

In traditional societies and in the nation-state regime of the Geneva Conventions, war was seen as an inevitable but containable departure from the usual state of nonwar that defined intergroup or international relations. Codes and conventions relating to war were introduced to confine the duration and impact of conflict so as to minimize cruelty, humiliation, and cycles of violence that might impede the return to peace (8). By defining who is the targeted victim and who is not, who is expendable and who is not, and how force is to be used against the enemy, war conventions set the terms of conflict transactions. One side pledges that it will avoid indiscriminate slaughter and adhere to other constraints in order that its enemy makes and keeps a similar pledge. Such conventions, and behaviors respectful of them, depend on a high degree of human connectivity and perceived equality of trust and risk of reprisal (9).

Erosion of civilian protection

This tradition of civilian protection rests on the assumption that it is in the best interests of the military mission to abide by humanitarian tenets. However, warfare over the course of the 20th century has slipped significantly from this version of rational interests. Since the end of World War II, civilians have constituted the overwhelming majority of total war casualties (10). The complex regional and civil wars of the 1990s reveal nonstate actors, relatively untrained and using light arms, attacking civilians in order to obtain significant military advantage from the destruction, terror, flight, and chaos that these attacks produce (11).

In the case of internal conflicts, civilian populations are now being caught in the crossfire between insurgents and state forces and are bearing most of the casualties. In extreme situations (Bosnia-Herzegovina, 1992–1994; Rwanda, 1994; and Kosovo, 1998–99), entire segments of the civilian population have been perceived as a primary military target on political, racial, or ethnic grounds. Civilian deaths in just these three wars can be summed — based on estimates of 800,000 dead in Rwanda; 300,000 dead in Bosnia-Herzegovina; and 10,000 dead in Kosovo — to over 1.1 million people. This number far exceeds any estimate advanced for the number of specific military casualties that have occurred in these wars. The current war in the Democratic Republic of Congo (DRC), which began as a civil war but has since become internationalized, has caused an estimated 2.5 million civilian deaths — a number that is massively disproportionate to the combatant injuries and deaths that so far have occurred (12).

Forced migration in the face of assault and terror is another significant outcome of a war strategy that targets civilians as a calculated means of achieving strategic goals. In the last decade, armed conflict or internal strife has forced, on average, 35 million people throughout the world into refugee status or the category of internally displaced (13). The consequences of such displacement are severe and include grave assaults on all three measures of the psychosocial domain of human security.

- *Relationships with location (a sustainable sense of home and safety; providing identity, recognition, and freedom from fear)*: Forced rupture of ties with home and production of chaotic situations puts civilians in the path of hostile combatant forces and places them at risk during all phases of flight and search for refuge.

- *Relationships with community (a network of constructive social or family support; providing identity, recognition, participation, and autonomy)*: Dispersal of families exposes women and girls to sexual violence and prostitution and enables forced military recruitment of children, sending those as young as the age of seven into armed combatant roles.

- *Relationships with time (an acceptance of the past and a positive grasp of the future; providing identity, recognition, participation, and autonomy)*: The breakdown of the social fabric, disintegration of community, and abandonment of home all hinder the return to normality and peace-building efforts.

Obliteration of humanitarian space

International aid to targeted civilian populations thwarts the anticivilian strategies of the warring parties and is seen as intensely political and partisan. These parties to the conflict defend their actions by appealing to the principle of national sovereignty in matters they deem essentially within their domestic jurisdiction. In their zones of influence, the warring parties block relief convoys, obstruct ambulance passage, invade hospitals, destroy clinics, and harass and terrorize national and international medical and other humanitarian relief workers. They create conditions that threaten or inflict grave harm on those who are obligated by professional and international laws to provide aid to civilians in need. The recent literature is replete with examples of such assault and obstruction in Somalia (14), Bosnia (15), Chechnya (16, 17), and Kosovo (18).

Human insecurity in war: the psychosocial impact of suffering

The impact of internal wars on civilian populations has not been systematically described from the perspective of those enduring them. In 1999 the International Committee of the Red Cross (ICRC) surveyed 12,000 people exposed to recent wars, conducting a formal randomized inquiry into the war experience and attitudes of ordinary people. Analysis of the questionnaire and focus group data from this effort yields a range of insights on the psychosocial dimension of war trauma (19). These insights have direct bearing on our understanding of human security. Key findings of relevance to this discussion come from Afghanistan, Bosnia, Somalia, Cambodia, South Africa, and Israel-Palestine.

Collective suffering and demoralization

In internal wars, states recede or fail, and there are no frontlines where men fight and die in heroic efforts to save the nation. There is no mention of the rear echelon, the zone where civilians might expect some protection from battle-related injury and provide material and moral support for the combatants. People testify to experiences that amount to more than a sum of their individual painful biographies. They describe the violence and loss in terms that evoke a societal dimension, an ecology of suffering (20) that affects all aspects of collective life, of being and acting together. The narratives of suffering are always related by 'we' and articulated as collective experience and collective fate. Violence has changed their entire world.

Respondents note the distinction between civilian and combatant only in the negative, observing with bitterness that the reality of events has betrayed their trust in this fundamental precept. The data from the ICRC survey show that although young men are more exposed to combat injuries, combatants and civilians are affected almost equally by assaults on their property and families, by group dislocation, and by all forms of attack that target people rather than armies.

When people speak of bereavement, it is without the solace of conviction that their loss has served some higher purpose. People report feeling that they have participated in something 'wrong,' yet they cannot make sense of what happened. They portray themselves as captives of an exclusive collective experience, which is either impossible or pointless to share with those who have not taken the same journey. What emerges from these accounts is a sense of collective failure and pervasive moral bewilderment about what has befallen entire populations. With varying intensity, the focus group respondents look at their immersion in epidemic violence as effecting a harmful transformation, impairing their capacity to reenter what they vaguely remember to have been a normal moral universe.

BETRAYAL OF COMMUNITY

The wars described by the respondents brought sweeping physical destruction. This aspect, most underscored in the Afghanistan study, leaves people with a sense of futility, anger, and despair. Everything beautiful, everything productive, everything that links people to their past or supports a path to the future has been broken or crushed. The devastation of landscape and infrastructure, the wiping out of farms, livestock, towns, and cities, cries out for some return, some rationale, some victory in the midst of such great loss. The question that people raise and answer in the same breath is, "To what end?" They see no reason for the destruction.

A core experience with many implications emerges from all the discussions: people realize with a mix of shame and disbelief that in these internal wars they had become utterly expendable in the minds of those they had thought were friends and neighbors. A human connection they had worked hard to sustain over the years had suddenly ruptured. Perceived as a betrayal of trust, this shift in relationships fueled intense feelings of anger and violence. At the group level, the collapse of social trust into communal violence led to levels of brutality that people had previously thought unimaginable.

When the state no longer exists, or can no longer act as an objective authority, proximity between groups poses dangers. An apparent characteristic of internal conflict is that it triggers and perpetuates this cataclysmic erosion of social trust, which, once lost, seems to consign all involved to protracted spasms of hatred and brutality. Feeling wronged, people become perpetrators who seek relief in progressively self-defeating cycles of vengeance. In so doing, they risk incurring their own self-hatred. Former combatants are particularly aware of being held captive in this way.

People view what has happened to their land and to themselves in terms that convey a complete destruction of meaning. Intrastate conflict inflicts such costs that people cannot retrieve the argument about why the war began. When asked why they were involved they reply only that they had no choice. This response reflects in part a strategic posture towards the outsider, but reveals as well a deeper truth. In these wars, no one could be trusted to take care of you; social contracts were shattered; the state, the army, and your neighbors betrayed your trust; your sense of right and wrong was violated by daily events; and you were helpless against the full assault of conflict. Survival was the best that could be achieved. Survival with meaning was too much to ask for.

GLOBAL FAILURE TO PERCEIVE THE PSYCHOSOCIAL DIMENSION

The data suggest that people in areas of conflict have great expectations with regard to the external world. The majority of respondents in all countries surveyed request more intervention from the outside, with the general sense that internal resources for dealing with the conflict have been exhausted, and the last and only hope must come from the international community.

The focus groups from regions where actual humanitarian operations are underway, however, reveal distinct layers of disappointment and criticism. International efforts are seen as chaotic, shortsighted, and governed by self-interest. The respondents note the fragmented approach of the many different organizations competing for visibility, purveying goods and services ill designed to address the continuum of suffering in their communities. Additionally, everyone recognizes the disparities in lifestyles between the wealthy outsiders and the local people. Many suggest that as the humanitarian workers continue their efforts, they increasingly (although unintentionally) sow distrust, anger, and envy.

The findings suggest that the international community, for all its good will, is not positioned to address the psychological and social issues of collective shame and demoralization found among respondents. By not dealing with these complex issues, while at the same time delivering material support in a clumsy and piecemeal fashion, humanitarian aid is destined to make the recipients restless and dismissive.

HUMAN SECURITY AND THE GENEVA CONVENTIONS

The findings from this study underscore the ways in which the erosion of civilian protection in war determines the persistence of social disarray in post-conflict settings. Reports from people trapped in war provide empirical detail to support our understanding of what happens when these conventions are ignored, when limits are exceeded and human connectivity is sundered. Once launched, internal wars can last for decades, throughout the lifetime of participants. Civilians are entrained in fighting that wipes out the distinction between the home front and the battlefront. Social, environmental, and economic destruction becomes extensive and severe. Combatants are ill trained, ill led, and forced into a spiral of violence, atrocity, humiliation, and rage. The ultimate psychological damage is inflicted upon those who fight, for they suffer the trauma of realizing how capable they have become of committing horrible acts, and how powerless they have become in protecting their families from the horrible acts of others.

In essence, these results suggest that the role of the Geneva Conventions is to protect people from atrocity so that the potential for a return to peace can be kept alive. The respondents overwhelmingly endorsed the principles of international law as the means to "prevent wars from getting worse." All those enmeshed in their own local conflict could see beyond it to know that another path might have been taken.

HUMAN SECURITY AND PROTECTION OF HUMANITARIAN SPACE

The changing nature of war has prompted recognition of the need to expand the scope of humanitarian concerns during war. As all aspects of civilian life have become potential strategic pawns in the conflict continuum, the international community has found it necessary to articulate and develop new guidelines and normative barriers to place in the path of attack.

The expanded role over the past decades of UN agencies and NGOs in humanitarian operations has increased considerably the number of humanitarian actors in conflict situations (21). This increase in number and diversity has had a direct impact on the perceived scope of protection, from one driven by IHL to one driven by the many concerns arising from the relief community who have witnessed the needs of specific groups of victims. Children need caring adults; terrified refugees need to feel safe; people from diverse cultures seek respectful space for religious practice; women in camps should not be forced into prostitution. Without specifying the rationale as such, a human security perspective has infused these initiatives and arguments.[6]

This needs-based expansion has sought legal confirmation by referring to a number of key human rights documents that the humanitarian community views as extremely relevant and applicable in conflict settings. By a slow process of insisting that key provisions of these documents do indeed apply in a state of war or conflict (22, 23), there is a growing recognition that just because people are trapped in war, they do not in any moral or legal sense lose the zone of protection they could claim were they living in a country at peace.

Reflecting the influence of aid workers, the time frame of humanitarian protection is also being extended. The horizon of applicability of international humanitarian law was traditionally assumed to conform to the duration of actual hostilities. From the perspective of public health and humanitarian aid, however, the early phases that lead up to a conflict and the extended post-conflict and reconstruction periods are of equal concern. The humanitarian time frame for civilian protection is thus much longer and encompasses a far more complex political terrain. Central and persistent concerns for the humanitarian community throughout the post-conflict period include the establishment of policing power and civil security (24), the repatriation of refugees (25), and the status of vulnerable groups such as women and girls (26).

To establish this expanded scope of humanitarian protection in the legal and operational sphere is a complex challenge. Recent initiatives, undertaken at international legal levels and pursued by many humanitarian and human rights organizations in a grassroots mode, have focused on protecting civilians against the use of anti-personnel landmines, protecting internally displaced persons, and prohibiting military recruitment of children.

Expanding humanitarian protection must also include efforts to maintain a dialogue with local people before, during, and after the course of war. In any conflict, the evolving rules of survival define what scholars have called the local morality (27). Ethics based on human rights and humanitarian principles are perceived as external and in many ways opposed to the dictates of the local set of norms. People engulfed in the local morality are still very capable of talking about these external norms as abstractions. It is in the application that the gap appears. The international humanitarian community occupies a curious position in this space between local morality and external ethics. When people request rules to prevent war from escalating, they are asking the international community to protect them, through practical, on-the-ground application of international humanitarian law. People seek concrete actions that save lives, not a simple reassertion of norms in UN deliberations.

HUMAN SECURITY AND HUMANITARIAN INTERVENTION

Media attention and substantive civil society dialogue, giving voice to humanitarian agencies and to local people, have contributed to the development of an increasingly nuanced and informed debate about the obligations of nation-states, in their collective security arrangements, to enforce these protections. In active evolution is the practical import of what has long been seen as an implicit, background responsibility of the international community. What should be done when states, or warring parties, fail to protect their citizens from grave human rights abuses and violations of international humanitarian law? Throughout the 1990s we have seen the rationale for international intervention move beyond the UN Chapter VII language (response to threats to global peace and security) to concern for maintaining international standards of civilian protection in conflict settings (28).

A human security perspective, advanced by the humanitarian community, would support the development of strategies and options to maximize the resources available within a given set of political and security constraints. In settings where consent of warring parties can be obtained and external force is not required, such options would include the establishment of humanitarian corridors, the delivery of targeted relief assistance, the planned safe exit of a population in an emergency situation, or the creation of protected areas. Where the consent of warring parties cannot be obtained or has broken down, and the civilian population continues to be at high risk, the international community must face the last resort option of deploying UN or regional forces to protect civilians — especially displaced populations and refugees in large settlements — against violent assaults.

These strategies and options pose complex issues in terms of humanitarian neutrality, protection of civilians from unanticipated or collateral consequences of armed intervention, and the reach of international engagement across borders of national sovereignty (29). Yet it is clear from recent past experience that allowing pervasive internal wars to assault civilian populations for years or decades incites grave regional instability and, from the human security perspective, fundamentally undermines the prospects for these societies to return to peace and integration of community. There is, it could be argued, a fairly direct line from a commitment to protect human security in war, to an interest in discerning options for humanitarian intervention.

Human security and the culture of impunity

An important focus of these efforts should be to strengthen international judicial institutions for the protection of civilian human rights in situations of armed conflict. A culture of impunity shelters individuals responsible for violent assaults against civilians; it is one of the most significant obstacles to the protection of civilians in most conflict situations. The unwillingness or inability of states to bring these people to justice undermines the effectiveness of the entire legal framework. An International Criminal Court (ICC) has been established as a remedy for such situations. The adoption of the Statute of the ICC in July 1998 constitutes a major first step in this ambitious but vital enterprise. The creation by the Security Council of the two ad hoc tribunals for the former Yugoslavia and Rwanda set valuable precedent in this regard.

The recognition that the continuum of suffering in internal wars ranges from victims to perpetrators adds complexity to resolution of issues of impunity. At some earlier stage, most perpetrators were victims. Entering the cycle of violence once it is established requires this acknowledgment in order to balance the assessment of violations and maintain a generative, inclusive perspective on how to move on from active hostilities.

To respond to the suffering of victims without addressing the needs, anger, and humiliation of the perpetrators may not be the most effective way to deal with societies caught in internal wars. Many of these cultures still designate men as the normative agents and the authority figures. It is important to enlist these men to influence interpretations of the war and attitudes toward reconstruction. This process will require granting them some dignity and refraining from humiliation, in parallel with the more familiar steps of establishing a path toward justice. Identifying and punishing the leaders and serious offenders can protect others from the pressure of collective stigmatization.

An understanding of these issues provides the psychosocial and humanitarian rationale for legal and operational efforts to sustain civilian protection in war. A human security approach would insist upon redoubled efforts to promote and enforce the Geneva Conventions, less from the perspective of playing by the rules than from the recognition that, absent adherence to norms, the people who have suffered throughout the long years of abusive war may find the return to a viable post-conflict society virtually impossible to accomplish.

HUMAN SECURITY AND HUMANITARIAN PRACTICE

The concept of human security, as an interesting way of examining populations in stressed circumstances, is just beginning to percolate among humanitarian agencies (nongovernmental organizations and the humanitarian units of international institutions and governments). However, one can track an implicit understanding of the basic tenets outlined here through the evolution of humanitarian practice since the 1994 genocide in Rwanda and the debacle of the Goma relief effort in 1994–1996.

Early warning failed in Rwanda and protection for those who fled into eastern Zaire (later DRC) was not adequate to forestall epidemic disease and grossly violent predation on unarmed refugees and surrounding host communities. A deeply influential assessment of the assistance response challenged the entire humanitarian community to consider ways to become more professional and more effective in carrying out the core mission of protection as well as relief (30).

This process of reflection and focus has infused The Sphere Project, a network of humanitarian actors established in 1996 who have since produced, with wide input from organizations and individuals around the world, a core statement of values and a set of standards for humanitarian action. In its latest edition, this group's publication aims explicitly to integrate principles of human rights and civilian protection (31). Building on what is known to be best practice in the delivery of aid — including process parameters such as transparency, accountability, and attention to local initiative and culture — The Sphere Project contributes to a growing self-awareness, resolution, and humility on the part of humanitarian relief workers. It is becoming increasingly evident, in multinational and multisectoral humanitarian efforts, that organizational readiness, disciplined attention to core competencies, and coordination with other stakeholders and actors in the region are essential attributes of a successful relief effort.

ESSENTIAL HUMAN SECURITY ELEMENTS

Applying the human security perspective to current strategies and policies of the humanitarian community in war and post-conflict settings yields broad thematic improvements and specific program recommendations.

Before the crisis

As indications of impending communal crisis or civil war begin to unfold, humanitarian workers should try to fulfill their potential role in providing early warning. Within the limitations of their own organizational mandates, and attending to their own security, relief agencies in the field can quietly provide information and alerts to responsible external institutions (the UN, the ICRC, and regional security bodies).

The content of these communications should include:

■ Indications of breakdown in group interactions

■ Escalation in actions that inflict humiliation and affronts to dignity

■ Influx and diffusion of small arms

■ Development of hate media

During crisis

During crisis, emergency relief objectives should provide basic survival inputs and seek to protect populations from short-run threats to individual and group safety.

Specific steps include:

■ Expand observance of the Geneva Conventions at all levels of society

■ Negotiate humanitarian zones under the parameters of international humanitarian law

■ Disarm and demilitarize refugee camps

■ Reduce the size of camps for refugees and displaced people

■ Identify and institute best practices for reducing sexual violence in camps

■ Develop protocols and agreements for possible evacuations of the seriously ill and injured

■ Introduce programs at the group level to cope with psychological distress

■ Build in support and training for local personnel

Post-conflict

In the immediate post-conflict period, interventions should guard against heightening tension between groups and focus on building habits of respect for dignity and fairness. Every effort should be made to avoid creating or magnifying existing social divisions. It is important to remain vigilant in this early post-fighting phase, as the key issues that led to the war still smolder (32). The post-conflict phase is truly a misnomer, in that the factors igniting the conflict have not yet been dealt with and events on the ground can quickly slip out of apparent control.

Specific steps include:

■ Establish an effective process for enforcing and monitoring the ceasefire or other peace agreement

■ Organize and deploy an effective police or security force to increase levels of safety for all local groups and expatriates

■ Introduce the rule of law by first establishing regime presence, stability, and consistency; then by building public confidence in due process and administrative coherence

■ Build infrastructure, particularly roads

■ Introduce essential services, such as health care

Common policies to pursue in all phases

At all times, agencies should focus on the three domains of psychosocial stability. They should encourage resettlement through disarming and demining initiatives, strengthen community ties through participatory and egalitarian service delivery, support a positive sense of the future by restoring the rule of law and the credibility of police authority, reconstruct infrastructure, and encourage investment. The common thread of resource infusion underscores the need for a consistent policy aimed at minimizing any accentuation of inequality among groups. There are five aspects to this common policy:

1. Emphasize egalitarian distribution of resources (including relief commodities and services such as health care)

2. Foster inclusion after identifying those who are marginalized and insecure

3. Shore up local capacities and coping strategies at all levels of society

4. Support attention to human rights at all phases of a response

5. Improve training and procedures for expatriate and national personnel

WHAT LIES AHEAD?

Coherence on these policies is evolving just as the nature of current wars and conflict is growing more complex and unpredictable. The rise of terrorism, the criminalization of fighting groups, and the dominant role of the U.S. in conflict and post-conflict regimes pose new challenges for humanitarian practice. The methods and tactics of warfare are shifting. HIV/AIDS, now assuming pandemic scope with unique mortality patterns, looms against all assistance and intervention. How does one establish priorities? What key competencies are still needed? With whom does one coordinate? How does one maintain humanitarian space and noncombatant distinctions for one's own staff, let alone for the local civilian population?

Evolving strategies implicitly invoke tenets of human security. There is mounting recognition that to protect people in crisis and conflict settings, the humanitarian community must engage many sectors and enterprises in a vigorous campaign of upstream prevention. Strategies include an international assault on the trade — in small arms, illicit drugs, and illegally extracted minerals — that funds the violence, as well as an international call to relieve debt burdens and revive agricultural economies. These strategies anticipate the need to develop new or more assertive roles for civil society in establishing collective responsibility for the human security of world populations (33).

Framed in a more positive light, the human security approach seeks to understand and support the ways in which human beings can be proud in their identity, at peace in their community, and filled with hope for the future. This stance must not be abandoned in times of conflict. Instead, insisting upon the enduring relevance of this approach to human populations in all phases of their communal life span holds the best promise for sustaining them through the worst of times.

NOTES

[1]   For history of the term 'human security,' see Leaning and Arie, 2001 (1).

[2]   These categories were designed for practical assessment and map to Amoo's concepts of basic human psychosocial needs for identity, recognition, and participation (2).

[3]   The world has become accustomed to the use of measurements and composite indices since the UN first introduced the Human Development Index (HDI) ten years ago. Tracking progress in key aggregate social and economic areas of education (adult literacy and school enrollment), health (life expectancy at birth), and economy (GDP per capita), the composite index has been used to rank countries and follow trends in human development over the past decade. In 1997, the UN introduced an inverse measurement, the Human Poverty Index (HPI), in order to measure deprivations along the same dimensions of education, health, and economic life (3).

[4]   For social dislocation, for example, one could use distance from home, years spent away from home, number of family ties broken, number of household heads forced into penury, number of landless laborers, or the number of dispossessed (4, 5, 6).

[5]　This distinction is at the core of humanitarian protection in International Humanitarian Law as described in Article 48, Basic Rule of Protocol I, which reads: "In order to ensure respect for and protection of the civilian population and civilian objects, the Parties to the conflict shall at all times distinguish between the civilian population and combatants and between civilian objects and military objectives and accordingly shall direct their operations only against military objectives." The provisions of humanitarian law aim to stress the civilian character of individuals (Article 50, Protocol I), specific premises such as hospitals (Article 52, ss. Protocol I), and activities such as relief operations (Article 68, ss. Protocol I) that should be spared from military interference or obstruction.

[6]　An expanded version of the legal arguments for this position can be found in Bruderlein and Leaning, BMJ (20).

References

1.　Leaning J, Arie S. *Human security in crisis and transition.* Working Paper Series, Volume 11, Number 8. Cambridge (MA): Harvard Center for Population and Development Studies; 2001.

2.　Amoo S. *The challenge of ethnicity and conflicts in Africa: the need for a new paradigm.* New York: United Nations Development Program Emergency Response Division; 1997.

3.　United Nations Development Programme. *Human development report 2000.* Oxford: Oxford University Press; 2000. p. 147.

4.　Drèze J, Sen A. *Hunger and public action.* Oxford: Clarendon Press; 1989. p. 5.

5.　De Soto H. *The other path: the invisible revolution in the third world.* New York: Harper and Row; 1989.

6.　Kaplan R. The coming anarchy. *The Atlantic Monthly* 1994 Feb;2:33.

7.　Webb, P. Drawing lines in water: the challenge of vulnerability analysis in developing countries. Medford (MA): Fletcher School of Law and Diplomacy. *Fletcher Forum of World Affairs* 2000;24(1):35–46.

8.　Kalshoven F. *Constraints on the waging of war.* Geneva: International Committee of the Red Cross; 1991.

9.　De Lupis ID. *The law of war.* LSE Monographs on International Studies. Cambridge (UK): Cambridge University Press; 1987. p. 339–52.

10.　Sivard RL, *World military and social expenditures 1996.* Washington: World Priorities; 1996.

11.　Kaldor M, Vashee B, editors. *Restructuring the global military sector.* Volume I: New wars. London: Pinter; 1997.

12.　Roberts L. *Mortality in eastern Democratic Republic of Congo.* New York: International Rescue Committee; 2001. Available from: URL: http://www.theirc.org, accessed on 2003 Aug 4.

13. International Federation of Red Cross (IFRC) and Red Crescent Societies. *World disasters report 2002*. Geneva, Switzerland: IFRC; 2002. p. 204–11.

14. Leaning J. When the system doesn't work: Somalia 1992. In: Cahill KM, editor. *A framework for survival: health, human rights, and humanitarian assistance in conflicts and disasters*. New York: Basic Books and the Council on Foreign Relations; 1999. p. 31–48.

15. Ramsbotham O, Woodhouse T. *Humanitarian intervention in contemporary conflict*. Cambridge (UK): Polity Press; 1996. p. 167–92.

16. Jean F. The problems of medical relief in the Chechen war zone. *Central Asian Survey* 1996;15:255–8.

17. Hansen G. Aid in war-ravaged Chechnya: a severe test for humanitarians. *Christian Science Monitor* 1997 Dec 31;19.

18. Physicians for Human Rights. Medical group documents systematic and pervasive abuses by Serbs against Albanian Kosovar health professionals and Albanian Kosovar patients. Preliminary report and press release. Boston: PHR; 1998 Dec 23.

19. Holleufer G, Briton N, Leaning J. Report on people in war. Overview and country reports prepared for the International Committee of the Red Cross. Francois Xavier Bagnoud Center for Health and Human Rights. Boston: Harvard School of Public Health; unpublished.

20. Das V, Kleinman A. Introduction. In: Das V, Ramphele M, Reynolds P, editors. *Violence and subjectivity*. Berkeley: University of California Press; 2000.

21. Bruderlein C, Leaning J. New challenges for humanitarian protection. *British Medical Journal* 1999;319:430–5.

22. Lubbers RFM. Humanitarian aid: redefining the limits. The Hague: Advisory Council on International Affairs, Government of The Netherlands; 1998.

23. O'Donnell D. Trends in the application of international humanitarian law by United Nations human rights mechanisms. *International Review of the Red Cross* 1998;324:481–503.

24. Kolb R. Relationship between international humanitarian law and human rights law: short bibliography. *International Review of the Red Cross* 1998;324:572–5.

25. Sifton J, Zia-Sarifi S. The lesson of Afghanistan: peacekeeping in Iraq. *International Herald Tribune* 2003 May 20. Available from: URL: www.iht.com/ihtsearch.php, accessed 2003 Aug 6.

26. Boutroue J. Missed opportunities: the role of the international community in the return of the Rwandan refugees from Eastern Zaire July 1994–December 1996. Rosemarie Rogers Working Papers Series. Cambridge (MA): MIT Center for International Studies, Massachusetts Institute of Technology; 1998.

27. Iacopino V, Rasekh Z, Yamin AE, Freedman L, Burkhalter H, Atkinson H, et al. *The Taliban's war on women: a health and human rights crisis in Afghanistan*. Boston: Physicians for Human Rights; 1998.

28. Kleinman A. Moral experience and ethical reflection: can ethnography reconcile them? A quandary for "the new bioethics." *Daedalus: Journal of the American Academy of Arts and Sciences* 1999;128(4):69–97.

29. United Nations Security Council. Report of the Secretary General to the Security Council on the protection of civilians in armed conflict. UN Doc. S1/1999/957. New York: United Nations; 1999.

30. Joint Evaluation of Emergency Assistance to Rwanda. The international response to conflict and genocide: lessons from the Rwanda experience. Copenhagen; 1996 Mar.

31. The Sphere Project. Humanitarian charter and minimum standards in humanitarian response. Oxford: Oxfam Publishing. In press 2003.

32. Holzgrefe JL, Keohane RO, editors. *Humanitarian intervention: ethical, legal, and political dilemmas.* Cambridge (UK): Cambridge University Press; 2003.

33. Leaning J. Human rights and conflict. *Health and Human Rights* 2003;6:3–12.

CHAPTER 3

HEALTH AND SECURITY IN HISTORICAL PERSPECTIVE

SIMON SZRETER

HEALTH AND SECURITY: TWINS RECENTLY PARTED

It is distinctly odd that such a primeval human concern as *security* should only recently be explicitly linked in the academic and policy literature with *health*, another of humanity's eternal preoccupations. This signifies nothing so much as the manner in which both the worlds of knowledge and of action may be divided by meaningless disciplinary fences and can be separated, instead of joined, by words. *Security* and *health* have been kept segregated from each other for several decades largely because they have each acted as major symbols for previously opposed — or at least mutually disinterested — sets of political interests, ideological dispositions, and networks of institutions. *Security* is undoubtedly long established as a key term in the lexicon of the defense establishment of most western liberal democracies, notably that of the U.S. *Health* has been adopted by many groups wishing to promote it in various contexts but most consistently in an academic or policy context by those studying and advocating public health.

However, the separate usage of these two terms in recent decades belies the fact that historically they have usually dwelled together. Sovereigns such as the French medieval kings swore in their coronation oaths to protect the frail and weak, widows and cripples. The power to afford such security was both symbol and justification of their divine right to rule. Successful generals, from the time of Alexander the Great, have long known that the effectiveness of their armies depends crucially on their health — summarized in Napoleon's celebrated dictum that an army "marches on its stomach." Naval surgeons and army doctors in the 18th century were important early exponents of the principles of preventive medicine and techniques of epidemiology (1). Much of the whole field of tropical (formerly imperial) medicine developed from the joint interests of the military and the medical professions (2).

But in the general public's discourse, too, there was a time until not so long ago when the explicitly twinned themes of security and health of the populace dominated attention. A good example is the era of debate over National Efficiency during the decade of imperialist rivalry that led to the outbreak of World War I in 1914 (3). Indeed, in England, the successful turning of this discourse by the medically trained leaders of the public health movement (away from its social Darwinist formulation, toward a more environmentalist understanding of the poor health of the urban masses) paved the way for the British state's belated conversion to a range of Bismarckian, insurance-based welfare and social security provisions (4, 5). This trend led eventually in 1919 to the establishment of the British public health movement's dream of a national Ministry of Health (6). Thus, the historical omens are not unpropitious. When the public health movement is able to ally its arguments with profound concerns for national security, great progress can be made in mobilizing resources and creating new institutions to promote health and human security.

It was the even more direct subsequent military threat to Britain's human security, the fight against aerial bombardment on the home front in World War II, that provided the context for the formation of the Emergency Medical Service, the forerunner for the National Health Service (NHS) (7). Indeed, the close affinity between the promotion of the nation's health and its security was semantically fused in the celebrated wartime Beveridge Report on *Social Insurance and Allied Services*, the 1942 blueprint for the nation's future welfare state and the NHS. At its heart was Beveridge's Plan for Social Security:

> "Social Security is defined as security for the individual, organized by the State, against risks to which the individual will remain exposed even when the condition of the society as a whole is as good as it can be made (8)."

Beveridge's plan for society's security consisted of several main elements: children's allowances; maintenance of full employment; national insurance and pensions; and, of course, a universal and free (at point of use) health service. There is, then, nothing new in the occurrence of periods of crisis, provoked by the perception of external threat to the nation's security, like the American public's shocked response to September 11, providing a galvanizing political opportunity for the promotion of ambitious new thinking about health, framed as an issue of national security. Indeed, when comparing the way in which the same vested interests — the insurance industry and the medical profession itself — were able to resist politicians' attempts to create a national health service in the U.S. in the 1940s while being unable to resist it in Britain, the absence in America of such a traumatic threat to citizens' personal security as the experience of the Nazi bombing campaign would seem to have been a politically decisive factor (9, 10).

Thus, although the words *security* and *health* have rarely appeared in public together during the last half-century, a little history reveals their secret: they are in fact — and always have been — twins. From an historical perspective, the interesting question is how the two terms could have remained apart for several decades recently in the academic and policy literature? There is, I believe, a revealing, somewhat paradoxical answer to this question. But before we can arrive at this answer, we must begin by establishing the historical correctness of a profoundly counterintuitive understanding of the relationship between economic growth, human security, and health.

ECONOMIC GROWTH AND THE DISRUPTION OF HUMAN SECURITY AND HEALTH

Economic growth has always been, by definition, a process that transforms and challenges all dimensions of human security: of individuals, states, even businesses. The more generally held, superficially optimistic view of economic growth and the expansion of markets — as synonymous with opportunity and as the source of all our creature comforts — has led to a blind reverence for maximizing national economic growth rates among political leaders and electorates alike.

As Amartya Sen has cogently insisted, development is not equivalent to rising per capita GDP, but relates primarily to enhanced freedoms and dignity (11). These benefits *may* flow from economic growth, but to portray them as if they were essential and integral to the process itself is a dangerous untruth. The growth process guarantees no net benefits, least of all to the general society. The only statement that is true about the process of economic growth is that it is thoroughly disruptive. It is as full of insecurities as it is of opportunities or risks.

The potential for economic growth, trade, capital accumulation, market competition, and cost-cutting to be of genuine long-term benefit to the great majority, rather than merely to a few successful individual competitors, depends entirely on the manner in which peoples and their governments adapt: how they negotiate, fight over, and decide to manage, tax, and distribute the wealth created. This process constitutes the political and constitutional history of economic and social change. Without any recorded exception known to this author, all current, successful, leading western societies that industrialized before 1945 (most of them before 1914), suffered a painful and difficult learning experience in coming to terms with the insecurities and health threats of full commercialization and economic growth (12). They all experienced at some point in their growth trajectory the severe 'demographic footprint' of the 'four Ds' of economic growth: disruption, deprivation, disease, and death (13). In some of the worst cases, such as Britain, the disruption for an entire half century was so great for large proportions of the national population that insecure, marginal, and deprived sections (the urban proletariat, in particular children, women, and the Irish in the British case) died prematurely and from preventable infectious and sanitary diseases in such numbers as to depress the national average health measures for decade after decade (14).

The process of constitutional and political adaptation to the turbulent demands of living with economic growth, so as to minimize its accompanying disruption of security and health, has taken these 'successful' advanced economies centuries to achieve — literally. This situation seems to be an extremely poorly understood and distinctly undervalued lesson of history and one which has, incredibly, been ignored if not entirely forgotten during the last two decades, with the separation of health from security in the policy literature as symptomatic of this amnesia.

We are repeatedly told that we now live in a world where economic growth is occurring within the novel context of globalization. What does this mean for health and human security if history tells us that economic growth entails disruption? The only prudent conclusion is to expect health and security problems on a global scale, unless the difficult historical lessons of adaptation are heeded.

What is globalization, and what is new about it? There has rarely been a society in recorded human history where economic change has not occurred. However, there is no doubt that the rate of such change and the geographic scale of its effects began to increase substantially as a result of the intercontinental commercial, mercantile, and industrial revolutions of the 17th and 18th centuries. For all the hype about the novelty of globalization, economic growth is a phenomenon that has been continuously transforming social, political, and natural relationships almost everywhere, on a truly global scale, for at least the last two centuries (15).

There are, however, three truths about historical novelty in the period since 1989 underlying the 'g-hype.' Each of these is largely the consequence of the information-acceleration effects of satellite plus fiber-optic communications and computing technology, allied to previous political decisions, taken at the behest of the world's financial elites, to free up international capital and foreign exchange markets. The three truths are: firstly, the rate and volume of short-term financial flows has increased significantly; secondly, with the end of the Cold War, there is something more like a single global system of trade and finance than at any time since the gold standard era preceding the Great War and the Bolshevik Revolution; thirdly, the most articulate and influential citizens of the richest democracies in the world are more immediately, frequently, painfully, and worryingly aware of the truly global nature of their interdependence with the fate of all the rest of humanity than ever before.

The latter in particular encapsulates the most important single paradox of humanity's long-term love affair with the post-Enlightenment project of economic growth, world development, and progress. The promise of security and health has been a primary aim and justification of all the effort that humans have devoted to contriving their economic growth during the last several centuries. Freedom from the caprices and misfortunes of fate and nature has been a motivating dream for a populace that can manufacture its own secure food supply, shelter, and protection from disease, weather, and other species. However, as the doyen of Polish economic historians, Witold Kula, has astutely observed,

> "The mastering of the forces of nature, the uncovering of its potentialities, the growing utilization of its wealth, all these do away with some manifestations of the dependence, but create new ones in their stead....The more of nature's inherent potentialities man learns to bring to the surface, the more, by mastering her, he comes to depend on her (16)."

To this premise we can add that our capacity to 'master' nature ever more elaborately is based on an increasing specialization and division of labor on a global scale. Hence, we become ever more dependent for the maintenance of our way of life on wider circles and networks of our fellow humanity. The pursuit of personal wealth and the promise of material security through market exchange thus brings with it an ever-greater dependency on nature, technologies, and institutions, and on all those myriad humans contributing to the global market, from which we draw the means to our material security and enhanced life expectancies.

Economic growth — the process whereby these expanding markets for diverse goods and services are brought into exchange — is an intrinsically disruptive and destabilizing process of change. It works firstly by converting into commodities aspects of the material environment not previously perceived to have commercial value; secondly, by imaginatively creating the market for entirely new goods and services; and thirdly, by cutting the price of existing commodities. All of these activities, as can readily be appreciated, are fundamentally transformative and necessarily associated with psychological, social, ideological, and cultural change. These challenges create tides of disruption and insecurity, especially for workers or owners of assets who find that their labor or property has been devalued by the ever-changing commodity markets.

Thus, if we live now in an age of more rapid and global economic change than ever before in human history, it is crucial in any evaluation of the current prospects for health and human security, that we commence our analysis with the clear-eyed understanding that economic growth does not directly enhance human security, and in fact, systematically jeopardizes it for many if not most people at some point during their lives. Although the accumulation over generations of productive physical capital and the construction of all the associated human and social capital undoubtedly gives both individuals and societies the capacity to live healthier, longer, and more fulfilled lives, the process whereby this potential is realized can be an extremely rough ride for all concerned. Economic growth is intrinsically a process of creative destruction, as the two greatest historians of industrial capitalism — Karl Marx and Joseph Schumpeter — would readily agree, from quite opposed ideological positions.

Paul Farmer's revealing analysis of the 'structural violence' of inequality has shown that the commercial and ephemeral values of newsworthiness mean that crises, such as famines, may be the only health threats to the world's poor that gain adequate public attention in the free presses of the First World's liberal democracies (17, 18). Yet it is the 'silent crises' of preventable infectious diseases such as malaria and tuberculosis, killing millions every year, that are much more quantitatively important. They remain unknown, however, to western public opinion, partly because their perennial nature renders them unnewsworthy. They also constitute guilty secrets, since they are 'orphan diseases,' that the commercial pharmaceutical industry has neglected because there is little prospect of any payment from impoverished individuals or debt-ridden governments, who have in any case been ordered to slash their health budgets in the structural adjustment programs of the International Monetary Fund (IMF) (19).

In thinking about the historical relationship of economic growth to human health and security, it may be helpful to invoke another geological metaphor, that of the volcano. Living with rapid economic growth is like living on the fertile lava slopes of an active volcano. The volcanic energy is the force of economic growth. Like the market, the volcano is extremely prolific in producing an accumulation of useful matter, which continually alters the living environment, indeed the very landscape.

There is much inconvenience and need for adaptation when living in the shadow of the volcano. However, given time, the inhabitants know that these disruptive flows of lava will provide them the most fertile soil, enhancing their living standards over the generations. But in the shorter term, the volcano's mode of operation is always somewhat threatening and can occasionally be disastrous. Over a period of many centuries, those peoples who have been encamped longest on and around the volcano of rapid economic growth have slowly and painfully learned the best ways to minimize the personal and collective risks of living with the disruptive processes of economic transformation in their midst.

The problem appears to be that, since 1989, people have suffered a collective attack of euphoria-induced amnesia. They have beckoned all sorts of newcomers to the vicinity of the volcano and suggested that they take up residence as near as possible to the rim. Indeed, they have decamped and moved in that direction themselves, failing to recall why, over the previous centuries, they had adopted a less exposed and more protected location. Now they profess surprise when the newcomers show anger at getting burned in the volcano's frequent eruptions, fight among themselves for a less exposed position, and even try to enter the safer encampments of the well-established.

Learning to live with the volcano comprises the conflict-ridden history of the developed western societies during the last several centuries. To illustrate some of the conflicts and adaptations that have been necessary, a brief overview of certain aspects of British history since the 16th century is offered below. This example shows the importance for health and human security, under conditions of economic growth, of constitutional, legislative, and institutional change — all of it highly contested and closely fought in the political arena. Without these developments, the forces of economic growth would rapidly have extinguished themselves in a holocaust of infectious and sanitary diseases in Britain's industrial cities, which no amount of in-migration could have matched.

After literally centuries of painful social, political, and international conflict, and tragic levels of mortality, western liberal democracies had, by 1945, gradually and with many setbacks along the way, inched their way toward establishing a constitutional form that dealt tolerably well — safely and securely for all — with the vicissitudes of continuous economic growth. This form combined a social democracy with institutional and political pluralism, strong individual rights and protection in law, a free press, and a market economy carefully regulated and taxed so as substantially and widely to redistribute the wealth it generated through a welfare state (20).

MAINTAINING HUMAN SECURITY AND HEALTH UNDER CONDITIONS OF ECONOMIC GROWTH: THE LESSONS OF BRITISH HISTORY

The constitutional changes required to adapt to economic growth while maintaining health and security comprise three related historical developments. Firstly, official registration of all individuals and acknowledgment of their rights to security and health, critically including respect for their diverse social, religious, and ethnic identities. Secondly, the formation by such diverse citizens of legally recognized civil associations and institutions to represent and campaign for their varied and changing interests. This notably includes elected local government, trade unions, professional and employers' associations, as well as a host of less directly political civic associations and, of course, an independent free press. Thirdly, the establishment of some form of welfare or social security state: the securing through the state of various forms of effective collective provision to ensure the promotion of citizens' aspirations for their own security and health.

In Britain, the evolution of these three essential provisions took centuries to accomplish and was disrupted by the process of industrialization. The inception in 1538 of the nationwide parochial registration of all births, deaths, and marriages by Henry VIII was a crucial step in creating a system to record and therefore recognize each individual's existence. By the end of the same century, the Elizabethan Poor Laws gave every person a right to claim sustenance from his or her community of settlement in times of hardship. Historians recognize these laws as having provided the institutional underpinning that ensured that the English (but not the Irish, where there was no such Poor Law) were the first nation in the world to cease to experience famine mortality (21, 22). Although in no way a voting democracy, the subjects of the British sovereign in the 17th and 18th centuries enjoyed advanced, state-guaranteed practical entitlements to security and health — functionings and capabilities in Amartya Sen's terminology — which facilitated the society's precocious economic development (11, 23).

However, in the absence of a democratic franchise to defend these privileges, individual rights were then rudely interrupted, paradoxically by the industrial revolution itself. The reason was very simple and has a parallel in virtually all of today's developing countries. Decades of extremely rapid and chaotic urban industrial growth through in-migration from the countryside produced a breakdown in the urban registration system by the late 18th century. As today in the shantytowns of India, Africa, or Latin America, many individuals were unknown to the authorities and had no recognized address.

Eventually, in 1836, Parliament legislated for a new civil registration system to keep full and accurate records of all births, deaths, and marriages in England and Wales, regardless of religion (Scotland and Ireland were granted such systems somewhat later). With the availability of this centrally collated registration data, the Victorian public health movement found its voice and began to publicize authoritatively the diseased state of the crowded cities and to explore and devise effective remedial policies (24).

But simultaneously in 1834, following the dictates of the then-new liberal ideology of the free market — the classical political economy of Adam Smith, Ricardo, and Malthus — the state radically curtailed its support for the poor, as has happened in many developing countries today under neo-liberal structural adjustment programs and also in the U.S. with welfare cuts. Access to sources of support in these circumstances became closely tied to membership in certain privileged groups, such as religious congregations, workingmen's mutual associations, or the paternalism of some large employers (25, 26, 27).

The subsequent period until 1914 was characterized by a gradual and conflict-ridden process of building up the second factor emphasized above: elected, representative, local government; trade unions; professional and employers' associations; and many other civil and voluntary organizations or forms of social capital. This process culminated in the beginning of a serious movement on the part of these institutions toward negotiation of the third element — collective provision of health and social security.

During the last three decades of the 19th century, the two rival municipalities of Glasgow and Birmingham led a nationwide provincial revolution in government, finance, and social capital, which amounted to a wholly new, collectivist, and municipal (but not yet national) model of delivering social security and health to their crowded urban populations. This system included administering a massive range of municipal schemes of regulation of the urban environment and food supply, preventive and public health measures, welfare and social services, and even the education system and public housing schemes (28, 29, 30). Interestingly, powerful businessmen heading leading international companies, such as Joseph Chamberlain in Birmingham — whose imagination was caught by the 'civic gospel's' promise to transform the lives of the poor — were integral to the practical success of this movement. It was a genuinely cross-class alliance, involving the electoral support of newly enfranchised working-class men, as well as the administrative and technical expertise of new and growing categories of public professionals, such as medical officers of health, and food and sanitary inspectors.

The longer-term product of the experience and momentum built up in this period was the British electorate's eventual acceptance after 1905 of the beginnings of collectivist, state-funded models of provision for health and social security (4, 5, 6). Following the further harsh learning experiences of two world wars, the fight for national survival, and the severe interwar crises of the international economic system, the ultimate result was the acceptance of the Keynesian principles of macroeconomic management and the Beveridge Plan for national social security of the 1940s (7, 8, 31).

HUMAN SECURITY AND HEALTH PROBLEMS IN LESS DEVELOPED COUNTRIES: HISTORICAL REFLECTIONS ON AN INVERTED MIRROR IMAGE

If there is one single foundational policy that the world's poorest states should be encouraged to undertake (and given financial grants to fund) in pursuit of their citizens' long-term health and security, it is to start at the democratic ground level by establishing a full and accurate registration and census enumeration of all their citizens from birth to death. This data must of course be protected (as it has been by strong confidentiality laws in the British case), so that it is used for public health and civil rights purposes only, and not for political surveillance and repression. But the possibility that it could be used for such negative purposes does not destroy its fundamental value, provided this abuse can be avoided. Indeed, without the legally sanctioned capacity to prove one's identity, most positive legal and civil rights are worthless, while the individual's capacity to function economically is severely constrained to a local context or a network of familiars. Correspondingly, in a fast-changing economy, the capacity of central or local governments (or NGOs) to devote scarce resources to effective promotion of social security and health is extremely limited without accurate, locally precise intelligence, derived from individual-level data, on demographic trends and epidemiological patterns.

Registration and enumeration of individuals — to become officially acknowledged, legal persons — comprise a crucially necessary development to facilitate the integration of the poor into property markets, which also function on their behalf in the world's poorest countries. In his pathbreaking analysis, Hernando de Soto identifies the failure of an appropriate formal property law system to develop in many countries, such as his native Peru, as a gross institutional disability preventing capital formation (32). This failure restricts the commercial usage to which all but the richest in society (who alone can afford the costs, bribes, and delays of the tortuous legal processes) can assign their assets — homes, land, businesses. For the rest, their inability to gain legal formal title to their assets means that these cannot be used as capital in the conventional economic sense, as a security to generate credit or funds for investment.

But de Soto's policy prescription is radically incomplete. He focuses on only one half of the problem of creating fixity and security of legal title, and omits the question of the legal personhood of agents themselves in many poor countries. As we have seen, from the 16th century onward in British history the two aspects worked together in the form of the common law's rules of property ownership and the Henrician parish register system — the nationwide registration through parishes of all births, deaths, and marriages — enabling British capital markets to develop sufficiently to drive the mercantile and industrial revolutions. The process was jeopardized by its own success but was then brought back into full working order with the creation in 1836 of the modern civil (secular) registration system.

When we consider today's less developed countries and continents — notably Latin America, Africa, and Southeast Asia — their histories since the 18th century (themselves very diverse of course) have been extremely different from Britain's when evaluated in these terms. The mercantile and industrial revolutions of western Europe affected and transformed these three other continental areas and their indigenous polities and peoples at least as much as they transformed Europe itself. But the relationship between the capital-accumulating European metropole and the southern and eastern trading partners was, as is well known, highly unequal. Many of the populations of these vast areas were subject to formal, colonial, or imperial domination or to practical dependency status (China) throughout much of the period from 1750 to 1945 or even until the 1960s. The main regional exceptions were the independent countries of Latin America. However, having precociously flung off their Spanish and Portuguese colonial rulers, most Latin American states fell prey to a vicious, nepotistic, post-colonial, neo-aristocratic elite who relied on primitive rather than industrial capital accumulation, often through slave-labor, to exploit their enormous continent's rich natural resources and agricultural potential.

Consequently, the three constitutional and institutional developments, identified above as crucial for societies faced with the challenges and disruptions of economic change to evolve the political capacity to pursue their own health and security agenda, never occurred in these three, continent-scale regions of underdevelopment. These crucial adjustments to law and the social relations between citizens and their government, taking decades or even centuries to negotiate in the histories of today's developed nations, were blocked at the source in Africa, large tracts of Asia, Latin America, and the Caribbean.

The possibility for such a set of changes to the constitution of social relations in a dependent or colonial society was inimical to the political requirements of the dominant colonial European political forces and the neocolonial plantation and ranch elites of Latin America. Individuals were not granted meaningful voting rights; they were permitted only carefully policed rights of civic association. The central state (the colonial government) mainly used local rulers or authorities as transmission mechanisms for its own centrally administered policies. Population registration was not primarily motivated to ensure a diverse citizenry's property rights or to devise the expense of effective public health measures, but was primarily a surveillance exercise for law and order purposes to keep the costs of policing under control. Hence in India the efficient registration of deaths was of much less pressing interest to the authorities than it was in England, where the relevant census official, William Farr, became the world's leading expert on the subject (33). In India, the geographical distribution of religions and castes was of much greater interest to the census authorities, especially following the trauma of the Indian mutiny in 1857, after which the British believed that specific Indian castes had to be watched carefully (34).

In the final analysis, the main goals of colonial rule were — and always have been — to benefit the colonizing country economically to the maximum. Europe's plutocratic class found it advantageous to exploit territories whose populace lacked the citizenship rights that their own middle and working classes increasingly enjoyed. Rates of profit and rent extraction could be highly lucrative in such unprotected labor markets. A convenient, evolutionary, racist ideology explained and justified the absence of civic rights for the colonized peoples (35). The governing interests of the imperial states firmly committed them to maintaining these dependent societies in a limbo of constitutional underdevelopment.

Thus, during the period from 1815 to 1945 in northwest Europe and those parts of the globe in which migrants from these states settled and suppressed the indigenous peoples (principally North America and Australia), citizenship/civil society/state relationships gradually evolved and adapted to the challenges of rapid economic growth in a manner that ultimately enabled human security and health to be preserved and maintained. But, through the direct and indirect influence of the formal and informal trading empires that these same states established throughout the globe, they simultaneously prevented virtually all other societies from adapting in similar ways to world economic growth.

When decolonization and independence came relatively suddenly in the two decades after 1945, world economic development did not stop to enable these societies — lacking a history of the development of state-recognized individual citizenship, civic associations, elected local self-government, and collective state provision — to catch up with a century and a half of missing adaptation. Their societies, having a long tutelage in dependence as the worst possible preparation, were immediately subjected to all the disruptions and demands of ongoing world economic growth.

In fact, in many ways, the period of tutelage was prolonged for most of these countries for a further three to four decades after 1945 because of the clientalist relationships eagerly sought by the two nuclear superpowers, the U.S. and the U.S.S.R. Thus the tendency, already marked under formal colonial regimes, for small, trusted (by the foreigners), subaltern elite groups and families to garner most of the power and economic resources, through their personal contacts at the very center of the state's administrative apparatus, was further emphasized in these initial decades of independence. At least this protracted period of Cold War clientage permitted the independent governments of many poor countries to enjoy a reasonably dependable flow of income. Although much went into private bank accounts, in most countries enough of it found its way into the state's investment programs so that roads, schools, and hospitals were built between the 1950s and the 1980s. And more importantly, precious human capital to staff the schools and hospitals was increasingly forthcoming, much of it initially trained through exchange programs set up by the nations of the rival liberal and socialist ideological blocs of the First and Second Worlds. There were also, of course, substantial helpful UNESCO educational and WHO-sponsored health programs during this period, such as the celebrated smallpox eradication program.

In calibrating the experience of many Third World countries in the 1945–1989 era against the historical model that has been set out here of the three constitutional developments that most First World countries achieved, and which, it is argued, are necessary to maintain security and health in the face of the disruptive challenges of economic growth, their most obvious weakness has been in the middle area of civic society: associations giving voice to groups — most importantly trade unions, representatives, elected local government — and bridging and linking social capital. Individual citizens certainly had a reasonable range of formal rights, including universal suffrage, in many of these newly independent states. There were also promising signs of collective provision by the state in terms of education, health, and social security. But now we see, given the tragic way in which many of these societies have buckled and some have virtually collapsed during the 1990s, how fragile and unviable formal individual rights and a relatively proactive central state are, without the vital range of middling civic institutions. These institutions took a long time to evolve, deepen, and multiply in the history of the west. They are important to making formal individual rights substantial and useful in practice and to giving the state and its resources the capacity for effective traction with the diverse, real society it both serves and guides.

THE SEPARATION OF SECURITY AND HEALTH FROM 1975 TO 2000: FORGETTING HISTORY

Tragically for the Third World and painfully for the socially excluded of the First World, the important historical lessons regarding the preservation of human security and health under conditions of rapid economic change have been progressively lost to the policymakers and leading opinion formers of the world's elite societies and global institutions during the 1980s and especially in the era of triumphalist 'free market fundamentalism' of the 1990s.

Historical developments — full citizenship rights, civil associations, a free press, and collective provision for human security and health — culminated in the mid-20th century with most of the advanced western liberal democracies assuming the form of pluralist societies with welfare states (20). This balanced pattern served the western democracies reasonably well for over a quarter century following the end of World War II, and also provided a helpful model for various client states in the Third World to emulate. Economic growth rates in both sets of states were consistently strongly positive, while rising average life expectancies confirmed that the fruits of such economic growth were being equitably distributed without undue disruption to the lives of the majority. But then, after a generation of relatively successful, well-adapted life on the slopes of the volcano (so successful that it has been referred to as the post-war 'golden age') (36), the inhabitants — or at least their political and ideological leaders — seem to have fallen into a fog of collective amnesia. They lost the plot.

The financial elite could no longer remember why they had agreed in the 1940s to set up an international system of strong currency controls and capital regulations, and could only see this system now as an encumbrance to their market-driven aspirations to earn greater profits from a larger, more globalized capital market. The libertarian right could no longer remember why, after the 1930s, they had agreed to provide generous collective welfare services. The intellectual left naively played into the hands of this New Right attack on the welfare state, since it now aspired to an unrealistic radical egalitarianism. It disparaged the welfare states for failing as yet to achieve equality, while ignoring the important evidence of the welfare state's effectiveness in dramatically reducing absolute poverty and health differentials between rich and poor in the space of a single generation (37). The Keynesian revolution's great policy gift to liberal market democracy of countercyclical government spending to maintain effective demand in the economy was subverted by lazy politicians into the practice of continuously increasing government spending to give the appearance of higher economic growth rates, figures which had come to assume a totemic electoral significance. In such an inflationary context, trade unions' and employers' negotiations were increasingly confrontational, leading to industrial strife between the two sides in many western democracies during the 1970s.

The ideological and political counterrevolution of the New Right was primarily an Anglo-Saxon initiative, whose main focus was the populist target of the supposedly bloated and inefficient high-taxing central state, aiming to reduce its welfare spending programs (the primary focus in the U.S.) and the range of publicly owned industries and services (mainly in the UK; there were almost none to privatize in the U.S.). It was an article of faith for the libertarian New Right that the world's ills were principally traceable to the overbearing and inefficient activities of unaccountable, bureaucratic central states, and that the general solution was to open up as much of the economy as possible and all spheres of life to the rigors of free market, commercial, competitive forces, incentives, and risk-takers.

After a generation of change since 1945, there was certainly much that needed reform and reinvigoration in the relationship between state, civic society, and citizenship in western liberal democracies by the 1970s. The prescriptions of the New Right offered partial diagnosis and a rather extreme form of medicine. The ensuing two decades have resulted in significant reforms along the lines advocated; however, considerable damage to human security and health also has been wreaked in these societies by the evangelical application of New Right ideology, resulting in sharply rising inequality and deepening poverty for the socially excluded in both developed and less developed countries.

In terms of the constitutional and civic underpinnings to ensure human security and health in a turbulent world of economic growth, it is arguable that the last thing the citizens of the poorest countries needed — emerging from centuries of dependence and decades of tutelage — was a generalized attack on the legitimacy of their state structures and nascent public goods and services. The neoliberal policies were originally devised in Chicago, Wall Street, and London by First World economists unhappy at the role played by a highly developed central state in their own economies. But these policies were soon applied as the 'Washington consensus' in many other contexts.

In developed western democracies, the ideologists of the New Right have had a fairer fight on their hands, facing a strong state and a well-developed range of civic associations able to argue for the continuing provision of collective services to ensure human security and health. Public services, so essential for the health and security of the poor, have been pruned but not eradicated. By contrast, in far too many ex-colonial countries, the IMF found that it could impose its strictures at will, through conditionality clauses to its loans, on relatively unconfident and young state bureaucracies and on civil societies lacking sufficient development in local government, trade unions, an independent press, or other civic associations capable of representing the poor and resisting the attack on their interests. In 1980, what all of these developing countries needed, and what was appropriate for the provisional state of development they had achieved by that point, was to expand and strengthen their nascent welfare states so as to boost significantly their nation's human and social capital. Instead, they received orders from Washington in the form of the structural adjustment programs to abandon the minimal welfare states they had begun to construct, and to open themselves up to western capitalism and trade.

It all looks very similar to these same countries' experiences under the European colonial powers before 1945. This is an era of U.S. neo-imperialism, backed by a similarly inhumane, rigid, self-righteous, and self-serving ideology and with the financial interests of the metropole as the principal beneficiaries. The evidence for this harsh judgment is found in Joseph Stiglitz's analysis of IMF policies in many countries. Stiglitz devastatingly observes that while using the justificatory rhetoric of promoting competition, in fact privatization was the goal most consistently pursued, which is not at all the same thing:

> "Economic theory says that for markets to work well, there must be both competition and private property....The IMF chose to emphasize privatization, giving short shrift to competition. The choice was perhaps not surprising: corporate and financial interests often oppose competition policies, for these policies restrict their ability to make profits (38)."

In order supposedly to boost the vigor and scope of free markets, the Washington consensus waged a messianic war throughout the 1990s on state capacity in the First World, on the Second World of the ex-Comecon transition countries, and on the Third World. This policy was based on an ahistorical and entirely sciolistic misunderstanding, which ignores the intimate relationship of interdependence between strong states and strong markets. For, as de Soto's historical reconstruction of the emergence of capital itself in the west demonstrates, only states strong enough to provide a universally available system of sanctions to guarantee individuals' legal titles to their diverse property holdings could provide the basis for markets in capital to develop, a theme that also emerges from the earlier Nobel prize winning work of D.C. North (39).

Without the state's capacity to guarantee the rule of law, interpersonal violence becomes commonplace, eroding the basis for public confidence, respect, and trust in others. Most societies are a diverse coalition of many kinds of 'others': strangers who learn to place a degree of trust in each other. This basic level of trust in the street is crucial for the practical functioning of a democratic citizenship of equal rights. In turn, this trust provides the social groundwork for all civic associations and representative bodies to form. They negotiate the pluralist democracy that liberal market societies require if they are to avoid degenerating into oligarchic plutocracies (the characteristic flaw of the capitalist system, first analyzed by Marx, being its inherent tendency toward monopoly).

Thus we come back to the central paradox of human security — its inherently collective and social nature — all the more so in a globalized world trading economy. Human security is conditional, negotiated, and dependent on the maintenance through appropriate behavior of respectful relations with others. This insight is one of the central tenets of social capital theory, with emphasis on its importance for development (40).

However, there is a powerful bias within the western, liberal, methodological, individualist, reductive, analytical tradition of thought, toward simplistically equating security with individual autonomy and household autarchy. To strive for the illusion of personal control over one's own destiny — elevated by Woodrow Wilson at the Versailles Treaty of 1919 to the principle of an individual nation's self determination when applied to the field of international relations — has been a consuming obsession in the western consciousness and in recent international political history. History repeatedly confirms that these are fantastically dangerous and self-defeating delusions. To elevate 'my' security or 'our nation's' security to the status of an absolute value that I/we have an absolute and unconditional right to defend and promote as only I/we see fit, is all too close to denying all rights of negotiation to others. It is the disposition of Fascist states. It directly implies a relationship of distrust to others and must look, in the eyes of others, like a threat to their security. This is a fundamental error, since it fails to perceive the intrinsically relational nature of security, succinctly summarized by Meddings, Bettcher, and Ghafele in this volume: "One cannot be secure if one's neighbor... is not secure (41)." This simple observation has profound implications.

Building faith in collective security in the face of the vicissitudes of disruptive economic growth is a difficult social and political accomplishment that the citizens of the advanced western liberal democracies gradually negotiated for themselves over a period of centuries, through a range of civil associations and in conjunction with their states, while simultaneously denying it to the supposedly inferior peoples of their imperial possessions. It requires simultaneously strong individual rights, upheld and rendered equal by a strong, redistributionist state, and strong civic institutions, including an independent free press. The strength of these three develops dialectically and unevenly, and the delicate balance between the three forces can unravel. If the state's legitimacy is brought into question, and its capacity to sustain individuals' equal rights is compromised, then citizens may rapidly turn from reliance on collective security and confidence in strangers in their society to more sect-like, defensive arrangements, reserving trust only for a carefully selected few. In social capital terms this scenario represents a retreat from a balance of bonding, bridging, and linking social capital to a predominance of bonding patterns only. This is certainly what happened in Britain's industrial cities during the first half of the 19th century; it also has been diagnosed as a current affliction of the U.S. during the last three decades (10, 42).

This trend is most unfortunate and ominous in the U.S., which is clearly the most powerful and influential state in today's globalized world. If American opinion leaders in this generation understand the pursuit of security as something most effectively achieved through finding and trusting only those recognizable as exactly like oneself (bonding social capital), while using the material technology available to create a supposedly impregnable homeland for oneself, then history indicates this approach is futile. Only the slow building of trust through negotiation of conflicts of interest with respected others and within agreed rules of law (including international law) can create any durable security between citizens or nations. The French Maginot line did not prevent German invasion in 1940, but the agreement of these two states and their citizens to participate in continual dialogue and negotiation through the European Union has now maintained peace between these two old enemies for the longest period in modern history.

History indicates that there are a number of critical issues to consider in pursuing strategies to promote human security and health in a globalized world in the 21st century. Firstly, a self-denying ordinance from the world's wealthiest nations and corporations will allow poor countries to develop their industries and economies at their own pace and follow their own domestic population's gradually rising demand levels for goods and services, rather than service the demand for a narrow range of goods that western consumers want at the lowest prices and for which the poor countries happen to have a comparative advantage (often little more than cheap labor costs because of the absence of unions and protective labor legislation). It is only in this gradual and organic manner that poor countries can build the all-important middle sector of civic institutions, which are necessarily intimately related to their capacity to develop a wide range of economic activities to supply their own needs.

Secondly, this means that the world's international organizations — such as the UN, WHO, ILO, World Bank, and even the IMF and WTO — must call for and work toward a new era of contingent protectionism. Despite its impeccable historical pedigree as the primary policy that the governments of the U.K., U.S., Germany, and Japan, for instance, each followed when it suited them to nurture their nascent industrial economies (43), the endorsement of any kind of protectionism will undoubtedly require a substantial alteration in the favorite assumptions of such important international bodies as the IMF and WTO. It should be noted that such contingent protectionism for poor countries will in fact have almost no aggregate negative impact whatsoever on international investment flows, for the simple reason that almost all such investment capital flows between developed nations only. It will, however, reduce the outlets for hot money gambling at the expense of the living standards of non-First World citizens, such as those in Argentina or Indonesia; and it will restrict the scope for highly profitable activity at the expense of poor countries' environments and labor forces, which many multinationals currently enjoy. These powerful vested interests cannot possibly be expected to change their practices without a protracted battle. Those who wish to promote global human security will necessarily come into conflict with these commercial interests, which are not acting in accordance with the ethics of human security.

Only the most developed economies with the most comprehensive social security protections in place should be exposed to the full competitive rigors of global free markets, since they alone have the constitutional and governmental machinery — their welfare states — to stand up to its disruptive effects. All the world's poorest societies should be granted general exemptions from free trade, with the restrictions gradually lifting as the constitutions and civic institutions of their societies (not simply their per capita GDPs) develop in strength and depth. This process is almost the opposite of the practical policies pursued throughout the 1990s by the WTO and especially the IMF, which have instead imposed open exposure to international capitalism and trade only on the poorest countries unable to resist the insistence on conditionality in return for life-saving loans. By contrast, the IMF remains impotent to force the richest countries, with their entrenched lobbying power of the producer interests, to drop their favored protections for large branches of the economy, such as agriculture in both Europe and the U.S.

The profound problems of the resistance to such desirable reforms of the vested interests of corporate and financial elites in the west bring us, thirdly, to the need for substantial constitutional changes. Individual voters and the rich inheritance of civic associations in western, liberal, pluralist democracies must push for anticorruption rules to better insulate their own political establishments and render their states more autonomous from the corroding and insidious influence of commercial interests and corporate entry into the processes of state policy formulation and execution. This problem is a mirror image to the one identified by the New Right philosophy of a generation ago, which decried all forms of government as sclerotic, inefficient, and intrinsically corrupt, and advocated reducing the role of the state or, where possible, running it more along the efficient, supposedly open, and competitive lines of the market. So successful has the New Right been in advancing the reach of the market that government in the U.S. and even in Britain has now become endemically prone to the market's own version of sclerosis: the corporate buying of influence (44, 45). The hubris of the business world, with no independent masters, no doubt also has contributed to the scale of the recent accounting scandals that have sent Wall Street into a bear market of distrust.

In the U.S., the far from impartial perspectives and vested interests of corporate America and Wall Street have become conflated with those of the U.S. government, as exemplified by the current occupant of the White House, George W. Bush, and his Vice President. This is also true of the international institutions dominated by the U.S., notably the IMF, where Wall Street financiers have frequently held the top post and the U.S. has veto power over its policies. This situation looks dangerously like a plutocratic system, the antithesis of democracy. The IMF represents probably the single most important and egregious case for reform among the international institutions, since it is so patently undemocratic in its constitution and has by now accumulated an unenviable record of policy mistakes, indefensible because of their dogmatic invariability, in the countries that have so little voice at its table.

There is nothing new here. Such corporate and financial interests undoubtedly managed to influence to their own advantage, both at a strategic level and in more specific ways, the state policies of the British government in London when it was the dominant world trading power in the late 19th century, as the important examples of the Opium Wars, the Suez Canal, and public health policy in India each illustrate in their different ways (46, 47). It is vital that other powerful nation blocs, notably the E.U., use their independent bargaining power today to oppose and criticize the policies and strategies of the dominant power, the U.S., and those institutions that it most directly influences, wherever it is reasonable and just to do so. It is the only conceivable hope for keeping honest the distorting and myopic force of U.S. financial and corporate elites who, like the British in the 19th century, will continue relentlessly to advocate the grand principle of free trade that is so evidently in their own self-interest.

Today, there is a vital need for both security and health to be visualized and understood in thoroughly global terms. It has been noted that in the past whenever the cause of health could be strongly linked to that of national security, it paid dividends to the public health movement; enhanced collective resources were consequently mobilized. But we need now to find the correct forms of political rhetoric and the compelling arguments to ally health with a more genuinely global conception of human security. History indicates that this scaling up from the national collectivity to the global, and the building of institutions for the global citizenship and civic forms necessary to accompany such a political entity, is going to be a heroically difficult task. It will be crucial for a portion of the world's leading businessmen to become genuinely motivated with this challenge, in the manner in which Chamberlain and leading British industrialists became fired by the civic gospel from the 1870s. Whether such activism is possible now hangs in the balance. It is vitally important for the future ecological security of the planet that the American nation and its business elite not be encouraged to perceive the appropriate response to the threat posed by September 11th merely in national security terms. Instead, they need to learn to embrace positively the truth of the dependence of their own security and health on that of their neighbors in this small globe of ours.

References

1. Haines R, Shlomowitz R. Explaining the mortality decline in the eighteenth-century British slave trade. *Economic History Review* 2000;53:262–83.

2. Curtin PD. *Death by migration: Europe's encounter with the tropical world.* Cambridge: Cambridge University Press; 1989.

3. Searle GR. *The quest for national efficiency: a study in British politics and thought, 1899–1914.* Oxford: Clarendon Press; 1971.

4. Szreter S. *Fertility, class, and gender in Britain, 1860–1940.* Cambridge: Cambridge University Press; 1996, ch. 4.

5. Hennock EP. *British social reform and German precedents: the case of social insurance, 1880–1914.* Oxford: Clarendon Press; 1987.

6. Hongisbaum F. *The struggle for the Ministry of Health, 1914–19.* London: G. Bell; 1970.

7. Titmuss R. *Problems of social policy.* London: HMSO; 1950.

8. Beveridge WH. *Full employment in a free society.* London: George Allen and Unwin; 1944. p.11.

9. Starr P. *The social transformation of American medicine.* New York: Basic Books; 1982. p. 280–9.

10. Szreter S. The state of social capital: bringing back in power, politics, and history. *Theory and Society* 2002;31:note 34.

11. Sen A. *Development as freedom.* Oxford: Oxford University Press; 1999.

12. Szreter S. The population health approach in historical perspective. *American Journal of Public Health* 2003; 93: 421–31.

13. Szreter S. Economic growth, disruption, deprivation, disease, and death: on the importance of the politics of public health for development. *Population and Development Review* 1997;23:693–728.

14. Szreter S, Mooney G. Urbanisation, mortality, and the standard of living debate: new estimates of the expectation of life at birth in nineteenth-century British cities. *Economic History Review* 1998;50:84–112.

15. Hopkins AG, editor. *Globalization in world history.* London: Pimlico; 2002.

16. Kula W. *The problems and methods of economic history.* Szreter R, translator. Aldershot: Ashgate; 2001. p. 371–2.

17. Farmer P. Social inequalities and emerging infectious diseases. *Emerging Infectious Diseases* 1996;2:259–69.

18. Farmer P. *Infections and inequalities: the modern plagues.* Berkeley: University of California Press; 1999.

19. Trouiller P, et al. Drug development for neglected diseases: a deficient market and a public-health policy failure. *The Lancet* 2002;359:2188–94.

20. Esping-Andersen G. *The three worlds of welfare capitalism.* Cambridge: Polity Press; 1990.

21. Slack P. *The English poor law 1531–1782.* London: Macmillan; 1990.

22. Outhwaite RB. *Dearth, public policy, and social disturbance in England, 1550–1800.* London: Macmillan; 1991, ch. 2.

23. Solar PM. Poor relief and English economic development before the industrial revolution. *Economic History Review* 1995;48:1–22.

24. Szreter S. The G.R.O. and the public health movement 1837–1914. *Social History of Medicine* 1991;4:435–63.

25. Gilbert AD. *Religion in Industrial Society: church, chapel, and social change 1740–1914.* London: Longman; 1976.

26. Roberts D. *Paternalism in early Victorian England.* London: Croom Helm; 1979.

27. Neave D. Friendly societies in Great Britain. In: van der Linden M, editor. *Social security mutualism.* New York: Peter Lang; 1996. p. 41–64.

28. Fraser WH, Maver M, editors. *Glasgow volume II: 1830–1912.* Manchester: Manchester University Press; 1996, chs.10–12.

29. Hennock EP. *Fit and proper persons.* Montreal: McGill-Queens' University Press; 1973.

30. Bell F, Millward R. Public health expenditures and mortality in England and Wales, 1870–1914. *Continuity and Change* 1998:13:1–29.

31. Addison P. *The road to 1945: British politics and the Second World War.* London: Cape; 1975.

32. de Soto H. *The mystery of capital.* New York: Basic Books; 2000.

33. Eyler JM. *Victorian social medicine: the ideas and methods of William Farr.* Baltimore: Johns Hopkins University Press; 1979.

34. Cohn B. The census, social structure, and objectification in South Asia. In: Cohn BS. *An anthropologist among the historians and other essays.* Oxford: Oxford University Press; 1987. p. 224–54.

35. Stocking GW. *Victorian anthropology.* New York: The Free Press; 1987.

36. Marglin S, Schor J, editors. *The golden age of capitalism.* Oxford: Clarendon Press; 1990.

37. Szreter S. Health, class, place, and politics: social capital, opting in, and opting out of collective provision in nineteenth- and twentieth-century Britain. *Contemporary British History* 2002;26:27–57, table 1.

38. Stiglitz JE. *Globalization and its discontents.* New York: Norton; 2002. p. 156.

39. North DC. *Structure and change in economic history.* New York: Norton; 1981.

40. Woolcock M. Social capital and economic development: toward a theoretical synthesis and policy framework. *Theory and Society* 1998;27:151–208.

41. Meddings DR, Bettcher DW, Ghafele R. Violence and human security: policy linkages. In: Chen L, Leaning J, Narasimhan V, editors. *Global health challenges for human security.* Cambridge (MA): Global Equity Initiative, Asia Center, Faculty of Arts and Sciences, Harvard University; 2003.

42. Putnam RD. *Bowling alone: the collapse and revival of American community.* New York: Simon and Schuster; 2000.

43. Chang H-J. The real lesson for developing countries from the history of the developed world: freedom to choose. Available at: URL: http://www.historyandpolicy.org/main/policy-paper-09.html, accessed on 2003 May 30.

44. Boggs C. *The end of politics: corporate power and the decline of the public sphere.* New York: Guilford; 2000.

45. Monbiot G. *Captive state: the corporate takeover of Britain.* London: Macmillan; 2000.

46. Davis M. *Late Victorian holocausts: El Nino famines and the making of the Third World.* London: Verso; 2001.

47. Watts S. World trade and world disease. Available at: URL: http://www.historyandpolicy.org/main/policy-paper-07.html, accessed on 2003 May 30.

CHAPTER 4

BIOETHICS, HUMAN SECURITY, AND GLOBAL HEALTH

GIOVANNI BERLINGUER

SECURITY FOR WHOM?

Security and freedom are primary needs of every human being. The tragedy of the Twin Towers on September 11, 2001 showed how evil international terrorism can be, the risks it creates, and why all available forces should be mobilized to fight it. Most people have become conscious that the world in recent years is more insecure and more unjust (one condition reciprocally influencing the other), so that even the richest and most powerful are now vulnerable. Terrorism must be rejected because it harms innocent people, threatens life, and reduces its quality; by reaction, it may stimulate hatred, self-defensiveness, discrimination, and racism, and lead to the restriction of liberties and the violation of human rights.

Following September 11, 2001, there have been increased concerns regarding terrorist activities for two reasons. The first is practical: the risk persists, involves other areas of the world, and in the Middle East, both individual and organized terrorism have become intolerable. The second has deep ethical implications: the current worldwide trend is to concentrate efforts almost exclusively on military solutions against terrorism.

This trend may lead us to overlook terrorism's links with poverty, oppression, and perceived cultural deprivation. Such underlying causes may be the result of "distributive justice arising from economic and political marginalization, ethnic and religious isolation, questions of identity, etc. Many have argued that the campaign against terrorism is more than just a 'battle of might,' but rather a 'battle of the hearts and minds.' In this regard, a human security approach that answers the question — Security for whom? — may offer an alternative approach to dealing with many of the problems facing us today" (1).

Restricting the broad spectrum of human insecurities prevalent today means that, instead of a pluralistic approach to multiple human needs and a response that mobilizes popular, intellectual, and political energies, the attention is focused on only one enemy, and only military instruments are taken into consideration. Philosophically, this limited view of the idea of security does not allow public authorities to include among their duties the task of facing other collective needs, which are equally urgent in order to provide each human being the opportunity to realize his or her essential capabilities, and to reconcile the universal need for security with personal and community necessities and choices.

Moreover, the decision by governments to use military and repressive power exclusively in their bid to achieve security restricts the spectrum of moral subjects who could contribute to creating human security. This restrictive approach to the issues, instruments, and subjects of human security may lead to a rigid separation and clash between those people, groups, or states considered 'good' and those considered 'evil,' thereby denying our individual consciousness the possibility of drawing distinctions and making personal judgments.

WHAT SECURITY?

In Walzer's theory of justice we find a concept of security and of the role of the state that is not concerned only with physical violence (2), as this would be unacceptable and shortsighted. A civil society — as well as an international community — is unlikely to survive if law and order are the only things guaranteed by the use of force, because the inequities may constantly lead to growing disorders.

It is true that national and international security were traditionally promoted (with ambivalent aims and results) to counter the threat of aggression across borders. Now the concept includes four new directions:

> "1) from the security of nations to the security of groups and individuals: it is extended *downwards* from nations to individuals; 2) from the security of nations to the security of the international system, or of a supranational physical environment: it is extended *upwards*, from the nations to the biosphere. The extension, in both cases, is in the sort of entities whose security is to be insured; 3) extended *horizontally*, or to the sort of securities that are in question. Different entities (such as individuals, nations, and 'systems') cannot be secure or insecure in the same way; the concept of security is extended, therefore, from military to political, economic, social, environmental, or 'human' security; 4) political responsibility for ensuring security (or for invigilating these 'concepts of security') is itself extended: is diffused *in all directions* from national states, including upwards to international institutions, downwards to regional or local government, and sideways to nongovernmental organizations, to public opinion and the press, and to the abstract forces of nature or of the market" (3).

In the 20th century, the language of security has acquired broader meaning through the experience of the welfare state, which includes collective or public activities to promote a higher level of health; to reduce (or compensate for) the risks of disease, disability, unemployment, and the conditions of maternity or retirement; and to make education accessible to everybody. Recent restrictions may lead us to ask whether the welfare state is still actually a system, or whether it should be considered merely a parenthesis in the history of mankind. At the same time, many new issues have been added in recent years, especially those concerning health, food, water, and environmental security, problems that are (or should be) faced on a global scale.

This broad and comprehensive idea of human security, which takes into consideration multiple threats and possibilities, represents one of the most difficult yet promising fields for human action and moral meditation, particularly when security thinking is broadened from military defense "to a 'people-centered' approach of anticipating and coping with multiple threats faced by ordinary people in an increasingly globalizing world" (4).

NEW TRENDS IN BIOETHICS

In recent years, bioethics, which is mainly concerned with the relationship between morality, biomedical sciences, and life, has become one of the most important fields of ethics. The sixth World Congress of Bioethics (Brazil, October 30 to November 3, 2002) indicated new trends, and many stimulating contributions were made to moral reflections on a people-centered concept of human security.

Following the indications of the fifth Congress (London, September 2000), according to which the highest bioethical priorities should be "the growing inequities in health throughout the world and the dramatic plight of women," the agenda of the Brazilian congress was concentrated on bioethics, power, and injustice.

This discipline was traditionally concerned with *frontier bioethics*, the emerging developments in biomedicine and genetics that were formerly unfeasible and sometimes even inconceivable, such as medically assisted procreation, organ transplants, artificial survival, cloning, the use of stem cells, guided mutations, and the creation of new species. This approach is sometimes transformed into *justificatory bioethics*, which may become the legitimization of any application of science, including those (like reproductive cloning) that may violate human rights and dignity. The former president of the International Association of Bioethics, A. Campbell, defined the prophets of justificatory bioethics as "bishops blessing warships."

Now the attention in journals, books, and meetings is focused on common individual and collective problems, which means the persistent conditions of human beings all over the world, and our moral reflections on birth and death, gender relations, disease, the environment, and on our responsibility to future generations. This field, which may be called *everyday bioethics* or *bioethics of everyday life* (5), chronologically represents the first chapter in the history of bioethics (because such issues have their roots both in the remote past and in present-day mores), and has a strong connection with issues of power and justice.

Contemporary bioethics, whose origins usually date to the 1970s and 1980s, is to a certain extent also concerned with such connections. Actually, "it was born largely as a revolt against the power of physicians to exert their will indifferent to the values and preference of the patients. But the word 'power' itself was rarely used...It is interesting to reflect on why bioethicists were by and large unwilling to confront directly the implications of power" (6).

One possible answer is that bioethicists were reluctant to go beyond the individual and personal interactions inherent in physician-patient relationships, and consider a series of power uses related more to public dimensions, to the presence of political institutions or economic agencies whose activities and powers influence the conditions in which many of the questions of daily life are presented and decided. The point of view emphasizing the approach to everyday bioethics may be considered a transposition of ideas introduced in a different context by John Dewey. He insisted repeatedly on the need for philosophic reflection so as not to lose sight of problems closely linked to people's everyday lives (7). It was in this context of the ordinary man's problems that Dewey developed his democratic philosophy, which may be viewed also as a point of reference for everyday bioethics.

Accordingly, *active bioethics* could play an important role. The subordination of bioethics to politics can be a dangerous operation, but at the same time the current *depoliticizing of moral conflicts* almost always leads to the passive acceptance of mainstream views, the endorsement of the power of the few, and the growth of injustice. Clearly, this is what is happening in the field of health.

SECURITY AND GLOBAL HEALTH

Since biomedical sciences have made possible, even in previous centuries, the recognition, prevention, and treatment of many diseases, human health has been acknowledged as one of the priorities of human security.

Health, which is at the same time an intimate process of each individual and a key component of community life, has a dual value on the moral plane: *intrinsic*, as the presence, limitation, or absence of vital capacity (ultimately, as the determinant between life and death), and *instrumental*, as a precondition for freedom. Freedom is substantially impaired when disease prevails because: a) the individual is substantially hindered in one or more decision making or action faculties; b) his or her destiny is entrusted to external powers (that may include physicians); and c) disease, when serious and persistent, often plunges the individual (and nations) into downward mobility, into the vicious circle of a regression that may become irreversible.

Health itself is a power, a fundamental capacity for the development or maintenance of all other capacities. Martha Nussbaum points out (8) that in the majority of modern nations, citizens accept the power of institutions to regulate their freedom in order to guarantee their access to health, the same way they accept the regulation of freedom in order to guarantee security.

Like other goods, health is unequally distributed among individuals, genders, communities, classes, races, and nations; health inequities, as we shall see, are growing almost everywhere, both within and between countries (9).

Unlike other goods, health justice cannot be sought in the form of better distribution of existing health, in zero-sum programs that take a certain amount of health from some to give to others. First, it would be difficult to find moral justifications and practical applications for such redistribution. Second, an alternative exists that is based on experience: the objective of a better health for all. In this context the attainment of health justice actually works as a multiplier of resources, achieves the best results, and contributes to increasing social cohesion. This is one of the reasons that makes the health of the world an indivisible good, and global health one of the main goals in any action for human security (10).

Global health does not mean the absence of all diseases, defects, or imperfections. The definition coined by the World Health Organization — "a state of complete physical, mental, and social well-being" — fails to say that health is not a state but a condition of changeable equilibrium, and is not perfection. Moreover, it is unlikely that human perfection can be attained through hygiene and medicine: sometimes such attempts lead people to commit excesses and nations to commit abuses. The target of health for all by the year 2000, launched by the WHO twenty years ago (and then postponed to 2020 or to the end of the 21st century), may also give rise to some discussion. It creates illusions and sidesteps the main goal, which is to guarantee for everybody health that is attainable by virtue of scientific knowledge and existing potential. It also may hinder the concentration of the necessary energy on an (apparently) limited vital core, based upon fundamental rights, essential capabilities, and absolute needs: this is the true meaning of health security.

FOUR STAGES OF HEALTH GLOBALIZATION

The global dimensions of health have a long history. I offer a brief outline of this history, describing it as a stage play with a prologue and four acts, and adding, for each part, some ethical considerations.

The Prologue is the microbial unification of the world. Until 1492, the New World had no smallpox, measles, yellow fever, malignant malaria, and probably no diphtheria, typhoid fever, scarlet fever, or influenza, due to different natural and human conditions (such as environment, nutrition, the absence of such germs or biological vectors), and Eurasia and Africa had no syphilis: a long list and a short one. With the discovery (or conquest) of America in 1492, the unknown diseases of the Old World spread in the New World, and vice versa with syphilis. The impact was devastating, especially on the American continent, whose population had no immunity against the Old World diseases (11). These diseases strongly contributed to the dramatic decrease in the population of the New World.

This unpredictable and uncontrollable phenomenon may be evaluated independently of any moral judgment. Humans had neither the knowledge nor the means to compensate for the 'economic virginity,' the unfavorable balance between the aggressiveness of the germs and the absence of natural antibodies. However, ethical consideration must be given to the synergy between the uncontrollable spread of disease and deliberate extermination: the deadly slave labor in mines; the breakdown in the food balance; the loss of identity, security, and power; the psychological and cultural collapse that weakened resistance to diseases and even led to outbreaks of suicide. Population extermination during the period following 1492 was the result of a combination of natural causes and human actions, and was certainly the greatest demographic tragedy experienced by the human species.

Act One represents the birth of international health policy. More than three centuries passed before humankind (populations, governments, culture, and science) realized the common risks of disease and began to make cross-border efforts to tackle them. Only in the nineteenth century did the three essential premises for effective action against diseases come together: knowledge of the causes, identification of preventive and therapeutic remedies, and the political will to take international action. The first steps in this direction were the establishment of International Health Conferences (the first was held in 1851), the quarantining of ships arriving in Europe from the East, and the internationalization of scientific knowledge with the parallel development of social policies (reduction of working hours, guarantees for pregnant women, limits to child labor, introduction of social insurance), which gradually contributed to better health for many.

The moral controversies, which also had a scientific and political background, were numerous. The first arose from the opposition of the British Empire to any rules that might hinder trade, including isolation and quarantine for ships, which is an ancient example of conflict between the free market and health measures. The second regarded the relative influence of microbes and of the social environment, nature, and culture in the origin and spread of disease (replacing the word 'microbe' with 'gene' would bring us to the present day). The third, which leads directly to the issue of global health, arose from the limited results of the *cordons sanitaires*, which many hygienists found 'perfectly useless.' Against these measures Robert Koch proposed the idea of fighting the diseases in the countries of origin: for instance, "to seize cholera by the throat and crush it forever" (12).

Act Two corresponds to the recognition of the right to health. This idea is embodied in many national constitutions (for example, in Italy, with the incisive formulation, "a fundamental right of the individual and interest of the collectivity"), and in the Constitution of the World Health Organization, signed on April 7, 1948. This concept emerged in industrial countries in response to different interests. Roy Porter mentions two facts, related to 20th century economics and politics: "the smooth and efficient functioning of intricate economy required a population no less healthy, literate, skilled, and law abiding; and in democracies where the workers were also voters, the ampler provision of health services became one way of pre-empting discontent" (13). The view of health as a right and a common interest became almost universal in the atmosphere of hope, fervor, and justice that accompanied and followed the end of World War II. The concept of 'equity in health' was formulated, in reference "to differences that are not necessary and that are avoidable; and at the same time unacceptable and unfair" (WHO), a concept that is at once descriptive and normative, and implies the possibility for each individual to pursue and attain his or her best potential health level.

The moral foundation of the right to health was affirmed as a kind of 'health citizenship' whose goal was health and whose dealings consisted of more than medical activities in the narrow sense, in order to deploy "all the factors of physical and mental improvement of the individuals and peoples," as stated in the WHO Constitution. In the following decades the WHO, which had been designated a 'world' organization rather than 'international' to signify that it was the result not only of an agreement among states but above all of a need felt by peoples, gained moral prestige and universal recognition, particularly through the worldwide eradication of smallpox and the Alma Ata Conference (1978), which affirmed the centrality of primary health care. In many cases, the improvement in health conditions became less selective and almost universal.

Act Three is characterized by a growing globalization of risks and a slow, partial, and insufficient response at the international level. The risks are evident in diseases or 'social pathologies' that have similar destructive consequences in different human beings, such as: a) the reappearance of old infections and the onset of new ones, which in some countries has become devastating; b) the implications of environmental degradation, both on present and future generations; c) the globalization of drugs, grown illegally in the South of the world or manufactured and marketed legally in the North; and d) the increase of different forms of violence, which has become the main cause of death in adolescents and young people (particularly males) and which threatens individual security, the collective consciousness, and the social cohesion. The global health indicators of the last fifty years point to progress, but social and national differences are increasing, and the inadequacy of the response is based upon the illusion that we can ignore the suffering of other peoples and live isolated from a common destiny.

From the practical and moral viewpoints, what features do these (and other similar) phenomena have in common? I emphasize three points. First, individuals, groups, or populations are harmed selectively, although not exclusively, with a severity inversely proportional to wealth, education, and power, thus reinforcing a condition of inequity. Second, the same rule applies to access to prevention or remedies, where these consist of treatment for illness, or security from violence or possible environmental catastrophes. Third, the risks no longer depend mainly on nature or on destiny: they are now largely *anthropogenic*, that is, created or aggravated by human decisions. Therefore they are not ineluctable; they may often be predicted, controlled, and modified.

Act Four may be defined as the trend towards regression of health paradigms. In the last two decades (paralleling the extraordinary development of biomedical sciences), the paradigms that had successfully guided public health and health services for a century were modified and even overturned. The formerly espoused truism that health is both a foundation and a primary objective of economic development has been replaced by the opposite idea that public health services and universal care represent an obstacle to the growth of wealth. The priority of the prevention-and-care model, based upon basic services accessible to everybody, has been supplanted by that of expensive high technology, even in countries with minimal resources. The agenda of health matters increasingly refers only to 'health care' instead of including 'health societies' and 'health systems.' Discussions on resources for health are downgraded from health to monetary aspects, while the effects of human resources and potential changes in the environment and workplace are underestimated. As a result, public health policies are no longer decided by health ministers but by economics ministers, and in the wider world the leadership has often been transferred from the WHO (which is still highly respected regarding technical issues) to the World Bank and to the International Monetary Fund.

These organizations may have moral obligations with regard to the financial assets of the world. They are frequently criticized for their methods and results, particularly in developing and underdeveloping countries (14), but surely they have no moral obligations with regard to the health of people, while the WHO does. The downgrading of health itself on the list of priorities for national governments may correspond to the fact that the privileged classes and countries appear less sensitive to other people's suffering; and that particularism may replace the idea — crucial and triumphant for more than a hundred years — that the health of the world is indivisible.

NEW OPPORTUNITIES

The question of why the previous humanitarian and scientific approach has been abandoned or neglected may have multiple answers. Here I underline some of the possible explanations. They include the swing in the pendulum of moral choices away from common interests and global solidarity. They include the idea that the virtuous combination of essential values like the free market and scientific progress could spontaneously extend its positive effects everywhere and to everybody; the growth of injustice frustrated this hope. They include — last in order but probably first in importance — the tremendous concentration of wealth and power in the world.

As a result of these and other factors, never before has the world enjoyed such healthy populations, so much knowledge, and so many possible remedies, and never before have so many diseases been preventable and curable. However, at the same time, there is little resolve to use the knowledge and remedies in the interest of all. For instance, in the past, the advantages of biomedical discoveries (such as antibiotics and vaccinations) were beneficial to almost everybody; now, their access is strongly conditioned by economic possibilities, and their selective distribution, paradoxically, aggravates the inequities in health. In other words, never before has our world enjoyed so much health and, at the same time, suffered from so many diseases. This may explain why the end of the nineteenth century (after the great discoveries and the early results in the fight against epidemics) coincided with a wave of excessive optimism, and the end of the twentieth century was characterized by doubt and pessimism.

Now, as underlined by Chen and Narasimhan in this volume, the idea of integrating health into human security can help to elevate health in political prioritization among a spectrum of competing public priorities, and in this process, the ethics of altruism as well as self interests should be harnessed, not simply charitable transfers among countries or groups. These ideas, far from being merely the expression of wishful thinking, are rooted in the positive developments of political and moral trends that began to emerge in the world at the end of the 1990s and are becoming culturally (although not yet politically) dominant in our time. They are supported by new opportunities that have appeared in the last few years. I will summarize some of them in a few interconnected items.

KNOWLEDGE, INFORMATION, AND INDIGNATION

All over the world, scientific studies — inspired either by the greater sensitivity of the researchers or by a stronger weight of evidence — have shown an increasing inequity in health and a growing gap between the potential and real situation. The first steps were made by the *Global Health Equity Initiative* (GHEI), which stimulated knowledge and action in many parts of the world (9) and was accompanied and followed by the flourishing of other studies echoed in the media.

Public opinion became more sensitive, probably for two reasons. One was underlined by Amartya Sen, at the close of one of the Asian meetings of the GHEI: "Information concerning discrimination, torture, poverty, illness, and abandonment helps coalesce the forces opposing these events by extending the opposition from the victims alone to the general public. This is possible because the people have the capacity and the willingness to react to other people's difficulties" (15). The other is that public opinion seems to be more sensitive to inequities in health than to other inequities, such as in income or property or material goods, probably because health inequities more directly affect life and death and therefore imply deep moral values.

HEALTH SECURITY IN THE INTERNATIONAL AGENDA

At the end of the 1990s health security returned, sometimes as a priority, to the political debate and to the attention of many governments. The stimulus came from different and sometimes opposing reasons, including the struggle against terrorism, problems of state security, economic evaluations, and strategic considerations. For instance, in April 2000, the U.S. National Security Council determined that the spread of AIDS in Africa, together with other factors of instability, "could jeopardize the national security and national interests of the USA in the world," and President Clinton doubled the amount of money appropriated to combat this disease on that continent.

History has shown interesting analogies. For instance, the birth of the international health policy (as described in Act One) was intended mainly to protect Europe from epidemics of Asiatic origin; only afterwards was it understood that prevention had to be universal. At the end of the nineteenth century, many discoveries related to germs (like *Plasmodium*), their life cycle, and their vectors (like *Aedes aegypti* for yellow fever) were made by army physicians, whose primary motive was the protection of colonial troops and investments against tropical diseases; these discoveries ultimately benefited everybody. A convergence of different forces and interests that multiplies the energies at work can be a powerful factor in favor of health security.

NEW SUBJECTS EMERGE

A new generation of young people and intellectuals have begun to blame stagnating international institutions, one-sided rules, and unbalanced powers for the detrimental effects they have on health, environment, poverty, justice, culture, and relations between science and society. A spreading wave of demonstrations and activities took place in the late 1990s; cities like Seattle, Genoa, and Porto Alegre became the symbols of their protest (like Berkeley in the late 1960s) and the focus of their debates. To a greater extent than the movements that began in Berkeley, these demonstrations expanded outside the universities and proposed alternative solutions — sometimes contradictory, but often more realistic than merely entrusting the destiny of the world to the spontaneous interactions between science and market. They were called *no-global*, an improper expression, because their activities are largely global in size and methods (16), and are increasingly becoming *new-global* in their projects. A similar role, and often a shared work, is assumed by many nongovernmental organizations (NGOs) that have an increasing influence on the decisions of governments and international institutions.

The contradiction that arose between patents and access to essential drugs in developing countries is one example of how the combined action of governments and the new subjects mentioned above can achieve success. In order to combat AIDS, nations like Brazil and South Africa decided to produce generic remedies (Brazil) or to buy drugs where they were produced at a cheaper price (South Africa) so as to bypass the patent-linked rules of pharmaceutical production and marketing. This action received broad international support and it was recognized that, in certain cases, saving human lives should take priority over other legitimate interests.

INTERNATIONAL AGENCIES AND WORLD HEALTH

I have already mentioned the role played by the International Monetary Fund (IMF) and the World Bank (WB) since the 1990s, in addition to or in place of the WHO, to orient national health policies. In the same years, G7 or G8 Summits began to make declarations concerning the health aspects of development (Lyon 1996, Denver 1997, Birmingham 1998, Köln 1999). The Okinawa Summit (July 2000) recognized that flexible and diversified targets must be selected, particularly against HIV/AIDS, malaria, and tuberculosis. It set out "to assign priority to the development of fair and effective health systems, to promote political leadership through high-level policy dialogue, to support the universal availability and affordability of essential drugs, vaccines, and preventive treatments." The Genoa Summit (June 2001) reiterated similar targets and suggestions, and created a *Global Fund for Health*, but the Summits never devoted sufficient attention to its achievements or the reason for its successes, difficulties, or failures. In addition, the activity of the World Trade Organization focused on the defense and strengthening of patents on drugs and attempted, through the General Agreement on Trade in Services (GATS), to extend the rules governing the *trading* of manufactured goods to the *delivery* of material goods (for instance, water, energy, and transport) and to *services* like health and education. This extension was questioned on the grounds that *services for persons* are considered rights essential for human life and development, and nations should decide freely how to guarantee them (with the contribution of private activities) to all citizens.

As the close of the century approached and the deep gaps and inequities became more evident, new global objectives were proposed by different international agencies, many of them directly related to the improvement of health. The IMF and the WB began to recognize the injustices caused or aggravated by their intervention in developing or underdeveloping countries; the many solemn appeals included reduction by three-quarters of maternal mortality before the year 2015, reduction by two-thirds of the mortality rates of children under five, and access through the primary health services to reproductive health care for all.

The most solemn event was the *Millennium Declaration*, approved in a special United Nations Assembly (New York, September 2000) by the heads of state and government, which repeated these targets and encompassed those concerning the struggle against epidemic diseases. The UN commitment included the intention to encourage the pharmaceutical industry to make essential drugs more easily available, to pursue development and the eradication of poverty, and to ask the industrial countries to grant more generous assistance. The negative reactions of many countries hinged on the fact that the proposed targets were not accompanied by any corresponding measures or by substantial and better targeted aid (including the abolition of barriers against the import of goods from developing countries).

CONCLUSION

In the previous section of this paper, I underlined some of the opportunities that may arise from the reintroduction of health into the political agenda and its links with security, from the emergence of new subjects, and from the growing role played by different international agencies, working in cooperation with a renewed World Health Organization (17). These trends are accompanied by promising debates concerning moral principles. Whatever impact philosophy and bioethics may have on the destiny of the world, the issues are now increasingly intertwined with the existing social conditions and new value systems. These issues may have a growing influence on the minds and behaviors of individuals and on the political decisions concerning health and human security.

REFERENCES

1. Caballero-Anthony M. Human security and primary health care in Asia: realities and challenges. In: Chen L, Leaning J, Narasimhan V, editors. *Global health challenges for human security*. Cambridge (MA): Global Equity Initiative, Asia Center, Faculty of Arts and Sciences, Harvard University; 2003.

2. Walzer M. *Sfere di giustizia.* Milano: Feltrinelli; 1987. Translated from: *Sphere of justice: a defense of pluralism and equality.* New York: Basic Books Inc.; 1983.

3. Rothschild E. What is security? *Daedalus* 1995;125(3):53–89.

4. Chen LC, Narasimhan V. *Human security: opportunity for global health.* Workshop on human security in relation to global health, Harvard University; 2002 October 14–15; Cambridge (MA).

5. Berlinguer G. Bioetica quotidiana e bioetica di frontiera. [Daily bioethics and frontier ethics.] *Rivista di teologia morale* 1988;78(2):63–76.

6. Murray T. Personal communication; 2002 May 31.

7. Dewey J. Problemi di tutti. Milano: Mondadori; 1950. Translated from: *Problems of men.* New York: Philosophical Library, Inc.; 1946.

8. Nussbaum M. *Women and human development: the capability approach.* Cambridge: Cambridge University Press; 2000.

9. Evans T, Whitehead M, et al., editors. *Challenging inequities in health: from ethics to action.* New York: Oxford University Press; 2001.

10. Berlinguer G. *Everyday bioethics: reflections of bioethical choices in daily life.* Amityville (NY): Baywood Publishing Company, Inc.; 2002.

11. Berlinguer G. The interchange of diseases and health between the old and the new world. *American Journal of Public Health* 1992;82(10):1407–13.

12. Koch R, quoted by Fantini B. La medicina tropicale: dalla medicina coloniale alla sanità internazionale [Tropical medicine: from colonial medicine to international health.] Symposium di storia della medicina; 1998 May 12; Bardolino, Italy.

13. Porter R. *The greatest benefit to mankind: a medical history of humanity.* New York: W. W. Norton; 1997. p. 631–2.

14. Stiglitz JE. *Globalization and its discontents.* New York: Allen Lane, Penguin Books; 2002.

15. Sen A. Closing address at the meeting of the Global Equity in Health Initiative; 1998 December 17; Dacca, Bangladesh.

16. Sen A. *Globalizzazione e libertà.* [Globalization and Liberty.] Milano: Mondadori; 2002.

17. Chen LC, Berlinguer G. Health equity in a globalizing world. In: Evans T, Whitehead M, et al., editors. *Challenging inequities in health: from ethics to action.* New York: Oxford University Press; 2001. p. 34–44.

CHAPTER 5

HEALTH AND SECURITY FOR A GLOBAL CENTURY

JONAS GAHR STØRE, JONATHAN WELCH, AND LINCOLN CHEN

INTRODUCTION

This chapter proposes that health and human security, which form a comparatively neglected linkage, drive many key domains of global health policy. Though the balance between military security and human security has waxed and waned historically, public concerns over health and security have risen dramatically in today's globalizing world (1, 2). Increasingly recognized is that many contemporary security concerns, both collective and personal, have strong health dimensions — for example, during conflict, devastating infectious epidemics, and bioterrorism in the aftermath of the September 11th tragedies. Moreover, some health threats, such as the HIV/AIDS pandemic, are threatening security by unraveling the cohesion and stability of vulnerable families, communities, and even nation-states (3, 4).

A second proposition is that health viewed through the prism of human security is inherently worldwide in scope. Although critical health actions continue to operate at the local and national levels, global dimensions of health are growing. Human security, too, must be viewed in global terms. Awareness of worldwide connections has been heightened by the revolution in information and communication, and health has been propelled onto the global agenda primarily due to the worldwide reach of health threats and the global nature of solutions necessary to address them. The HIV/AIDS pandemic, for instance, is a global challenge, even as control of the virus requires action at the individual, community, and national levels. Likewise, the recent SARS epidemic that began in East Asia illustrates the capacity of new epidemics for rapid global transmission, underscoring the increasing global health interdependence.

To secure the health of all individuals, global health policies and institutions must be strengthened. Our third proposition is that 'global health' is rapidly overtaking the paradigm of 'international health' as the organizing principle for health cooperation. While the latter term focuses on relations among sovereign nations, the concept of global health encompasses health affairs within and among nation-states, as well as transnational challenges not defined by political borders. Global health thus recognizes multiple actor groups in the production of health, including but not limited to national governments. Based on this concept of global health, this chapter sets forth the rationale for a global health architecture for the 21st century.

GLOBALIZATION OF HEALTH AND SECURITY

Globalization, an acceleration of many types of transnational flows, has produced numerous benefits. However, many individuals have also been left behind, and people everywhere, especially the poor and marginalized, are experiencing unprecedented worries over human insecurities, both old and new (5). Infectious diseases have emerged or reemerged, sometimes in stunning form (6). New technologies and lethal forms of warfare have placed civilians at great peril (7). Oftentimes there is minimal — even nonexistent — access to basic health services in the midst of pervasive poverty. Consequently, global health and development confront deeply troubling ethical challenges, since most of humanity lacks access to the simple benefits of medical and scientific progress (8). While average life expectancy in richer countries approaches 80 years, many people in poorer regions, especially in AIDS-ravaged sub-Saharan Africa, face falling life expectancies of 40 years or less. The poor continue to experience insecurities from devastating hazards and health crises.

More than ever before, global health must address these opportunities to provide health, security, and social justice. The free flow of information has exposed the stark contrast between reality and potentiality in world health. Disparities in global health have become increasingly recognized; indeed, avoidable deaths due to a lack of access to life-saving drugs are, to say the least, ethically disturbing. The greatest health disparities exist from insecurities created by preventable morbidity and mortality. Clearly, a renewed, fundamental commitment to health for all people is urgently needed, and the prevention of disease and the empowerment of people to generate health should be a top global priority. During the Brundtland era (1998–2003) at the World Health Organization (WHO), these challenges were frequently introduced into the global political discourse. Continuing on this path, the current WHO Director-General, Dr. J. W. Lee, underscored in his inaugural address, "The world today needs leadership in the ongoing struggle for security from infections, and justice for those worst affected by diseases of poverty" (9).

The spectacular health advances of the past 100 years have evolved historically from local to national to international action. A century of experience has validated that good health is 'knowledge based' and 'socially driven' (10). The knowledge base includes improved understandings of disease causation and the application of new technologies for disease control. 'Social knowledge' too has been important, for example, in the spread of primary education that has enabled individuals to produce their own health.

The concept of socially driven health refers to advances in living conditions such as clean water, food, and housing, as well as social institutional arrangements to organize people for collective health action. The most obvious social organization is health care systems, traditional and modern. Institutional arrangements, however, also refer to the organized contribution of government, business, civil society, and the press and media.

Historically, such arrangements have also included the health impact of social movements (11). In 19th century Britain, social activism played an important role in the sanitary movement, anti-poor laws, and the emancipation of child labor. Arguably the most important public action for health, however, is the assumption of responsibility by the nation-state for the health of all citizens. Indeed, the first national health legislation requiring compulsory taxation for public action, led by Edwin Chadwick, was the British Public Health Act of 1848 (12). In the 19th century, local and municipal governments in Britain contributed greatly to health advances. In Germany and Japan, the central government assumed a more leading role than local government. By the early 20th century, nationally organized health services were established in many, albeit not all, economically advanced societies.

The past century also witnessed increasing international cooperation. Through a series of sanitary conferences beginning in the mid-19th century, international health cooperation steadily grew among sovereign states. Stimulated in part by four waves of devastating cholera that swept from Asia through Europe into North America, interstate cooperation was sought to control contagious diseases while minimizing unnecessary disruption to free trade and travel, a balance that mirrors contemporary concerns. Formal international organizations began to be established by the beginning of the 20th century — the Pan American Health Organization in 1902, the Health Office of the League of Nations in the interwar years, and the WHO in 1948. Richard Cooper, in his study of international health cooperation, concluded that treaty negotiations improved when the mutual benefits of health cooperation became increasingly clear due to advances in the understanding of disease causation (13).

FROM INTERNATIONAL TO GLOBAL HEALTH

Over the last several decades, international health among sovereign states has begun to shift to global health, initially in small steps but now rapidly accelerating. The change is not simply one of nomenclature, but rather reflects a fundamental shift in the nature of health threats and their globally based solutions. Global health recognizes that today's health threats include yet extend beyond the reach of sovereign governments and incorporate the growing role of nonstate actors.

Many of today's health threats originate in one locale yet subsequently spread rapidly around the globe. Solutions are based, in part, on the transnational diffusion of knowledge, involving diverse global institutions and actor groups — government, industry, academia, nonprofit institutions, and the media. Local and national health actions increasingly call for global reinforcement, engaging many actors beyond nation-states. For example, more than two-thirds of reports of new epidemics now come from unofficial sources such as newspapers and nongovernmental organizations. These unofficial reports of disease outbreaks are scanned daily from newspapers and Internet websites. That the intergovernmental WHO investigates and coordinates subsequent monitoring and control of these reports demonstrates the complementary roles among an intergovernmental body and the diverse constituents of our global civil society (3).

The dramatic demographic and health transitions around the world have also underscored the importance of global approaches. Throughout the 20th century, most of the world's populations have progressed from high birth and high death rates to low birth and low death rates. Demographic and epidemiological dynamics therefore shape those who are at risk to health insecurities. For instance, high fertility within populations is associated with a younger age structure, which gives preeminence to diseases of childhood. Lowered fertility and lowered mortality at the completion of the demographic transition lead to a more stable population size as well as a shift in the age structure toward a more elderly population. Consequently, geriatric health problems increase. Development has presented other health challenges, including urbanization and changing health-related behavior. Nearly half of the world's population now resides in urban conglomerates, and intensified rural-to-urban migration has spawned slums, sometimes facilitating the spread of disease.

Paralleling demographic changes are health transitions generating great epidemiologic diversity (10). The world's privileged have mostly moved beyond the first generation of poverty-linked diseases, such as common infectious diseases, malnutrition, and maternity-related hazards. However, this transition has been highly uneven, varying by social status and geographical region. Pockets of poverty-linked diseases continue to persist among the disadvantaged within even the wealthiest countries. The biggest global burden of disease now is a second generation of chronic and degenerative diseases. Heart diseases, cancer, hypertension, and diabetes — afflicting adults of both the poor and the middle classes — have become the predominate cause of death in economically advanced countries, Eastern Europe, Latin America, and large parts of Asia (14).

A new configuration of epidemiological threats centers on emerging infections, environmental threats, and behavioral pathologies. These so-called 'third wave' diseases often assume global scope and afflict all people, wealthy and poor alike. Infectious diseases, some quite devastating, have emerged and reemerged due to drug resistance, ecological change, and human behavior. Since the appearance of HIV in the early 1980s, dozens of new bacteria and viruses have been identified. Since more than two million people travel internationally by air every day, these pathogens can reach new locales with unprecedented speed. The recent SARS epidemic demonstrated vividly this growing health interdependence.

In addition to the basic environmental amenities (clean drinking water and household sanitation) that are still inaccessible to millions of the world's poor, many people are increasingly exposed to chemical and other pollutants. Many of the new environmental hazards — such as ozone depletion, global warming, and toxic wastes — are fundamentally global with transnational reach. No country can escape these hazards because they extend beyond political boundaries: for example, pollution of the atmosphere. Behavioral pathologies — mental illness, abuse of addictive substances, unsafe sexual behavior, violence and injury — are other major causes of health and insecurity. These underlying risk conditions accelerate urbanization, joblessness, homelessness, and gender inequality. Violence comes in many forms, including road traffic and industrial accidents, gender-based sexual abuse, sexual harassment against women, self-inflicted suicides, and violence due to organized crime. Like infectious diseases, many of these harmful behaviors are 'socially contagious' — transmitted through imitative behavior, promoted by the mass media, and perpetrated by transnational criminal networks.

HEALTH POLICIES AND INSTITUTIONS FOR THE 21ST CENTURY

The 21st century challenges mentioned above have moved health onto the global human security agenda. Global health here is defined as health threats and responses that, while inclusive of national governments, go beyond the action of nation-states. The concept crosses geographical and political boundaries and is a true population-based approach. A recent example is the UN Millennium Development Goals (MDGs), which set time-bound targets for development achievements as part of a global compact to provide a minimal threshold of health and development in all societies. Another example is the new powers bestowed upon the WHO at the 2003 World Health Assembly. The assembly approved a resolution permitting the WHO to dispatch teams into countries for independent investigation of epidemics *without the invitation of governments*. The impetus for this action was the perceived need to correct for weaknesses exposed by the SARS epidemic, where some governments were accused of suppressing or distorting health information that hampered global control efforts (15).

After languishing for a decade, the WHO was indisputably revitalized under the leadership of Dr. Gro Brundtland (1998–2003). One of her major accomplishments was to present global health in terms that political leaders beyond the health sector could understand. The WHO's earlier history had confined the organization to medical and public health constituencies. Under Dr. Brundtland, health was vitally interjected into key global political forums, including to the G8 heads of state, the European Union, and the international financial institutions. In January 2000, another success occurred when the UN Security Council recognized the security threat from the AIDS pandemic, followed by the creation of the Global Fund to Fight AIDS, Tuberculosis, and Malaria. Dr. Brundtland noted the need to "[convince] presidents, prime ministers, and finance ministers that they are health ministers themselves." In doing so, Dr. Brundtland highlighted global health as a critical dimension of "hard politics," and recognized its moral and human rights dimensions (16).

The 2003 election of a new WHO Director-General, Dr. J. W. Lee, stimulated rich public dialogue on global health's institutional priorities (17, 18). Many parties explored the mandate and responsibilities of the WHO as part of the gradual but steady evolution toward more effective global health governance (19, 20). Most of the functions identified and debated may be considered core functions necessary for effective global health governance. For the sake of clarity, we have simplified these functions into four major groupings: evidence, laws, development, and partnerships.

EVIDENCE AND KNOWLEDGE MANAGEMENT

Since health is knowledge based, what is the role of global institutions in knowledge and research? We believe that global institutions do not belong in the role of directly producing biomedical knowledge, but rather in the critical role of effectively managing the validation, synthesis, and application of global health knowledge.

Today production of biomedical knowledge is a modern industry conducted by academia, industry, and governments, which combined deploy activities and budgets exceeding $100 billion annually. The scale and sophistication of these efforts are clearly beyond the pursuit of any single international organization. The WHO's annual budget, for example, is at most 1% of this annual turnover; only a miniscule proportion of the WHO's budget is devoted to research. However, there is a critical need for global health institutions to serve as mediators, catalysts, and evaluators of shared work and evidence. Their role should be to manage knowledge to advance world health, especially to bridge the equity gap. In the environmental arena, for example, data and knowledge on causalities helped propel the activism of the 'green' movement to the elaboration of national and international environmental law. In health, given the lack of commercial incentives for research on 'orphaned diseases of the poor,' there will be a continual need for a global health institution to generate and apply knowledge in the interest of global health equity. The institution's catalytic, intermediary, and management roles may be grouped into the categories of statistics, technical standards, improved practices, and health policies.

The foundation of evidence is global health statistics on health, illness, mortality, and health systems. Health statistics provide a clearer picture of global health situations, monitor and track trends, and identify causes and consequences of health change. Statistical information can be analyzed for patterns of disease and mortality at local, country, and global levels. Global statistical bodies also need to maintain and modify standardized systems of disease classification. Exercises such as the global burden of disease have pioneered for the first time an internally consistent picture of the global health situation. No other body beyond the WHO has the scientific credibility or capability to manage these essential tasks. A politically neutral intergovernmental body facilitates voluntary reporting by member nation-states. The WHO, thus, is the undisputed leader in this field. It has also recently taken the lead to launch world health surveys in some 70 countries, an unprecedented compilation of global health statistics.

An international organization like the WHO mobilizes technical expertise for the standardization and validation of health technologies and procedures. Such technical work supports and harmonizes the diverse work of various national bodies. Technical tasks include assessment of technologies — diagnostics, vaccines, drugs, and devices — by evaluating their safety, efficacy, performance, and cost effectiveness. Global institutions would certify laboratory procedures and diagnostic techniques, such as pharmaceutical bioavailability testing. Given the growth of the food trade, regional or international organizations are also needed to establish food safety standards. Many of these functions can and should be conducted by regional organizations like the OECD, the European Union, the Association of Southeast Asian Nations, and the North American Free Trade Area. Under Dr. Brundtland, the WHO renewed its agreements with OECD and the European Union in order to strengthen cooperation and exchange information. The WHO, the premier organization for world health, should neither replicate nor duplicate the work of such national or regional bodies. Rather, it should operate as a clearinghouse and harmonizer to make national and regional tasks more efficient and effective. Such work is best conducted through consultative committees convened by the WHO and consisting of members from national and regional bodies backed by independent scientific expertise.

A most dynamic and vital role in knowledge management is the promotion of best public health practices. The aim is to reduce local reinvention of the wheel by documenting and disseminating the best knowledge available for the advancement of health. The challenge is to provide not only technical information but also 'know-how'; for example, how best to improve the operations of health systems in diverse locations. There are many examples where best practices established by the WHO helped countries accelerate health progress. Spectacular health advances were achieved in Oman due in part to wholesale adoption of WHO best practice guidelines (21). In a span of 25 years, Oman, a comparatively small country, was able to accelerate health gains through the application of strategies that were scientifically tested elsewhere. Other practical examples have been the formulation and delivery of oral rehydration therapy and directly observed therapy (DOTS) for treatment of tuberculosis. Countries employing these strategies have shown impressive health improvements. In Bangladesh, for instance, a national nongovernmental organization, BRAC, was able to educate female members of every household in a country of 130 million people on oral rehydration therapy (22). In Peru, where a DOTS program has been operating for a decade, 91% of tuberculosis cases have been treated successfully; since 1995 more than 10 million patients have been successfully treated worldwide (23).

Promoting best practices can advance global health equity by bridging the gap between knowledge potential and reality in diverse real-world situations. In this regard, the relationship between global headquarters and country and regional offices of an international organization is critically important. Smoothly functioning relationships between these layered units are critical for learning best practices and disseminating them to all countries. Excessive centralization leads to omitting lessons learned from local situations and also runs the risk of rigidly imposing nonapplicable practices imported from elsewhere. Too much decentralization forfeits the learning that can be harnessed from horizontal communication among diverse groups. Striking the right balance between the center and the periphery is a key aspect of good global health governance.

The WHO's role in health policies has recently generated much debate. The Brundtland era assigned health policy high priority by creating a cluster of evidence and information for policy. The cluster produced the World Health Report 2000 (WHR2000), aimed at improving health systems performance, responsiveness, and financing by ranking nearly 200 countries according to national performance (24, 25). Some have objected to quantitative approaches or comparative national rankings. Yet, inspired by the experiences of the Human Development Index, presented annually by the UNDP, this unprecedented effort elevated the political attention paid to health systems performance and sparked an international political process for strengthening health systems in and among countries. Despite these worthy intentions, however, the WHO work has come under intense criticism. Some disagreements are undoubtedly due to the newness of the framework for assessment, and some to the political implications for certain member governments. There are others who have argued that the evidence base was weak, based on imputed and not real data, and that the methodologies employed for policy analysis were neither transparent nor widely agreed upon (26). To resolve the dispute, a distinguished review group recently completed a high-quality examination of the WHR2000 policy processes (27).

Academic debate on new methods is healthy, and political debate should be expected as an inherent part of any policy development process. Among the major considerations are the political nature of ranking health systems performance and the vast lacunae of knowledge on how to improve health systems performance. While important, 'policy' should be recognized as an inherently political process based on social values. 'Hard evidence' can be used objectively or subjectively to describe various health situations. But applying such descriptive data for policy formulation requires acceptance of selected assumptions that carry social, political, and ethical implications. The political nature of evidence-based policy becomes particularly intense if policy is employed to guide resource allocations. Proscriptive policy processes would be improved, however, if the data and analytical processes were transparent and the fundamental political nature of policy explicitly acknowledged. Policy formulation can never be an entirely technocratic process. For example, policy recommendations should make clear whether the desired outcomes emphasize efficiency (cost-effectiveness) or fairness (equity). Policy processes also must be perceived as inclusive. A key question is whether those affected by policy decisions are brought into the consultative process as a matter of democratic practice.

LAWS, CONVENTIONS, AND REGULATIONS

Much attention on globalization has been focused on the expansion of private markets. Yet many do not appreciate that global health and security are preconditions for efficient trade and the functioning of private markets. A well performing global private economy depends upon the control of contagious diseases. Indeed, the earliest international health regulations emerged from the imperative to control infectious diseases that could potentially impede trade. Today, the disruptive effects of SARS, AIDS, bovine spongiform encephalitis, and hoof-and-mouth disease illustrate the powerful economic impacts of epidemics. As a result of the recent SARS epidemic, international organizations no doubt will acquire stronger powers to control contagious diseases. For this reason the International Health Regulations, the longest ongoing international agreement in health, are currently undergoing revision after last being revised in 1969 (28). The Regulations list notifiable contagious diseases in an effort to reduce the spread of infections while minimizing disruption to international trade and travel. It is possible to visualize over time additional international regulations for noninfectious health hazards such as certain addictive substances.

'The Convention on Tobacco Control represents one of the biggest breakthroughs in global health during the Brundtland era. The Convention, the first international treaty negotiated under the auspices of the WHO (2003 WHA), employs a strategy developed by environmental groups. It requires countries to impose restrictions on tobacco advertising, sponsorship, and promotion; establishes new labeling and clean indoor air controls; and strengthens legislation to clamp down on tobacco smuggling (29). To come into full force, the Convention must be ratified by 40 member states, a feat achieved during the first week it was open for signature. As the Convention is enforced, many nations will employ it as the basis of national tobacco-control legislation. Arduous, contentious, and full of political pitfalls, negotiations of the Convention illustrate the global character of reaching consensus among diverse interest groups possessing 'asymmetrical power' — mixing the legitimacy of governments, the financial influence of industry, the social activism of nongovernmental organizations, and the scientific contributions of academia. The negotiations were successful because they were able to harmonize these diverse actors around a core set of health-related guidelines.

Health laws and conventions will shape several other arenas of global health. The proposed intellectual property regime of the World Trade Organization's Trade-Related Intellectual Property agreement (WTO/TRIPs) has important implications for affordable access to essential drugs. Because the management of intellectual property rights (IPR) has ramifications for health, a global health organization should ensure that health and human security concerns are vitally integrated into the formulation of the regime. Intellectual property rights for health must not be housed solely in a trade and commerce organization; the world's premier global health institution also must be engaged. Already public concerns, protests, and campaigns over restrictive clauses in TRIPs have resulted in some relaxation of rigid patent rules by allowing compulsory licensing and parallel importing exceptions for governments. At stake are global health and human security on the one hand and incentives for vitally important commercial research on the other. The role of global health institutions should be to interject forcefully their global health mandates and interests in the negotiations of such international agreements.

Another potentially contentious arena is WTO negotiation on trade in social services, including health (30). Liberalization of trade is likely to be accelerated under the General Agreement on Trade in Services (GATS). As international trade in health services expands, the WTO's influence and impact upon health services will correspondingly increase. Looking to the future, new WTO ground rules may impose pressures upon some countries to open up health service markets to private foreign competition. The GATS agreement could also, at least theoretically, force reductions of publicly financed and publicly operated health services, based on the charges of unfair competition due to public subsidy. While still in the early stages, the implications for many national health services could be significant.

Finally, just as regulations are needed to level the playing field for private markets to function domestically, there is a case for health regulations to modulate the effective functioning of the global market. Precisely which ground rules should be addressed is beyond the scope of this chapter, but one area worthy of investigation is the global labor market that some say is leading to massive 'brain drain' of highly skilled professionals from southern to northern countries. Medical migration is a complicated subject with causes and consequences that are still unclear. Simply erecting barriers to voluntary migration would be ineffective and, in any case, would compromise the basic human right of movement. But many poor countries (and internal poor regions in all countries) are unable to attract highly skilled medical professionals because these workers seek better opportunities in the global labor market. The health implications of workers' mobility are unclear, since many of the key services required by the poor and marginalized can be provided by paraprofessionals. An inequity in the current unregulated mobility regime, however, is the loss of public subsidy for higher medical education in poorer countries as educated health workers move to richer countries. Rather than trying to stop migration altogether, a goal should be to enhance fairness between sending and receiving countries to advance mutual health and human security in an increasingly interdependent world.

Health and development

Since health is a key dimension of overall socioeconomic development, global health institutions should interject health onto the global development agenda. Health after all is socially driven, and overall development and social arrangements are central to health production. Therefore, while the WHO should retain primacy as an international health organization, it must not become 'medicalized' — isolated from broader aspects of development. The foregoing examples of IPR and WTO negotiations illustrate the importance of health perspectives in development. Conversely, many if not most development activities would benefit from stronger health inputs on poverty alleviation, primary education, gender equality, and sustainable development.

A formidable challenge for health and development is the mobilization of political support and financial resources to produce global public health goods. In this regard, the recent WHO Commission on Macroeconomics and Health raised the political visibility of health. The Commission reported that "extending the coverage of future health services, including a relatively small number of specific interventions, to the world's poor could save millions of lives each year, reduce poverty, spur economic development, and promote global security" (31). To reach high-level policymakers, especially in finance ministries, the Commission offered an overarching assessment of the links between investment in health and economic development. Poverty and health are linked in a two-way interactive relationship. The Commission emphasized the causal linkages between disease and a lack of economic growth; there is equally compelling evidence for the reverse linkage, as poverty increases the risk of illness and premature death. Although the scientific validity of the Commission's work will surely undergo major scrutiny in the future, it has already exerted major policy impact. Follow-up at the country level is aimed at forging partnerships between ministries of health, finance, and other stakeholders.

The Millennium Development Goals have also placed health prominently on the global development agenda. The MDGs address key elements of human development and are a set of ambitious social targets to be reached by 2015. Of the eight goals, three (plus part of a fourth goal on hunger) specifically address health. They are: Goal 4 — reduce by two-thirds the mortality rate among children under five; Goal 5 — reduce by three quarters the maternal mortality rate; Goal 6 — halt and begin to reverse the incidence of HIV/AIDS, malaria, and other diseases; and Goal 1 — eradicate extreme poverty, hunger, and malnutrition. These are priority global challenges, and the MDGs bring political attention to these development issues.

The MDGs represent an important piece in a more structured global infrastructure, with health and human security as core elements. They have the potential to mobilize political will with powerful legitimacy, providing clearer focus to donor governments and aid agencies, and encouraging governments and civil society of poor countries to attend to the causes of poverty. The MDGs will stress an ensuing, coordinated campaign to achieve these goals. They also represent a global compact among poorer and richer countries for mutual responsibility in global health and development. In sum, the MDGs provide an important political framework for policymakers at national and international levels as well as for global institutions.

INSTITUTIONAL PARTNERSHIPS

In recent decades, the number and type of global health stakeholders has grown enormously — international agencies (UN, WHO, UNICEF, UNDP; the World Bank and IMF), bilateral donors from OECD countries (Norway, Sweden, France, UK, Germany, Japan, U.S.), private foundations (Rockefeller, Gates, Wellcome, Atlantic, Ellison), large and powerful private pharmaceutical companies, the private sector health care industry, nongovernmental organizations including faith-based groups, and the press and mass media. The emergence of multiple actors has necessitated more nuanced institutional arrangements in global health. After all, no single institution, however mandated or well intentioned, can hope to fulfill all global health functions. Thus the concept of one gigantic, monolithic bureaucracy for global health appears to have receded. A more desirable goal may be to welcome the various health actors, complementing vertically organized formal institutions with supplementary horizontally linked networks and coalitions. The WHO as the premier organization can take the lead in shaping these social and institutional arrangements. It must develop a coherent strategy of working with others in global health governance.

Under Dr. Brundtland's leadership, these novel arrangements, often called private-public partnerships (PPPs), increased markedly. In her inaugural address, Dr. Brundtland sought partnerships through 'reaching out' (16). This approach was controversial, especially with respect to internal WHO concerns over the erosion of its mandate and weakening institutional control of funds, programs, and staff. Brundtland's articulated rationale was two-fold: true leadership is never given, it must be earned; and partnerships can lead to win-win cooperative arrangements, impossible with a unilateral approach. Of course, many partnerships began before the Brundtland era; for example, drug donations by pharmaceutical companies were implemented by international agencies and nongovernmental organizations. Such was the partnership arrangement for the use of donated ivermectin by Merck in the control of onchocerciasis, or river blindness.

The past decade has witnessed a proliferation of partnerships. The Global Alliance for Vaccine Initiatives (GAVI) — perhaps the largest coalition of agencies, foundations, governments, and industry — aims to deliver basic vaccines to all eligible children around the world. Similar arrangements were structured around malaria (Roll Back Malaria) and tuberculosis (Stop TB Initiative). Especially energetic have been partnerships in research and development (R&D) to produce vaccines and drugs against 'orphaned diseases' of the poor. Drugs against these diseases are not profitable for commercial investments and thus their absence represents market failures. To address this situation, new R&D partnerships have emerged, including the International AIDS Vaccine Initiative (IAVI), the Global Alliance for TB Drug Development (GATBD), Medicines for Malaria Venture (MMV), the Global Program to Eliminate Lymphatic Filariasis, and the Global Vitamin A Alliance. These partnerships bring together a variety of stakeholders pooling resources and skills and working toward common goals. While promising in theory, these PPPs face many daunting challenges, including generating useful products, sustaining financing, and harmonizing diverse interests and power imbalances among partners. Organizationally, they take many different forms, some as private participants in intergovernmental operating units, and others as independent nonprofits with board membership for intergovernmental entities.

Conceptually, partnerships with multiple actors constitute a piece of the mosaic system of global health governance. Many novel types of partnerships or arrangements will emerge in the coming decade. It is appropriate to inquire about the optimal balance between horizontal profusion of new initiatives and coherence and sustainability. It remains a paradox that those nations that gathered to set up the Global Fund for AIDS, Tuberculosis, and Malaria insisted on safeguarding the fund's independence from the UN and the WHO. The long list of independent initiatives and institutions raises the risk of duplication and the danger of fragmentation. At the same time, this mosaic adds complexity to the burden of poor nations struggling to handle a myriad of aid institutions. It is also not clear when and how a particular initiative will be deemed nonperforming. A necessary approach is to achieve consensus among actors as well as to overcome political and bureaucratic bottlenecks. "Gaps and duplications will naturally emerge, but these flaws may not be fatal if the sub-systems are adaptive, flexible, and responsive to changing demands. A major challenge is how these new organizations will be assessed or should be closed after they complete their mission. There are also issues of proliferation beyond affordability or effectiveness" (8).

AN ARCHITECTURE FOR GLOBAL HEALTH: THE WAY FORWARD

Piece by piece, these core functions of global health governance are being put into place. Consolidation of these functions will generate an increasingly coherent global architecture for health and human security. Reforming large global institutions will not be easy; indeed, many consider these large bureaucracies beyond reform. More important is to change the institutional culture of established organizations so that they remain adaptable to changing circumstances. The severity of some global health crises and the imperatives for health, security, and justice will generate many powerful forces for institutional change. In such shifts, no single organization is guaranteed a future. The creation of a coordinating body such as UNAIDS and an independent organization like the Global Fund for AIDS, Tuberculosis, and Malaria illustrates how external demands can generate pressure either for institutional reform or a new organization altogether. The same holds true for major bilateral initiatives such as the U.S. billion-dollar initiative to fight AIDS in Africa. Sometimes difficult obstacles are bridged by unforeseen events, just as the SARS epidemic will enable a wholesale revision of the International Health Regulations that had earlier been dormant. It seems inevitable that the HIV/AIDS epidemic will increasingly focus pressure on international institutions to develop more effective responses. All these elements will contribute to an evolving global health governance system that will require consideration of three factors — political commitment, astute institutional management, and new modes of financing.

Leadership and vision are required for successful global health solutions. Political interest in global health has increased markedly, though not enough to accord global health the political and economic priority needed. The closing decades of the 20th century were largely disappointing. There was failure to achieve Health for All by the year 2000, a concept promulgated at the Alma Ata conference. Health care systems weakened, struggled, and even collapsed in many of the poorest countries. HIV/AIDS and other health challenges created virtual health crises in some of the world's poorest communities. No doubt, key obstacles to better performance were political instability and weak economic development in many countries. But political will was also lacking. Health needs to be recognized as a global public good. In many emerging welfare states, health services are viewed as public goods, and there is every reason to view global health as an essential global public good (8). Such an approach can form the basis for stronger political commitment vital for generating global health and human security.

Translation of political commitment to action will require astute management of organizations — from service delivery to nongovernmental organizations to global health agencies. One aspect of institutional management is clear. An era of vast bureaucracies conducting business like world government is unlikely; so too are the overly privatized structures now under consideration, which are based on the false premise that the model of private corporations can be applied to social sectors. It is therefore important that institutional partnerships be crafted to shape the mosaic of global health governance. For some purposes, a particular institutional form can function better than others; no single organizational form can serve all roles. In this chapter, we have presented some roles that we believe should constitute core functions of world health governance. In such an architecture, there is space for many actors and functions — research by academia, advocacy by nongovernmental organizations, national health systems by governments, and so on. Therefore the process is more a pragmatic trial and error approach rather than one that follows a blueprint or grand design. The process is guided throughout by the universally shared desire for good health.

Achieving these ambitious goals will require new modes of financing. The WHO today operates on about $1 billion per year. There is increasing projectization of its work by donors and consequent fragmentation, lack of stability, and weak sustainability. There is a growing need to develop new mechanisms for financing global health that go beyond the fickleness and charitable culture of foreign aid. One proposal is to establish a set of fee-based services. A 'health security' fee of, say, U.S. $1 could be charged per international air traveler. Since September 11th, $2.50 has been added to all U.S. air tickets to cover the extra cost of security checking. Therefore, a modest fee could be reasonably considered for health security. Given the economic impact of SARS and other epidemics on air travel, the airline industry might be an enthusiastic supporter of such a fee. With about 700 million cross-border air travelers annually, this fee would generate nearly the same amount of funds as the annual WHO budget. Fees could be pooled for oversight by a joint IATA (International Air Transport Authority) and WHO board. Part of the fee would be allocated to directly improving the health security of air travelers (through health screening and tracing contacts), but the bulk of the fee would be allocated to combating global health threats through the improvement of surveillance systems and global health infrastructure. Additionally, a modest portion of the fee could be directed toward subsidizing national health security infrastructure in the poorest countries. After all, new epidemics often erupt in such environments because the proximity of humans to domestic livestock enables new viruses to cross over into human populations.

Establishing a global health architecture for the 21st century will ultimately depend upon ethics, values, and political will. In the end, global health functions serve both altruism and the self-interest of all global citizens. Unnecessary suffering evokes human empathy, but global health with human security represents enlightened self-protection in a highly interdependent world. Increasingly, universal access to basic modern health technologies and services is recognized as a basic human right. Ultimately, global health reaffirms the unity and indivisibility of health and human security among all world citizens.

REFERENCES

1. Rothschild E. What is security? *Daedalus* 1995;124(3):53–98.

2. Rothschild E. Globalization and the return of history. *Foreign Policy* 1999;115:106–16.

3. Heymann D. Evolving infectious disease threats to national and global security. In: Chen L, Leaning J, Narasimhan V, editors. *Global health challenges for human security*. Cambridge (MA): Global Equity Initiative, Asia Center, Faculty of Arts and Sciences, Harvard University; 2003.

4. Shisana O, Zungu-Dirwayi N, Shisana W. AIDS: a threat to human security. In: Chen L, Leaning J, Narasimhan V, editors. *Global health challenges for human security*. Cambridge (MA): Global Equity Initiative, Asia Center, Faculty of Arts and Sciences, Harvard University; 2003.

5. Chen L, Fukuda-Parr S. Special issue on new insecurities: editor's introduction. *Journal of Human Development* 2003;4(2):163–6.

6. Wilson M. Health and security: globalization of infectious diseases. In: Chen L, Leaning J, Narasimhan V, editors. *Global health challenges for human security*. Cambridge (MA): Global Equity Initiative, Asia Center, Faculty of Arts and Sciences, Harvard University; 2003.

7. Leaning J, Arie S, Holleufer G, Bruderlein C. Human security and conflict: a comprehensive approach. In: Chen L, Leaning J, Narasimhan V, editors. *Global health challenges for human security*. Cambridge (MA): Global Equity Initiative, Asia Center, Faculty of Arts and Sciences, Harvard University; 2003.

8. Chen L, Evans T, Cash R. Health as a global public good. In: Kaul I, Grunberg I, Stern M, editors. *Global public goods: international cooperation in the 21st century.* New York: Oxford University Press; 1999. p. 284–304.

9. Lee JW. Speech to the fifty-sixth world health assembly. 2003; Geneva, Switzerland. Available from: URL: http://www.who.int/dg_elect/wha56_jwlspeech/en/, accessed on 2003 Aug 2.

10. Chen L, Berlinguer G. Health equity in a globalizing world. In: Evans T, Whitehead M, Diderichsen F, Bhuiya A, Wirth M, editors. *Challenging inequities in health: from ethics to action.* New York: Oxford University Press; 2001. p. 35–44.

11. Szreter S. Health and security in historical perspective. In: Chen L, Leaning J, Narasimhan V, editors. *Global health challenges for human security.* Cambridge (MA): Global Equity Initiative, Asia Center, Faculty of Arts and Sciences, Harvard University; 2003.

12. Porter R. *The greatest benefit to mankind: a medical history of humanity.* New York: W.W. Norton; 1998.

13. Cooper R. International cooperation in public health as a prologue to macroeconomic cooperation. In: Cooper R, Eichengreen B, Henning CR, Holtham G, Putnam R. *Can nations agree: issues in international economic cooperation.* Washington: Brookings Institution; 1989. p. 178–254.

14. Murray C, Lopez A, editors. *The global burden of disease: a comprehensive assessment of mortality and disability from diseases, injuries, and risk factors in 1990 and projected to 2020.* Cambridge (MA): Harvard School of Public Health; 1996.

15. Stein R. WHO gets wider power to fight global health threats. *The Washington Post* 2003 May 28;p. A15.

16. Brundtland GH. Speech to the fifty-first world health assembly. 1998 May 13.

17. Horton R. WHO: the casualties and compromises of renewal. *The Lancet* 2002;359:1605–11.

18. McCarthy M. What's going on at the World Health Organization? *The Lancet* 2002;360:1108–10.

19. Binka F, Cash R, Chen L, et al. An open letter to the executive board of WHO. *The Lancet* 2002;360:1797.

20. Lee K, editor. *Health impacts of globalization: towards global governance.* New York: Palgrave Macmillan; 2003.

21. Chen L, Hill A. *Oman's leap to good health.* Muscat, Oman: World Health Organization/United Nations Children's Fund; 1996.

22. Chowdhury AMR, Cash RA. *A simple solution: teaching millions to treat diarrhoea at home.* Dhaka: University Press Ltd.; 1996.

23. What is DOTS? 2003. Available from: URL: http://www.who.int/gtb/dots/whatisdots.htm, accessed on 2003 Aug 2.

24. Almeida C, Braveman P, Gold M, et al. Methodological concerns and recommendations on policy consequences of the world health report 2000. *The Lancet* 2001;357:1692.

25. World Health Organization. *World health report 2000 health systems: improving performance.* Geneva: World Health Organization; 2000.

26. Musgrove P. Judging health systems: reflections on WHO's methods. *The Lancet* 2003;361:1817–20.

27. Scientific Peer Review Group on Health Systems Performance Assessment. *Report of the scientific peer review group on health systems performance assessment.* 2002. Available from: URL: http://www.who.int/health-systems-performance/sprg/report_of_sprg_on_hspa.htm, accessed on 2003 Aug 2.

28. Cash R, Narasimhan V. Impediments to global surveillance of infectious diseases: consequences of open reporting in a global economy. *Bulletin of the World Health Organization* 2000;78:1358–67.

29. World Health Organization. *World health assembly adopts historic tobacco control pact.* Geneva: World Health Organization; 2003. Available from: URL: http://www.who.int/mediacentre/releases/2003/prwha1/en/, accessed on 2003 Aug 2.

30. Lipson D. The world trade organization's health agenda. *British Medical Journal* 2001;323:1139–40.

31. World Health Organization, Commission on Macroeconomics and Health. Report of the commission on macroeconomics and health: investing in health for economic development. Geneva: World Health Organization; 2001. Available from: URL: http://www3.who.int/whosis/cmh/cmh_report/e/report.cfm?path=cmh,cmh_report&language=english, accessed on 2003 Aug 2.

SECTION 11

GLOBAL EPIDEMICS

CHAPTER 6

HEALTH AND SECURITY: GLOBALIZATION OF INFECTIOUS DISEASES

MARY E. WILSON

INTRODUCTION

Infectious diseases kill, disable, disfigure, stigmatize, and cause terror. They remain a substantial cause of mortality globally, disproportionately affecting the poorest and most vulnerable populations. They have the capacity to destroy, destabilize, and profoundly alter populations. Because of the abundance, resilience, and mutability of pathogens, infectious diseases can change rapidly and in unexpected ways. Current attributes of the world's population — including size, density, mobility, vulnerability, and location — have increased the risks for many infectious diseases, despite the availability of an unprecedented array of tools to prevent, diagnose, treat, and track them. Some humans may employ infectious disease agents to kill, consume resources, and spread fear, but even without this potential menace, infectious diseases in the world today pose a serious security threat (Table 1). Infectious diseases of animals and plants also have major economic consequences and affect human health and security.

Approximately a quarter of all deaths in the world today are due to infectious diseases, but the burden weighs most heavily on the developing world. HIV, *Mycobacterium tuberculosis*, and malaria parasites remain the three pathogens that inflict the greatest toll in deaths. The diseases they cause also have major economic and demographic consequences. For example, it has been estimated that malaria has slowed economic growth in African countries by as much as 1.3% per year. Respiratory and diarrheal infections, caused by a number of different pathogens, cause more than six million deaths annually (1). Globally, infectious diseases and parasitic infections account for about 23% of the loss of disability-adjusted life years (DALYs), but in some populations in sub-Saharan Africa they account for over 50% of the loss of DALYs. In many countries in Africa, more than 20% of deaths in children less than five years of age are thought

Table I.   Ways that infectious diseases destabilize a community

Fear of spread or panic (especially severe when origin of infection, mechanism(s) of transmission, or consequences are not well defined)

Rejection of or discrimination against infected individuals or groups

Demographic shifts; creation of large numbers of orphans; loss of age groups; decreased life expectancy

Loss of capacity to produce (e.g., food, other goods), to educate, and to maintain economic stability

Loss of trust in government; political unrest

Poverty; lack of food, water, shelter, medications

Diversion of medical resources from preventive services, such as basic immunizations, prenatal care, etc.

Loss of hope

to be due to acute respiratory infections (ARI). This is in contrast to most industrialized countries where less than 5% of childhood deaths is due to ARI (2). Of the 40 million persons living with HIV at the end of 2001, 95% were in developing countries; 70% of persons with HIV/AIDS are in sub-Saharan Africa. Among the estimated 300 million annual malaria cases, 90% are in sub-Saharan Africa; 97% of malaria deaths occur in sub-Saharan Africa, primarily in children. In seven African countries — Botswana, Lesotho, Namibia, South Africa, Swaziland, Zambia, Zimbabwe — more than 20% of people between the ages of 15 and 49 years are infected with HIV (3).

This chapter reviews the influence of infectious diseases in today's world, specifically in the milieu and events associated with global interconnectedness and the transnational flow of people, goods, information, and resources. It addresses the following specific questions:

1. What events or processes associated with globalization impinge on the appearance, spread, and control of infectious diseases?

2. What is the backdrop (socioeconomic, environmental, demographic) against which these processes are occurring?

3. What are the characteristics of infectious diseases that can spread globally?

The chapter also briefly discusses the potential impact of antimicrobial resistance on the control of infectious diseases.

Question 1: What processes are associated with globalization of infectious diseases?

Processes relevant to infectious diseases can be discussed under three broad headings: 1) movement of humans and associated biological material; 2) trade; and 3) flow or sharing of ideas, social mores and values, information, policy, technology, materials, and other resources.

MOVEMENT OF BIOLOGICAL MATERIAL

The scale, speed, and reach of movement of people and goods today is unprecedented and shapes the appearance, spread, and distribution of infectious diseases in humans, plants, and animals (4). International travel and commerce facilitate rapid, massive, and global dispersal of biological material, including microbial genetic material. Travel, trade, and the wide availability of mass transport have vastly expanded the movement of this biological material that occurs naturally via migration of animals, flight of birds, movement of species such as insects, plant seeds, and marine life — over land, in winds and air currents, and in streams and oceans.

Each day more than 1.4 million people cross international borders on airplane flights. In 2002 more than 700 million international tourist arrivals were registered (5). By the 1990s more than 5,000 airports had regularly scheduled international flights. This means that dense urban centers throughout the world are linked by a steady flow of humans. But air travel is only one link. For example, an estimated 400 million international travelers entered the U.S. in 1999 by air, land, or ship. Modern technologies have expanded the number of easily accessible destinations and allow travelers to enter and survive in more extreme environments. Although most travel occurs along well established corridors, more travelers are reaching remote areas where they may have contact with potentially pathogenic microbes that are not yet well characterized in animals or environmental reservoirs.

Humans have a long history of travel and migration, and history books are filled with examples of the role of travelers (soldiers, merchants, explorers, refugees, others) in the introduction and spread of infectious diseases (6, 7, 8). The difference today is the scale, speed, and reach of interconnection. A human may be considered an interactive biological unit, carrying an assemblage of microbial genetic material and immune responses and capacity that reflect past exposures (9). Long distance travel typically involves spending time in sequential shared environments (e.g., bus, train, terminal, plane, ship, etc.), which potentially link the traveler to a wide network of contacts. Although travelers who are ill have often been the focus of study when considering the introduction of infections into new populations, all travelers are likely affected by exposures both in transit and at their destination. Travelers can acquire, process immunologically, carry, and transmit microbial genetic material during and after travel — in some instances long after travel. Microbes transmitted from person to person (especially respiratory pathogens and sexually transmitted infections) can be carried to any part of the world by travelers. A prominent contemporary example is HIV. Although transmission of HIV from mother to child and via blood and blood products does occur, the predominant mode of spread around the world has been via humans who carried HIV and transmitted it to others through sexual contact.

Humans may carry pathogens and transmit them to others in the absence of symptoms. Examples include asymptomatic infection with HIV and hepatitis B virus. Pathogens that regularly colonize mucosal surfaces (e.g., *Neisseria meningitidis*, *Streptococcus pneumoniae*, *Staphylococcus aureus*) may be carried (often transiently) and transmitted by healthy people who have no symptoms or awareness that they carry these potential pathogens (10). It is now clear that humans can also carry resistance genes, sometimes found in commensal bacteria of the gut or skin, that may be transferred to others (11, 12). A carrier who introduces a pathogen, a new clone, or a resistance gene into a community may never experience any illness. With infections such as HIV, which can remain asymptomatic for prolonged periods, transmission may occur repeatedly, over a long period of time, and in places remote from the site of acquisition. People with active tuberculosis may have minor symptoms allowing them to continue to work and travel — and transmit infection.

Travel may be brief or followed by settlement in a new country. As of March 2000, the estimated size of the foreign-born population in the U.S. was 28 million. Many of these people carry microbial material or immunologic consequences of past exposures. Immigrants typically remain connected with their country of origin, and so provide linkages through repeated visits in both directions.

Several specific types of travel and migration — and their consequences — are worth highlighting.

The numbers of environmental and political refugees have soared. An estimated 35 million people currently are fleeing war or persecution (13). This is the highest number since World War II. Large numbers of troops and associated staff are regularly deployed to foreign countries where they can introduce infections into local populations, pick up locally prevalent infections, and become a source for outbreaks when they return home.

Sexual tourism provides a mechanism through which microbes may be carried transnationally and reach wide, loosely connected networks. HIV is the most common, lethal infection spread sexually. Other genital infections facilitate the spread of HIV and are associated with infertility, perinatal loss, and other serious consequences.

A cruise ship may be likened to a floating city with passengers and crew of diverse origins who have periodic encounters with mainland populations. At the terminus, they disperse widely, usually via multiple airplane flights to various regions or countries. Many cruise ships now carry loads of more than 3,000 passengers and crew. This floating habitat provides abundant opportunities to share indoor spaces and pathogens. Cruise ships globally have the capacity to carry 47 million passengers per year. Outbreaks, including massive ones, have been documented on ships, caused by a wide range of pathogens including influenza, rubella, noroviruses, previously known as Norwalk-like viruses, and many other gastrointestinal pathogens (14). Ships used to transport cargo carry all types of biological life in ballast water and have been the source of introductions of invasive, exotic species into ports around the world (15).

TRADE

Imported food now comprises a substantial part of the diet for many populations, especially in North America and parts of Europe. For example, the U.S. imports more than 30 billion tons of food per year, including fruit, vegetables, meat, and seafood (16). Although the food chain has become very long, it often links microbial composition of produce in the field, at harvest, and during processing with the gastrointestinal tracts of large populations of consumers hundreds or thousands of kilometers away. Mass processing of many foods and wide distribution networks mean that microbial contamination at the production site or during processing may reach thousands or millions of people in multiple countries. Contamination occurs because of human ignorance or error, breakdown in equipment, or it may be introduced intentionally.

The following is an indication of the volume of trade coming into the United States. In 2001 the U.S. Customs Service received imports of 2.3 million rail cars, 11.2 million cargo trucks, 5.7 million sea containers from ships, almost a million aircraft — and whatever goods and biologic life they all contained (17).

In Miami alone, more than 30 million imported animals arrived in 1996. This number only includes legally imported animals at one port. Among the arrivals were 28.6 million fish, 1.1 million reptiles, 108,000 amphibians, 70,000 mammals, and 1,400 birds.[1] In 1999, the year that an outbreak of West Nile virus (WNV) was first identified in the U.S., with its epicenter in New York, 2,770 birds legally entered (were imported into) the country through JFK International Airport in New York. In addition, almost 13,000 birds passed through in transit (18).

Multiple wildlife species, many of them exotic and rare, are often collected from diverse, remote areas and kept in close proximity in zoos or wildlife conservation parks, adjacent to large human populations. These captive wildlife populations undergo inconsistently intense observation and monitoring. They are occasional sources of infection but can also serve as sentinel populations for new events. In the WNV outbreak in New York, testing of stored and newly collected sera suggested that birds newly introduced to the Bronx Zoo were not the source of infection, that WNV infection had not been present before 1999, and that it spread widely in the zoo bird population and to a lesser extent in mammals (19).

As an example of the dominance of trade pressures over good sense, distributors of exotic animals export prairie dogs from the U.S. to multiple other countries even though prairie dogs can be infected with the bacteria that cause tularemia, plague, and other potentially life-threatening infections in humans. A recent outbreak of tularemia in prairie dogs at a distribution center in Texas, which exported these animals to at least 10 states and seven countries, highlights this risk. Microbes in imported animals can be a source of human pathogens and may also threaten domestic and local wildlife populations (20).

Arthropods that serve as vectors of human, animal, and plant diseases are regularly transported by vehicles, including aircraft, and sometimes successfully become established in new geographic regions (21, 22). Historically, water tanks in boats provided a suitable environment for the survival of mosquitoes traveling across oceans. Infestation of a region with a vector competent to transmit human pathogens places that region at risk for the relevant vector-borne infections. *Aedes albopictus,* a mosquito competent to transmit dengue fever virus and other viral pathogens, was introduced into North America in the 1980s, probably via used tires imported from Asia. It was first identified in Texas and spread to 678 counties in 25 states within 12 years (23). Of note, its dispersal followed interstate highways. As of 2002, it had also been introduced into Brazil, the Dominican Republic, Guatemala, Honduras, Panama, Mexico, Nicaragua, Cuba, Bolivia, El Salvador, and Colombia, and it continues to spread.

Recent studies suggest that insects resistant to insecticides may also disperse and transfer resistance genes to pests in other areas (24, 25). Insects can directly damage plants and can also spread infections among plants, including important food crops.

Exotic or alien species threaten local populations and ecosystems. Infectious diseases also threaten plants and animals and thereby have a major economic impact. Examples include bovine spongiform encephalopathy (BSE) in the UK and subsequently in many other countries, and foot and mouth disease, especially in the UK. Infectious diseases in plants and animals may also have both direct and indirect consequences to human health. The appearance of fatal variant Creutzfeldt-Jakob disease (vCJD) in humans in the UK, and subsequent scattered cases in other countries, has been linked to BSE in cattle. Interventions have cost billions of dollars and have undermined the credibility of the government and panels that initially announced that no risk existed from consuming beef products. Of note, the extensive global trading links, cross links, and exportation of animals and animal products (including food) from the UK requires a global response. The long latency period between exposure and development of symptoms and difficulty in diagnosis (requires study of tissue) have complicated efforts to assess the magnitude of the problem. Recent findings that genetic differences may affect susceptibility — and perhaps incubation period — in humans further complicate the process of making informed projections.

The transnational movement of people and goods facilitates the introduction of plant pathogens and their vectors into communities. Infectious diseases of plants — such as Karnal bunt of wheat, potato late blight, and citrus tristeza — affect large, commercially important crops (26). The destruction by disease of major food crops such as rice, wheat, and potatoes, could affect food security.

A report published by the USDA (1998, revised in 2001) analyzed the potential for international travelers to transmit foreign animal diseases to U.S. livestock or poultry (27). The report listed infections that are considered List A diseases ("transmissible diseases with potential for very serious and rapid spread, ...of serious socioeconomic or public health consequence, ...and of major importance in the international trade of animals and animal products"). Among the listed diseases were Newcastle disease, swine vesicular disease, avian influenza, foot and mouth disease, African swine fever, vesicular stomatitis, and Rift Valley fever. Humans may carry pathogens either mechanically (e.g., on shoes or clothing) or biologically (human infected).

In Africa, the establishment of networks, improved infrastructure, and especially the building of roads for logging and other development have facilitated the spread of the bushmeat trade (28). Simian immunodeficiency viruses (SIVs) are widespread in primate species. In one study in Cameroon of blood and tissue samples from 788 monkeys (bushmeat and pet animals), 16.6% of plasma samples tested strongly positive for HIV antigens (29). There is good evidence that HIV in humans originated from introductions of related SIV viruses from primates to humans (30, 31). Contact with primates as pets or with primate tissue through butchering animals could allow transfer of SIVs to humans.

FLOW AND TRANSFER OF KNOWLEDGE; SHARED TECHNOLOGY AND MATERIALS

The global community has shared technical and scientific data for centuries; with the availability of the Internet, exchange has expanded. Several examples show the benefits and problems associated with shared information.

Global surveillance networks, though still rudimentary, exist and are improving. Ideally, knowledge of a specific disease in a particular geographic area would generate needed assistance from the global community to minimize impact, halt spread, and prevent recurrences (32). It would also alert those who might have been exposed to the risk so that steps could be taken to prevent infection or to intervene at an early stage. The study of outbreaks can identify risk factors; sharing this knowledge may help others to prevent outbreaks (33).

It is now easier, faster, and cheaper to communicate than ever before. A wide range of networks exists, some focusing on a specific infection (e.g., salmonella infections, Legionnaires disease, influenza, leptospirosis), others on specific populations (such as travelers, immigrants) and others on antimicrobial resistance patterns. Regional or area networks can identify laboratories or facilities with resources and expertise in diagnosing or treating specific diseases. Clinical or environmental samples can be sent to specialized laboratories for additional testing, and teams can be mobilized to assist local health care workers in dealing with an outbreak or unknown disease. Increasingly, technology that is shared or transferred allows local laboratories to extend capacity by sharing reagents or organizing workshops to train local laboratory workers. Despite availability of scientific information, a major hurdle is lack of resources in many parts of Africa and developing countries in Asia and Latin America, which manifests in lack of training, inadequate equipment, and absence of suitable reagents and testing kits.

Thanks to global communication networks, panels or organizations such as WHO have played a role in defining, naming, and characterizing some infectious diseases. However, social perception, response, and attributed cause may vary widely from one country or population to another. Uniform diagnostic criteria and laboratory approaches have been defined for many diseases to facilitate communication and scientific exchange across countries. This may lead to homogenization and consistency of approaches, treatment options, and interventions, and perhaps greater efficiency. A remaining question is whether a uniformly applied intervention is more vulnerable to failure. Would application of more diverse interventions offer greater resiliency to a system, for example, slowing the development rate of resistance in instances where antimicrobials or pesticides are part of the intervention?

Sharing knowledge of infectious disease outbreaks with international audiences has had perverse economic outcomes in many instances because of the profound impact on travel and trade. Examples include plague in India (34), and cholera in parts of South America. Some infectious diseases evoke fear and anxiety that is out of proportion to real risk (e.g., plague, cholera, Ebola) (35). Ebola has caused global concern, but no scientific data suggest a serious risk of global spread of the virus (unless used for bioterrorism).

Shared technology has led to enormous benefits and some disasters. The availability of widely disseminated injection devices has resulted in the spread of bloodborne infections — such as hepatitis B, hepatitis C, and HIV — to large numbers of people in areas where there are resources to buy some needles, but not to adequately sterilize them or discard them after one use (36, 37). A prominent example is the spread of hepatitis C in Egypt during a program in place from 1961 through the 1980s that used injectable medications to treat schistosomiasis (38). Each year an estimated 12 billion injections are administered. It has been further estimated, based on models of available epidemiological data, that each year unsafe injections result globally in 8 to 16 million infections with hepatitis B, 2.3 to 4.7 million infections with hepatitis C, and 80,000 to 160,000 infections with HIV.

Nosocomial infections occur wherever medical care is delivered, but appear at especially high rates in developing countries where barrier protections (such as gloves, gowns, and masks), good ventilation, sterilization of medical equipment, and isolation facilities are lacking. Nosocomial spread has been an important amplifier in local outbreaks of Ebola in Africa. Multiple drug resistant (MDR) tuberculosis has spread in hospitals in many areas (as well as in prisons and other congregate settings).

Transfusion technology has been adopted widely and saves lives. Transfusions have also been a source of infections in areas without adequate testing of donors and donated blood for bloodborne pathogens, such as HIV, hepatitis C, hepatitis B, and syphilis. Regionally specific infectious diseases may also be spread by transfusions, in some instances in a time frame and place far removed from acquisition. Cases of *Trypanosoma cruzi* (American trypanosomiasis) and malaria related to transfusions have been reported in nonendemic areas. In some locales, donors of blood or blood products have become infected with HIV because of improper use of equipment. Many bloodborne infections have a long latency and can be transmitted to sexual contacts or household members. Technology adopted without sufficient resources or infrastructure (or without adaptation to local conditions) may become a source for transmission of infections.

Knowledge of a disease in another geographic location changes local practice. For example, the reach of malaria extends far beyond endemic areas. Because people visit and migrate from malarious areas, clinicians everywhere must be aware of malaria and have clinical training and knowledge of preventive strategies, diagnosis, and treatment. The economic consequences of the disease extend beyond the malarious areas.

Nations now are sharing the technology for making vaccines and drugs. However, because serotypes, serogroups, or strains of a particular microbe (e.g., HIV, *Streptococcus pneumoniae*, among others) may vary by geographic region, a vaccine that works in one population may not perform optimally in another. Economics also plays a role. A country with the greatest resources to develop a vaccine may have no incentive to produce one that will be effective against strains in developing countries, where the need may be great but the market is limited due to economic constraints.

QUESTION 2: WHAT IS THE CULTURAL BACKDROP AGAINST WHICH THESE PROCESSES OCCUR?

Key factors include population size, urbanization, low latitude location of large population centers, demographic shifts, environmental degradation, scarcities, and inequities (39).

The world population reached six billion by late 1999. The population is growing faster in developing than in industrialized countries. Six countries — India, China, Pakistan, Nigeria, Bangladesh, and Indonesia —

account for half the global growth of 77 million persons annually (40). Most of the population growth in the coming decades is projected to be in developing countries.

More people live in urban areas than ever in history, and urbanization is projected to continue to increase. Currently about half of the world's population lives in urban areas; the global urban population is expected to reach five billion by 2030. Urban populations are growing at four times the rate of rural populations. Migrants account for about 40% of growth in urban areas. In Latin America about 75% of the population lives in urban areas, in contrast to 37% in Asia and Africa in 2000. The most rapidly growing segment in the world is the urban population in developing countries.

The number of megacities, defined as urban areas with a population greater than 10 million, has increased from five cities in 1975 to 19 in 2000. The new megacities are mostly in low latitude areas and in developing countries (among them Lagos, Mumbai, Delhi, Dhaka, Karachi, Jakarta, Manila, Cairo). Tokyo, at 26.4 million, was the most populous urban area in 2000. Many of the rapidly growing urban areas are surrounded by periurban slums characterized by poor infrastructure, absence of clean water, inadequate waste disposal and sanitation, poor housing, and close contact between human and animal populations. Many migrants to these periurban slums have families in rural areas, and frequent contact with them offers the opportunity for passage of microbes to and from the city. Public health infrastructure and diagnostic capacity is often lacking in these settings. Many have limited access to medical care and routine immunizations. Infectious diseases may go untreated, allowing them to spread unrecognized.

If, on average, those living in urban areas have regular contact with a larger number and variety of people than those living in rural areas, then this situation has potential implications for the spread of infectious diseases that spread from person to person. Those living in urban areas are more likely to obtain food and water from shared sources (municipal water supplies, mass processed foods). When food or water is contaminated with microbes, it is more likely to affect a large number of people, rather than just a family or local community.

Factors that increase host vulnerability to infection — such as poor nutrition and micronutrient deficiencies — remain prominent in some developing areas. Ezzati et al. identified undernutrition as the single leading global cause of health loss. Globally 9.5% of the disease burden (as measured by DALYs) is attributed to childhood and maternal underweight, and 6.2% to deficiencies of iron, vitamin A, zinc, or iodine (41). Today's world population is also increasingly vulnerable to infections related to two other factors: AIDS and aging. The population is older than ever in history. In many countries the most rapidly growing age segment is those over 80 years. In Europe 15.5% of the population was 65 years and older in 2000. The percentage of those over 65 is expected to increase in all countries, including developing countries. The elderly are more susceptible to a number of infectious diseases, even in the absence of underlying diseases, and are also more likely to have cancers and other diseases that require treatment with immunosuppressive drugs, radiation, and other interventions that place them at increased risk for infectious diseases. An increased global population of elderly people is likely to translate into an overall greater burden from infectious diseases.

The presence of HIV increases risk for many infections, some of them easily transmitted from person to person, such as tuberculosis. Because of the difficulty in clearing infections, HIV-infected individuals may continue to shed organisms longer, such as *Cryptosporidia*, than someone with a normal immune system. Globally the interaction between HIV and tuberculosis is the most important synergy because each has an adverse impact on the other infection. Because TB is transmissible, the consequences extend to both HIV-infected and uninfected individuals.

QUESTION 3: WHAT ARE THE CHARACTERISTICS OF INFECTIONS THAT CAN SPREAD GLOBALLY?

It may be useful to define the characteristics of infections that are globalizable — meaning those that can spread widely in today's world. Which infections can be controlled by local interventions? Which ones cannot? Which infections require a global response to control? The following examples describe key characteristics of infections that have or could spread widely (Table 2). It is notable that the pathogens come from several different classes of organisms and have different means of transmission.

RESISTANCE AND ITS IMPACT ON CONTROL OF INFECTIONS

A phenomenon that may have a profound influence on the future burden of infectious diseases is the development of resistance, broadly defined (43, 44, 45). Resistance of pathogens (including viruses, bacteria, fungi, protozoa, and helminths) to antimicrobials that have been the mainstay of treatment is increasing. Resistance of arthropods to pesticides also limits options in the control of vector-borne infections. Multidrug resistance in major pathogens, such as *Mycobacterium tuberculosis* and *Streptococcus pneumoniae*, is spreading. Resistance has reduced therapeutic options and is influencing specific treatment recommendations for major human pathogens, including *Mycobacterium tuberculosis*, *Plasmodium* spp., *Streptococcus pneumoniae*, *Staphylococcus aureus*, and HIV (although globally most of those infected with HIV do not have access at present to treatment). In North America, where anti-HIV drugs are widely available, the proportion of newly acquired HIV infections that involve drug-resistant viruses is increasing (46, 47, 44). In general, drugs used to treat resistant

Table 2.   Key characteristics of infections that spread widely

HIV

Zoonotic origin; probable multiple introductions of related viruses into human population

Spread from person to person with no need for animal reservoir or vector

Long period without symptoms during which infection can spread

Spread by sexual activity, childbirth and breastfeeding, IV drug use, contaminated needles, blood and blood products

Interaction with many other infections, including tuberculosis, which is common in areas where HIV is common; contributes to faltering control efforts for other diseases

Stigma associated with infection means delay in diagnosis

Resistance to antiviral agents used to treat infection is already emerging

Infected individuals can be infected with a different strain of the virus

Meningococcus W135 (33, 42, 10)

Can be carried by humans without symptoms; spreads from person to person

Clonal spread (specific strains may be more virulent, more transmissible)

Spread facilitated by crowded living conditions

Other risk factors for disease include smoking, coincident respiratory infections

Vaccine may reduce but does not eliminate carriage

Vaccines used widely in the past protected against one or two serogroups, not including W135

Annual hajj (pilgrimage to Mecca) provides opportunity for mass gathering and subsequent dispersal of population from multiple countries (about two million people from about 140 different countries)

Selective pressures from vaccine? Meningococcal serogroup W135 has caused epidemic disease in populations who have received vaccines that did not protect against W135

Avian influenza, spread to humans

Direct transmission of avian H5N1 to humans in 1997 in Hong Kong

Virus had high pathogenicity in humans and poultry (in 1998–1999, direct transmission of avian H9N2 viruses to humans in Hong Kong and China was documented)

Unexpected crossing of species barrier contributed to delay in diagnosis and recognition (although avian influenza strain could infect humans, it did not spread efficiently from person to person)

Live bird markets; multiple avian species; contact with migratory birds

Proximity of large populations of humans and birds

Massive size of poultry farms; movement of live chickens

Dengue

Increasing population size and density, especially in low latitude areas

Expansion of areas infested with *Aedes aegypti*, other competent vectors

Storage of water in or near homes

Abundance of nonbiodegradable containers for breeding sites

Increasing air links of all urban areas with tropical areas

Growing populations with past infection with at least one dengue serotype

Increasing viral diversity (number of dengue lineages has increased roughly in parallel with the growing human population over the last two centuries)

Recombination events in humans and mosquito vector, also leading to viral diversity

Transovarial transmission of virus in mosquitoes

Although the spread of the dengue virus is restricted to tropical and subtropical areas because of the temperature requirements of its mosquito vector, the large size of the human population living in and visiting tropical and subtropical regions means that a large population is at risk (currently estimated at 40% of the world's population)

Hepatitis C

Many chronic infections cause no symptoms

Person-to-person spread especially via injections, transfusions

No animal reservoir or arthropod vector

Spread widely through parenteral drug use

Diagnostic test not available until relatively recently

Technology to test blood and blood products not commercially available in the U.S. until May 1990; still not used in parts of the world due to lack of resources

Widespread use of injections for vaccine delivery and treatment of many diseases (including schistosomiasis in Egypt); injection without adequate sterilization still widely practiced in developing countries

vCJD (variant Creutzfeldt-Jacob disease)

Lack of awareness that prions in cattle with BSE could cross species barrier to humans

Long latency

Potential to spread from human to human via tissue transplantation

Limited knowledge of extent of spread among animals via animal feed containing animal parts

West Nile Virus in Western Hemisphere

Delay in diagnosing initial cases because transmission of virus had never been previously reported in Western Hemisphere

Despite bird deaths, poor communication between those involved with animal and human health

Limited knowledge of behavior of virus in New World hosts; gaps in knowledge of competency of local vectors to transmit

Limited knowledge about migration habits of birds, especially if viremic

Wide host range, including migratory birds, which may be important in spread to new areas

Potential for transmission by several different kinds of mosquitoes infections are typically more expensive, may be less effective, and often are more toxic, causing more adverse effects. Resistance may make an infection operationally untreatable if alternative drugs are unavailable or too expensive for the patient or the community.

Clonal spread is important for many infections (48). Resistance can be dispersed, as noted earlier (49, 11); resistance that emerges locally may not remain localized. New molecular tools allow tracking of microbes across oceans and continents (50, 51). Many examples exist of the acquisition of multidrug resistant tuberculosis by an individual in one geographic location and its transmission in another. Resistance of the malaria parasite *Plasmodium falciparum* to chloroquine appears to have emerged from foci first detected in Colombia and at the Cambodia-Thailand border in the late 1950s. Resistant strains spread from those foci through South America, Southeast Asia, and India in the 1960s and 1970s (52). Recent study of malaria in five regions in South America suggests that mutations in *P. falciparum* leading to resistance to sulfadoxine-pyrimethamine (relatively inexpensive antifolate combination commonly used to treat malaria in regions where the parasite had become resistant to chloroquine) probably had a common origin. Results of haplotyping and microsatellite analysis of the parasite support the conclusion that multidrug resistant *P. falciparum* most likely emerged in the lower Amazon and then spread north-northwest across the continent (53).

With one major exception — HIV/AIDS — newly identified infectious diseases and newly characterized microbes have not had a big impact on global infectious disease mortality but have been notable for their large number and visibility. These microbes include Nipah virus, metapneumovirus, many newly recognized hantaviruses, prions causing variant Creutzfeldt-Jacob disease, West Nile virus in the Americas, the novel coronavirus causing SARS, and avian influenza viruses (in humans). It is worth noting that many of these viruses and prions have animal reservoirs and are zoonoses. Influenza virus in particular deserves continued close attention. An avian influenza strain unexpectedly spread to humans in Hong Kong, killing about a third of those with the identified infection, but the virus did not spread efficiently from person to person. Because of influenza's potential to undergo genetic drift and shift, and the huge reservoir of avian influenza genes that can lead to new variants of virus, the likelihood of another influenza pandemic remains high. Even in the absence of a new strain, the ongoing, year in–year out toll from influenza is substantial.

Conclusion

Today many factors converge to increase the risk of appearance and spread of infections, including those not previously recognized in humans. The large size and high density of many populations, especially in areas of extreme poverty, the linkages of diverse peoples through travel and trade, plus the capacity of microbes to mutate and undergo change through acquisition of new genetic material, create an unstable situation.

NOTE

[1]   Stephanie Ostrowski, Division of quarantine, CDC; verbal communication.

REFERENCES

1.   World Health Organization. *World health report 2002.* Available from: URL: http://www.who.int/whr/2002/whr2002_annex2.pdf, accessed on 2003 Mar 12.

2.   Williams BG, Gouws E, Boschi-Pinto C, Bryce J, Dye C. Estimates of world-wide distribution of child deaths from acute respiratory infections. *Lancet Infectious Diseases* 2002;2:25–32.

3.   Steinbrook R. Beyond Barcelona — the global response to HIV. *New England Journal of Medicine* 2002;347:553–4.

4.   Wilson ME. Travel and the emergence of infectious diseases. *Emerging Infectious Diseases* 1995;1:39–46.

5.   World Tourism Organization. World tourism in 2002. Available from: URL: www.world-tourism.org/, accessed on 2003 Mar 12.

6.   Berlinguer G. The interchange of disease and health between the old and new worlds. *American Journal of Public Health* 1992;82(10):1407–13.

7.   Bruce-Chwatt LJ. Movements of populations in relation to communicable disease in Africa. *East African Medical Journal* 1968;45(5):266–75.

8.   Crosby AW Jr. *The Columbian Exchange.* Westport (CT): Greenwood Press; 1989.

9.   Wilson ME. The traveler and emerging infections: sentinel, courier, transmitter. *Journal of Applied Microbiology.* In press 2003.

10. Wilder-Smith A, Barkham TMS, Earnest A, Paton NI. Acquisition of W135 meningococcal carriage in Hajj pilgrims and transmission to house contacts: prospective study. *British Medical Journal* 2002;325:365–6.

11. O'Brien TF. Emergence, spread, and environmental effect of antimicrobial resistance: how use of an antimicrobial anywhere can increase resistance to any antimicrobial anywhere else. *Clinical Infectious Diseases* 2000;34(Suppl 3):S78–84.

12. Okeke IN, Edelman R. Dissemination of antibiotic-resistant bacteria across geographic borders. *Clinical Infectious Diseases* 2001;33:364–9.

13. Editorial. Tougher policies on refugees. *The New York Times.* 2002 Feb. 19.

14. Centers for Disease Control and Prevention. Outbreaks of gastroenteritis associated with noroviruses on cruise ships – United States, 2002. *Morbidity and Mortality Weekly Report* 2002;51(49):1112–5.

15. Carlton JT, Geller JB. Ecological roulette: The global transport of non-indigenous marine organisms. *Science* 1993;261:78–82.

16. Murphy FA. The threat posed by the global emergence of livestock, food-borne, and zoonotic pathogens. In: Frazier TW, Richardson DC, editors. *Food and Agricultural Security*. New York: Annals of the New York Academy of Sciences 1999;894:20–7.

17. Fields G. For U.S. customs, trade and security clash on the dock. War on terror has inspectors examining more ships, delaying more deliveries. *Wall Street Journal*, 2002 Sept. 12. p. 1–2.

18. Rappole JH, Derrickson SR, Hubalek Z. Migratory birds and spread of West Nile virus in the Western Hemisphere. *Emerging Infectious Diseases* 2000;6(4):319–28.

19. Ludwig GV, Calle PP, Mangiafico JA, Raphael BL, Danner DK, Hile JA, et al. An outbreak of West Nile virus in a New York City captive wildlife population. *American Journal of Tropical Medicine and Hygiene* 2002;67:67–75.

20. Daszak PA, Cunningham AA, Hyatt AD. Emerging infectious diseases of wildlife — threats to biodiversity and human health. *Science* 2000;287:443–9.

21. Bram RA, George JE, Reichard RE, Tabachnick WJ. Threat of foreign arthropod-borne pathogens to livestock in the United States. *Journal of Medical Entomology* 2002;39:405–16.

22. Lounibos LP. Invasions by insect vectors of human diseases. *Annual Review of Entomology* 2002;47:233–66.

23. Moore CG, Mitchell CJ. *Aedes albopictus* in the United States: ten-year presence and public health implications. *Emerging Infectious Diseases* 1997;3:329-34.

24. Daborn PJ, Yen JL, Bogwitz MR, Goff GL, Feil E, Jeffers S, et al. A single P450 allele associated with insecticide resistance in *Drosophila*. *Science* 2002;297:2253–6.

25. Denholm I, Devine GJ, Williamson MS. Insecticide resistance on the move. *Science* 2002;297:2222–3.

26. Bandyopadhyay R, Frederiksen RA. Contemporary global movement of emerging plant diseases. In: Frazier TW, Richardson DC, editors. *Food and agricultural security*. New York Academy of Sciences; 1999:892:28–36.

27. Centers for Epidemiology and Animal Health. The potential for international travelers to transmit foreign animal diseases to US livestock or poultry. USDA:APHIS:VS;1998; revised 2001.

28. Nisbett RA, Monath TP. Viral traffic, transnational companies and logging in Liberia, West Africa. *Global Change & Human Health* 2001;2(1):18–9.

29. Peeters M, Courgnaud V, Abela B, et al. Risk to human health from a plethora of simian immunodeficiency viruses in primate bushmeat. *Emerging Infectious Diseases* 2002;8:451–7.

30. Hahn BH, Shaw GM, De Cock KM, Sharp PM. AIDS as a zoonosis: scientific and public health implications. *Science* 2000;287:607–14.

31. Sharp PM, Bailles E, Chaudhuri RR, Rodenburg CM, Santiago MO, Hahn BH. The origins of AIDS viruses; where and when? *Philosophical Transactions of the Royal Society of London Series B* 2001;356:867–76.

32. Freedman DO, Kozarsky PE, Weld LH, Cetron M. GeoSentinel: the global emerging infections sentinel network of the International Society of Travel Medicine. *Journal of Travel Medicine* 1999;6:94–8.

33. Aguilera J-F, Perrocheau A, Meffre C, Hahne S, W135 Working Group. Outbreak of serogroup W135 meningococcal disease after the Hajj pilgrimage, Europe, 2000. *Emerging Infectious Diseases* 2002;8(8):761–7.

34. Cash RA, Narasimhan V. Impediments to global surveillance of infectious diseases: consequences of open reporting in a global economy. *Bulletin of the World Health Organization* 2000;78:1358–67.

35. Wilson ME. The power of plague. *Epidemiology* 1995;6:458–60.

36. Drucker E, Alcabes PG, Marx PA. The injection century: massive unsterile injections and the emergence of human pathogens. *The Lancet* 2001; 358:1989–92.

37. Simonsen L, Kane A, Lloyd J, et al. Unsafe injections in the developing world and transmission of blood borne pathogens: a review. *Bulletin of the World Health Organization* 1999;77:789–800.

38. Frank C, Mohamed MK, Strickland GT, et al. The role of parenteral antischistosomal therapy in the spread of hepatitis C virus in Egypt. *The Lancet* 2000;355(March 11):887–91.

39. Wilson ME. Infectious diseases: an ecological perspective. *British Medical Journal* 1995;311:1681–4.

40. United Nations Population Division. World population prospects: The 2000 revision. ESA/P/WP.165.2001. New York: United Nations; 2001.

41. Ezzati M, Lopez AD, Rodgers A, et al. Selected major risk factors and global and regional burden of diseases. *The Lancet* 2002;360:1347–60.

42. Shlush LI, Behar DM, Zelazny A, Keller N, Lupski JR, Beaudet AL, et al. Molecular epidemiological analysis of the changing nature of a meningococcal outbreak following a vaccination campaign. *Journal of Clinical Microbiology* 2002;40:3565–71.

43. Trape JF. The public health impact of chloroquine resistance in Africa. *American Journal of Tropical Medicine and Hygiene* 2001; 64(1, 2) Suppl:12–7.

44. Trachenberg JE, Sande MA. Emerging resistance to nonnucleoside reverse transcriptase inhibitors: a warning and a challenge. *Journal of the American Medical Association* 2002;288:239–41.

45. World Health Organization. Anti-tuberculosis drug resistance in the world. Report No. 2: Prevalence and Trends. The WHO/IUATLD Global Project on Anti-tuberculosis Drug Resistance Surveillance. Available from: URL: http://www.who.int/gtb/publications/dritw/index.htm, accessed on 2003 Mar 12.

46. Grant RM, et al. Time trends in primary HIV-1 drug resistance among recently infected persons. *Journal of the American Medical Association* 2002;288:181–7.

47. Little SJ, et al. Antiretroviral-drug resistance among patients recently infected with HIV. *New England Journal of Medicine* 2002;347:385–94.

48. Dufour P, Gillet Y, Bes M, Lina G, Vandenesch F, Floret D, et al. Community-acquired methicillin-resistant *Staphylococccus aureus* infections in France. Emergence of a single clone that produces Panton-Valentine leukocidin. *Clinical Infectious Diseases* 2002;35:819–24.

49. Manges A, Johnson J, Foxman B, et al. Widespread distribution of urinary tract infections caused by a multi-drug resistant *E. coli* clonal group. *New England Journal of Medicine* 2002;345:1055–7.

50. Oliveira DC, Tomasz A, de Lancastre H. The secrets of success of a human pathogen: molecular evolution of pandemic clones of methicillin-resistant *Staphylococcal aureus*. *Lancet Infectious Diseases* 2002;2:180–9.

51. Sa-Leao R, Tomasz A, Santos Sanches I, Brito-Avo A, Vilhelmsson SE, Kristinsson KG, et al. Carriage of internationally-spread epidemic clones of *Streptococcus pneumoniae* with unusual drug resistance patterns in children attending day care centers in Lisbon, Portugal. *Journal of Infectious Diseases* 2000;182:1153–60.

52. Wellems TE, Plowe CV. Chloroquine-resistant malaria. *Journal of Infectious Diseases* 2002;184:770–6.

53. Cortese JF, Caraballo A, Contreras CD, Plowe CV. Origin and dissemination of *Plasmodium falciparum* drug-resistance mutations in South America. *Journal of Infectious Diseases* 2002;186:999–1006.

CHAPTER 7

Evolving Infectious Disease Threats to National and Global Security[1]

David L. Heymann

Introduction

The deliberate use of anthrax to incite terror, which quickly followed the events of September 11, 2001 in the U.S., changed the profile of the infectious disease threat in a dramatic and definitive way. Prior to these events, the emergence of new diseases — and, most especially, the devastation caused by AIDS — had sharpened concern about the infectious disease threat as a disruptive and destabilizing force, and given it space in national security debates. The reality of bioterrorism immediately raised the infectious disease threat to the level of a high-priority security imperative worthy of attention in defense and intelligence circles. In so doing, it also focused attention on several features of the infectious disease situation that make outbreaks — whatever their cause — an especially ominous threat. As smallpox again became a disease of greatest concern, both politicians and the public began to comprehend problems long familiar to public health professionals. These have ranged from silent incubation periods that allow pathogens to cross borders undetected and undeterred, through the finite nature of vaccine manufacturing capacity, to the simple fact that outbreaks have a potential for international spread that transcends the defenses of any single country.

Perhaps most important, this heightened concern has clearly identified a central principle of global public health security: strengthened capacity to detect and contain naturally caused outbreaks is the only rational way to defend the world against the threat of a bioterrorist attack. If, for example, the world's public health community can respond to the needs that will arise when the next major shift in the influenza virus occurs — pandemic planning, addressing insufficient vaccine supplies, the need for antivirals to treat infected cases, and the surge capacity in health facilities to manage a major influx of patients — these accomplishments will show the way forward for better preparedness for bioterrorism.

This principle has evolved in response to three concurrent trends. First, the highly publicized resurgence of the infectious disease threat illustrated the vulnerability of all nations to outbreaks and epidemics, often of new or unusual diseases. Second, the impact of AIDS on sub-Saharan Africa demonstrated the capacity of an emerging disease to destabilize a large geographical region in ways that undermine the very infrastructures needed for governance. Third, a reconsideration of the determinants of national security broadened the perception of what constitutes a security threat in the post-Cold War era, making space to accommodate infectious diseases — at least in their most internationally disruptive forms. Each of these trends is discussed in detail.

THE RESURGENCE OF THE INFECTIOUS DISEASE THREAT

During the past 30 years, the infectious disease threat has diverged considerably from previous patterns of epidemiology, drug susceptibility, geographical distribution, and severity (1). Such divergence arises from the naturally volatile behavior of the microbial world, amplified by recent ecological and demographic trends. Continual evolution is the survival mechanism of the microbial world. Infectious disease agents readily and rapidly multiply, mutate, adapt to new hosts and environments, and evolve to resist drugs. This natural propensity to change has been greatly augmented by the pressures of a crowded, closely interconnected, and highly mobile world, which has given infectious agents unprecedented opportunities to exploit (2).

The result has been an equally unprecedented emergence of new diseases, a resurgence of older diseases, and a spread of resistance to a growing number of mainstay antimicrobials (3). Vulnerability to these threats is now seen to be universal. As adversaries, microbial pathogens have particular advantages in terms of invisibility, mobility, adaptability, and silent incubation periods that render national borders meaningless. Infectious agents, incubating in symptomless air travelers, can move between any two cities in the world within 36 hours and slip undetected past any border. They can also be transported over long distances by migratory birds. Disease vectors, concealed in cargoes or riding in the cabins or luggage holds of airplanes, can likewise enter new territories undetected and become endemic. Such theoretical vulnerability has been amply demonstrated in practice.

New diseases, which are poorly understood, difficult to treat, and often highly lethal, are emerging at the unprecedented rate of one per year (4). Ebola hemorrhagic fever in Africa, Hantavirus pulmonary syndrome in the U.S., Nipah virus encephalitis in Southeast Asia, and the SARS virus in southern China, are just a few examples. Older diseases have reemerged in dramatic ways. Cholera, now in its seventh pandemic, returned to Latin American in 1991 after an absence of almost a century. Within a year, 400,000 cases and 4,000 deaths were reported from 11 countries in the Americas (5). Yellow fever is poised to cause massive urban epidemics in sub-Saharan Africa and Latin America. An urban outbreak in Côte d'Ivoire in 2001 necessitated the emergency immunization of 2.9 million persons in less than 2 weeks, depleting the international reserve of vaccine stocks (6). Urban yellow fever promptly returned in 2002 in outbreaks in Senegal that again caused frantic efforts to secure sufficient emergency vaccine supplies (7). The 1998 epidemics of dengue and dengue hemorrhagic fever were unprecedented in geographical occurrence and numbers of cases, and the epidemics of 2002 have continued this alarming trend (8, 6). A new strain of epidemic meningitis, W135, emerged in 2002, defying emergency preparedness in the form of stockpiled vaccines against conventional strains (9, 6). New and more severe strains of common foodborne pathogens, including *Escherichia coli* O157:H7, *Campylobacter*, and *Listeria monocytogens*, have made the profile of foodborne diseases distinctly more sinister (10, 11, 12). The invariably fatal variant Creutzfeldt-Jakob disease, first recognized in 1996 and probably transmitted to humans through beef, has added considerably to this concern (13). Year by year, the highly unstable influenza virus is a reminder of the ever-present threat of another lethal influenza pandemic (14).

Disease vectors are equally resilient and adaptable. Some anopheline mosquito species that transmit malaria have developed resistance to virtually all major classes of insecticides. Others, such as the tsetse fly that transmits African sleeping sickness, have returned to areas where they had previously been well controlled. The *Aedes aegypti* mosquito that transmits both yellow fever and dengue, originally confined to tropical jungles, has adapted to breed in urban litter. The diseases carried by vectors have likewise spread to new continents or returned to former homes. Rift Valley fever is now firmly established on the Arabian peninsula. West Nile virus, first introduced on the East coast of the US in 1999, has now been detected in 43 states across the U.S. and in five provinces of Canada as well (15, 16, 17).

The threat posed by drug resistance is particularly ominous and universal. Health care in all countries is now compromised by the shrinking number of effective first-line antimicrobials and the need to resort to more costly, and often more hazardous, alternative drugs, when available. Fueled by coinfection with HIV, the return of tuberculosis as a global menace has been accompanied by the emergence of multidrug-resistant forms costing up to 100 times more to treat (6). Malaria may soon be resistant worldwide to all currently available first-line drugs (6). Drug resistance to common bacterial infections is now so pervasive that it raises the specter of a post-antibiotic era in which many life-saving treatments and routine surgical procedures could become too risky to perform (18).

These developments have eroded past confidence that high standards of living and access to powerful medicines could insulate domestic populations from infectious disease threats abroad. They have also restored the historical significance of infectious diseases as a disruptive force — this time cast in a modern setting characterized by close interdependence of nations and instantaneous communications (19). Within affected countries, the disruptive potential of outbreaks and epidemics is expressed in ways ranging from public panic and population displacement to the interruption of routine functions that occurs when containment requires the emergency immunization of populations numbering in the millions. Disruption can also be measured in economic terms. Outbreaks are always expensive to contain. Affected countries can experience heavy additional burdens in the form of lost trade and tourism — estimated at U.S. $2 billion during the 1994 outbreak of plague in India, and currently being estimated for the outbreaks of SARS and the resulting decreases in global travel and business (20). At the global level, some of the most telling efforts to measure economic consequences, in terms of international relations and foreign affairs, have centered on determining what the AIDS epidemic in sub-Saharan Africa means for the economies of wealthy nations. At one extreme, the high mortality caused by this disease and the particular age group it affects has been interpreted as the cost to industrialized countries of lost export markets (21). At the other extreme, the economic costs of AIDS to the international community have been expressed in terms of the price of drugs and services needed to rescue a continent (22). The human suffering caused by this disease defies calculation in any terms.

AIDS: A CLEAR THREAT TO NATIONAL SECURITY

Of all diseases, AIDS provides the most dramatic and disturbing example of the capacity of a previously unknown pathogen to rapidly spread throughout the world, establish endemicity, and cause social and economic upheaval on a scale that threatens to destabilize a large geographical area. Although the disease has a global distribution, its impact is overwhelmingly concentrated in sub-Saharan Africa, where approximately 3.5 million new infections occurred in 2001. This brings the total number of people living with HIV/AIDS in sub-Saharan Africa to 28.5 million, accounting for 71% of the global total. In sub-Saharan Africa, an estimated 9% of all inhabitants between the ages of 15 and 49 carry the virus. In one country, HIV prevalence among pregnant women in urban areas now stands at 44.9%. The region as a whole is home to an estimated 11 million AIDS orphans (23).

Prior to the events of September and October 2001, AIDS already provided a strong case for considering infectious diseases as a security issue. At the most obvious level, any agent with such high rates of mortality — whether infectious or otherwise — that directly threatens to kill a significant proportion of a state's population constitutes a direct threat to state security (24). In this respect, few would argue against the proposition that

AIDS is a direct security threat to countries in sub-Saharan Africa. Recent analyses by experts in international security and foreign affairs have defined the nature of this threat in more explicit terms (25, 26, 27). In Africa, AIDS poses an immediate threat to the organization of many different societies as well as to the security of political institutions, the capacity of military operations, and the performance of the police force (27). Evidence from several sources indicates that AIDS has already begun to diminish the operational efficiency of many of Africa's armed forces while also escalating the social costs of ongoing wars to new levels (26). Other immediate effects on state capacity include the loss of high-level government officials, an overwhelming of the health care system, and an erosion of traditional systems of social support (27). Studies of the long-term security impact predict a significant decline in the economic performance of many countries due to absenteeism, the loss of skilled workers, reduced foreign investment, increasing government expenditure on health care, higher insurance costs, and a paucity of teachers to train the next generation of workers (28, 27). More, not less, state failure and insecurity is projected, and this is expected to translate into new forms of transnational security threats (28).

CHANGING PERCEPTIONS OF SECURITY

Efforts to understand the security implications of AIDS have taken place within the context of a reconsideration of what constitutes a security threat in the post-Cold War era. In its traditional meaning, 'security' has long been a strictly national pursuit aimed at defending territorial integrity and ensuring state survival. It is intrinsically self-centered, focused on shielding state citizens from external danger in an international system ruled by anarchy (29). Traditional approaches to the defense of national security are military functions: protecting borders, fighting wars, and deterring aggressors (30, 31).

Two events have challenged these traditional views. First, the end of the Cold War meant an end to security issues polarized by the ideological conflict and geopolitical interests of the superpowers, and kept on edge by the nuclear arms race. As old threats subsided, more attention focused on threats arising from civil unrest, internal conflicts, mass migration of refugees, and localized wars between neighboring countries, particularly when these had the capacity to undermine state stability or contribute to state failure (32, 33, 34, 24). The absence of a bipolar power system magnified these threats considerably, as intervention to prop up a failing state of geopolitical strategic interest was no longer assured (35, 36, 37). As a result, security issues became broader and more complex, and attention began to focus on ensuring the internal stability of states by addressing the root causes of unrest, conflict, and mass population movement rather than defending national borders against external aggressors (38).

In the wake of these changes, a number of factors — from environmental conditions to income, education, and health — were put forward as determinants of internal state stability and therefore of potential relevance to the evolving security debate (27).

In a second event, the forces of globalization demonstrated the porous nature of national borders and eroded traditional notions of state sovereignty. In a closely interconnected and interdependent world, the repercussions of adverse events abroad easily cross borders to intrude on state affairs in ways that cannot be averted through traditional military defenses (30). For example, in the world's tightly interrelated financial system, a crisis in a distant economy can rapidly spread to affect others (39). Many other transnational threats — whether arising from environmental pollution or tobacco advertising — were recognized as having an effect on internal affairs that went beyond the control of strictly national actions. Emerging and epidemic-prone diseases qualified as a transnational threat for obvious reasons: they easily cross borders in ways that defy traditional defenses and cannot be deterred by any state acting alone (30). In the broadened debate, their disruptive potential gave them added weight as a possible security concern, although this potential differs considerably between industrialized and developing countries (33, 40).

In industrialized countries, global pandemics such as influenza, where supplies of vaccines and antivirals are clearly insufficient, have the capacity to destabilize populations, and the panic that they incite could cause great social disruption. In developing countries, where economies are fragile and infrastructures weak, outbreaks and epidemics are far more directly disruptive. In these countries, the destabilizing effect of high-mortality endemic diseases, including malaria and tuberculosis as well as AIDS, is amplified by emerging and epidemic-prone diseases, as they disrupt routine control programs and health services, often for extended periods, due to the extraordinary resources and logistics required for their control (3). For example, outbreaks of epidemic meningitis, which regularly occur in the African 'meningitis belt,' disrupt normal social functions and bring routine health services to the brink of a standstill as containment depends on the emergency vaccination of all populations at risk (6). During the recent SARS outbreak in China, programs for childhood immunization, AIDS, and tuberculosis were halted for months as all staff and resources were diverted to SARS control. The resurgence of African sleeping sickness, which is also a disease of livestock, has disrupted productive patterns of land use and jeopardized food security in remote rural areas (6). Recent outbreaks of dengue in Latin America required the assistance of military forces, sometimes from neighboring countries, for their containment. Outbreaks of new or unusual diseases can cause public panic to a degree that calls into question government's capacity to protect its population. For example, management of the SARS outbreak jeopardized political careers in several countries. In addition, the dramatic interruption of trade, travel, and tourism that can follow news of an outbreak places a further economic burden on impoverished countries with little capacity to absorb such shocks (3).

HIGH PRIORITY ON THE SECURITY AGENDA?

Several recent events suggest that emerging and epidemic-prone diseases are being taken seriously as a threat to national and global security. In an unprecedented step, a U.S. government-supported study concluded in 1995 that emerging and reemerging infectious diseases, especially AIDS, constituted a national security threat and foreign policy challenge (41). In 1996, the U.S. Department of Defense established the Global Emerging Infections Surveillance and Response System, based on a network of domestic and overseas military laboratories, as an explicit acknowledgment that emerging diseases can threaten military personnel and their families, reduce medical readiness, and present a risk to U.S. national security (42). The threat posed by microbial agents to the security of the U.S. was further acknowledged in 2000 by an equally unprecedented report from the U.S. Central Intelligence Agency's National Intelligence Council (40). Citing the 'staggering' and 'destabilizing' number of deaths caused by AIDS in sub-Saharan Africa, the report documented specific consequences in the form of diminished gross domestic product, reduced life expectancy, weakened military capacity, social fragmentation, and political destabilization. The report also addressed the growing threat posed by infectious diseases in general, and drew attention to the contributing roles of rapid urban growth, environmental degradation, and cross-border population movements (40). A further acknowledgment that microbial 'foes' could threaten international peace and security came in 2000 when the UN Security Council, in its first consideration of a health issue, concluded that the AIDS pandemic had moved beyond a health crisis to become a threat to global security, the viability of states, and economic development (43).

Although the creation in January 2002 of the Global Fund to Fight AIDS, Tuberculosis, and Malaria gives cause for hope, the magnitude of the response falls far short of what is needed to rescue Africa and other areas from a humanitarian crisis of historic proportions (22, 44). In many ways Africa has become increasingly marginalized as a player in global economics and politics, with the possible exception of South Africa (25). At the same time, the reality of the industrialized country response to Africa's AIDS crisis brings into question the extent to which AIDS and other emerging diseases — even if formally acknowledged to be a security threat — rank as an absolute priority in national security agendas.

The events of September and October 2001 changed this situation dramatically, as the prospect of bioterrorism brought infectious disease agents into direct intersection with national security imperatives. It has also brought into sharp focus many of the difficult problems faced by public health on a daily basis. For example, the anthrax incident demonstrated the difficulty of quickly identifying an unfamiliar disease. This difficulty arises with almost all outbreaks, particularly in the developing world, that do not follow a predictable geographical or seasonal pattern. It also arises with the thousands of cases of imported malaria and other tropical diseases that occur each year in temperate countries having large international airports, which are frequently misdiagnosed. It also occurred following the unexpected arrival of West Nile virus in the Western hemisphere, where the disease was initially misdiagnosed as St. Louis encephalitis and a full three weeks lapsed before the causative agent was correctly identified. The rapid determination of whether a disease might be deliberately caused is likewise notoriously difficult. Plague in India, dengue in Cuba, Hantavirus in New Mexico, and West Nile virus in New York are just some examples of diseases initially considered to have a deliberate origin in the recent past.

Also in connection with the anthrax incident, the question of whether a country experiencing a public health emergency has the right to override the patent of a vital drug, such as ciprofloxacin hydrochloride, has been vigorously debated, primarily within the context of the AIDS humanitarian crisis, since shortly after the Agreement on Trade-Related Aspects of International Property Rights was signed in 1994. Concerning the particular problems posed by the sudden demand for smallpox vaccine, the difficulty of quickly building an adequate vaccine reserve as preventive defense is experienced on a daily basis in efforts to contain outbreaks of epidemic meningitis and urban yellow fever, where the finite nature of vaccine manufacturing capacity frequently jeopardizes emergency containment operations (6). In the case of yellow fever, the situation is a particularly disturbing example of the impact of poverty. Because of the expense, few high-risk countries practice routine childhood immunization against yellow fever, although this option is ten times more cost-effective and prevents more cases and deaths than emergency immunization campaigns (6). Vaccine shortages have also, on occasion, threatened the effectiveness of National Immunization Days during the end stage of the drive to eradicate poliomyelitis. Nor is smallpox the only severe infectious disease for which no effective treatment exists. Dengue, yellow fever, Japanese encephalitis, rabies, and the Ebola, Marburg, and Crimean-Congo hemorrhagic fevers are just some of the diseases of major public health importance that lack effective treatments. In this sense, some of the terror incited by the prospect of a bioterrorist attack in industrialized countries is a constant feature of life in the many developing countries prone to outbreaks of these diseases.

As a final example, the question of how the world can best defend itself against the threat of a bioterrorist attack has also been addressed in a series of practical actions that date back to at least 1997 (45). On September 5, 2001, the U.S. Senate Committee on Foreign Relations, at a hearing on 'The threat of bioterrorism and the spread of infectious diseases,' heard testimony explaining how systems set up to detect and contain naturally caused outbreaks provide global defense against the threat posed by bioterrorism (46).

'DUAL USE' DEFENSE

Efforts to prevent the international spread of infectious diseases have a long history. In the 14th century, ships that were potential carriers of plague-infected rats were forcibly quarantined in the harbor of the city-state of Venice to prevent importation of plague (47). A series of international health agreements between the newly industrialized countries, elaborated during the 19th century, culminated in the adoption of the International Health Regulations in 1969 (48). The regulations are designed to maximize security against the international spread of infectious diseases while ensuring minimum impact on trade and travel. Administered by the World Health Organization (WHO), these are the only international regulations that require reporting of infectious diseases. At the same time, they provide norms and standards for airports and seaports designed to prevent the spread from public conveyances of rodents or insects that may be carrying infectious diseases, and describe best practices to be used to control the spread of these diseases once they have occurred.

The regulations are currently being revised to serve as an up-to-date framework for global surveillance and response in the 21st century. To support the revision process, the World Health Assembly has endorsed a series of resolutions aimed at ensuring a global surveillance and response system, operating in real time and under the framework of the International Health Regulations, that facilitates rapid disease detection and rational responses (49, 50, 51, 52). The WHO is also now authorized by the Health Assembly to utilize information sources other than official notifications submitted by governments (48).

The WHO has long argued that the most important defense against the infectious disease threat in all its forms is good intelligence and a rapid response. Intelligence is gleaned through highly sensitive global surveillance systems that keep the world alert to changes in the infectious disease situation. Routine surveillance systems for naturally occurring outbreaks enhance the capacity to detect and investigate those that may be deliberately caused, as the initial epidemiological and laboratory response techniques are the same. Adequate background data on the natural behavior of known pathogens provide the epidemiological intelligence needed to recognize an unusual event and to determine whether suspicions of a deliberate cause should be investigated (3, 53, 45). A global surveillance system, operating in real time, facilitates rapid and rational responses. It ensures that the necessary laboratory and epidemiological skills are kept sharp, since the call-out for natural outbreaks at the global level is almost daily. It provides a mechanism for sharing expertise, facilities, and staff. The performance of routine systems in detecting and containing naturally occurring outbreaks provides an indication of how well they would perform when coping with a deliberately caused outbreak, although the scale of a deliberately caused outbreak would probably be much larger. Strong public health systems are vital, as public health plays the initial and leading role in the response to a deliberately caused outbreak (54).

The mechanisms for global surveillance and response are in place and operational, on a daily basis, in the Global Outbreak Alert and Response Network (3). Under development since 1997, this overarching network interlinks electronically, in real time, 110 existing laboratory and disease reporting networks. Together, these networks possess much of the data, expertise, and skills needed to keep the international community constantly alert and ready to respond.

The network, which was formalized in April 2000, is supported by several new mechanisms and a customized artificial intelligence engine for real-time gathering of disease information. This tool, the Global Public Health Intelligence Network (GPHIN) (55), maintained by Health Canada, heightens vigilance by continuously and systematically crawling websites, news wires, local online newspapers, public health email services, and electronic discussion groups for rumors of outbreaks. In this way, the network is able to scan the world for informal news that gives cause for suspecting an unusual event. Apart from its comprehensive and systematic search capacity, the GPHIN has brought tremendous gains in time over traditional systems in which an alert is sounded only after case reports at the local level progressively filter to the national level and are then reported to the WHO. The network currently picks up — in real time — more than 40% of the outbreaks subsequently verified by the WHO. However, outbreaks of some diseases, including Ebola hemorrhagic fever, frequently occur in very remote rural areas that fall outside the reach of electronic communications, thus necessitating continued reliance on other sources, including reports from countries.

Additional sources of information linked together in the network include government and university centers, ministries of health, academic institutions, other United Nations agencies, networks of overseas military laboratories, and nongovernmental organizations having a strong presence in epidemic-prone countries. Information from all these sources is assessed and verified on a daily basis. 'Suspected accidental or deliberate release' is one of six criteria used to determine whether an outbreak is of international concern, and is routinely considered (3).

Once international assistance is needed, as agreed upon in confidential proactive consultation with the affected country and with experts in the network, electronic communications are used to coordinate prompt assistance. To this end, global databases of professionals with expertise in specific diseases or epidemiological techniques are maintained, together with nongovernmental organizations present in countries and in a position to reach remote areas. Such mechanisms, which are further supported by a network of specialized national laboratories and institutes located throughout the world, help make the maximum use of expertise and resources — assets that are traditionally scarce for public health. Surge capacity, insufficient vaccine supplies, and expensive drugs are issues that must be dealt with on a regular basis in order to keep the world ready to respond — issues similar to those needed for preparedness for bioterrorism. Chronic shortages of vaccines for epidemic meningitis and yellow fever are being addressed through international collaborative mechanisms, also involving manufacturers, that stockpile vaccine supplies and pre-position them in countries at greatest risk of epidemics. The highly unstable influenza virus is kept under close surveillance by a WHO network of 110 institutes and laboratories in 83 countries. The network determines the antigenic composition of each season's influenza vaccine and keeps close watch over conditions conducive to a pandemic.

From July 1998 to August 2001, the network verified 578 outbreaks in 132 countries, indicating the system's broad geographical coverage. The most frequently reported outbreaks were of cholera, meningitis, hemorrhagic fever, anthrax, and viral encephalitis. During this same period, the network launched effective international cooperative containment activities in many developing countries — Afghanistan, Bangladesh, Burkina Faso, Côte d'Ivoire, Egypt, Ethiopia, Kosovo, Sierra Leone, Sudan, Uganda, and Yemen, to name a few (3). Responding in February 2003 to reports of an unusual pneumonia in Vietnam, Hong Kong, and southeastern China, the WHO activated this network to provide an unprecedented collaborative epidemiological investigation of what proved to be the SARS virus.

The work of coordinating large-scale international assistance, which involves many agencies from many nations, is facilitated by operational protocols that set out standardized procedures for the alert and verification process, communications, coordination of the response, emergency evacuation, research, monitoring, ownership of data and samples, and relations with the media. By setting out a chain of command and bringing order to the containment response, such protocols help protect against the very real risk that samples of a lethal pathogen might be collected for later provision to a terrorist group.

A RATIONAL RESPONSE TO A SHARED THREAT

The source of the evolving infectious disease threat is a microscopic adversary that changes and adapts with great speed and has the advantages of surprise on its side. The possibility that biological agents might be deliberately used to cause harm is yet another divergence of the infectious disease threat. Its capacity to incite terror builds on the fears aroused by the resurgence of naturally caused outbreaks and epidemics. Its significance as a security threat is readily appreciated in light of the well-documented ability of naturally caused infectious diseases to invade, surprise, and disrupt. The issues that require attention and resources — vaccine production, stockpiling of antibiotics, and protective clothing — are vital.

The dramatic change in the profile of infectious diseases, which followed the deliberate use of anthrax, has focused high-level attention on features of the infectious disease situation that make all outbreaks especially ominous events, often with international as well as local repercussions. The challenge is to manage this new threat in ways that do not compromise the response to natural outbreaks and epidemics, but rather strengthen the public health infrastructure, locally and globally, for managing both threats. Increasing vaccine manufacturing capacity to counter the bioterrorism threat should also work in the long term to increase the supply of vaccines needed to control naturally occurring infectious diseases.

In the U.S., the initial response to the anthrax incident concentrated almost exclusively on the strengthening of domestic public health capacity, with very little attention given to the international dimensions of either the threat itself or the measures needed to ensure protection (54). More recent developments indicate a growing awareness of the inadequacy of a strictly national response. They also indicate a growing willingness to view improved global capacity to detect and contain naturally caused outbreaks as the most rational — and the most reliably protective — way to defend nations, individually and collectively, against the threat of a bioterrorist attack (56).

In November 2001, a meeting of G7 + Mexico health ministers culminated in agreement on the *Ottawa Plan for Improving Health Security* (57). The plan acknowledged bioterrorism as an international issue requiring international collaboration, and launched a series of collective efforts aimed at improving international preparedness and capacity to respond. Additional emergency preparedness and response plans and exercises have moved forward quickly. By the time of its third meeting, held in Mexico in December 2002, the concerns of the group had expanded to include plans for increasing the WHO emergency reserve of smallpox vaccine to manage cases of an outbreak occurring in any country lacking the resources to purchase and stockpile vaccine in advance. The meeting established a working group to address problems surrounding influenza and other epidemic-prone diseases, including insufficient vaccine supplies and preparedness planning for the management of massive numbers of patients. The meeting also launched a global collaborative network of high-security laboratories as a strategy for improving global capacity to rapidly and accurately diagnose diseases "whether naturally or intentionally occurring."

In another significant development, the proposed U.S. *Global Pathogen Surveillance Act 2002* acknowledged the universal nature of the infectious disease threat and frankly admitted that "domestic surveillance and monitoring, while absolutely essential, are not sufficient" to combat bioterrorism or ensure adequate domestic preparedness. The Act singled out the role played by the Global Outbreak Alert and Response Network, and further noted the inability of developing countries "to devote the necessary resources to build and maintain public health infrastructures," thus underscoring the need for foreign assistance. Finally, the Act treated natural and intentionally caused outbreaks as closely related threats and recognized that strengthened capacity to monitor, detect, and respond to infectious disease outbreaks would offer dual dividends in the form of better protection against both threats (58).

The acceptance of the infectious disease threat as a high-level security imperative has been sudden, ushered in by an equally sudden and previously unthinkable event. Within a year, the repercussions of the anthrax incident have led to an unprecedented appreciation of problems that have long hindered efforts to improve the detection and containment of naturally occurring outbreaks. Although public health has struggled — with little success — for decades to have these problems acknowledged, it can take some satisfaction from the fact that its experiences and advice are now guiding the way forward in a joint public health and security policy endeavor. Recent developments provide encouraging evidence that political leaders have a better understanding of the issues facing public health and — above all — appreciate both the need to strengthen public health infrastructures and the universal benefits of doing so. Equally important is the understanding that strong national and international public health must be considered as elements of national security, and that increased funding for strengthening national and international public health must come from government sectors that go beyond health to include national security, defense, and international development aid. Only then can the world begin to move toward a degree of security that sees the volatile infectious disease threat matched by a stable, alert, and universal system of defense. The lasting benefits for the daily work of outbreak detection and control could be enormous for both industrialized and developing countries.

Infectious diseases and human security

This chapter has largely focused on the threat to global health security posed by emerging and epidemic-prone diseases. It has also pointed out that other infectious diseases, such as AIDS, impose a constant and unacceptable burden on individuals and communities, and are a recognized impediment to the achievement of human health security. According to the latest WHO estimates, infectious diseases caused 14.7 million deaths in 2001, accounting for 26% of total global mortality. Most of these deaths could have been prevented through existing drugs and vaccines and simple access to food and drinking water free of fecal contamination (6).

Three diseases — AIDS, tuberculosis, and malaria — continue to account for a large share (39%) of deaths attributed to infectious diseases. Total deaths from these three diseases amounted to 5.6 million in 2001. When deaths from diarrheal disease and respiratory infections (5.8 million) are added, these five diseases alone are responsible for approximately 78% of the total infectious disease burden.

Perhaps the most powerful acknowledgment that these diseases compromise human security and impede development is inclusion of the control of HIV/AIDS, malaria, and other diseases as one of the eight time-bound and measurable Millennium Development Goals (59). These goals, along with the report in December 2001 of the Commission on Macroeconomics and Health, and the establishment in January 2002 of the Global Fund to Fight AIDS, Tuberculosis, and Malaria, give health a higher place on the global development agenda and underscore its fundamental importance to human health security (22, 60).

Other signs indicate the willingness of the international community to take unprecedented steps to combat infectious diseases, especially those that disproportionately affect poor populations in remote areas of the developing world — the so-called 'neglected diseases.' In just the past few years, partnerships, often involving open-ended donations of high-quality drugs and strongly supported on the ground by nongovernmental organizations, have formed to eliminate or control, by a specified date, seven severely disabling diseases of the poor: African sleeping sickness, Chagas disease, guinea worm disease, leprosy, lymphatic filariasis, onchocerciasis, and trachoma. Progress has been strong and results, especially when elimination or eradication targets are met, can be permanent. For lymphatic filariasis, which seriously disables an estimated 40 million people in 80 countries, the annual number of people treated has rapidly risen from 2.9 million (in 12 countries) in 2000, to 26 million (in 22 countries) in 2001, to 65 million (in 34 countries) in 2002.

Growing concern over the issue of global health security, the main focus of this paper, has resulted in heightened vigilance, better disease intelligence, and strengthened capacity to respond when outbreaks occur. Populations in all countries will benefit from this strengthening of basic public health functions. While this trend can be seen as anchored in the enlightened self-interest of nations, the commitment and energy now focused on other diseases that are endemic in the developing world and concentrated among the poor are good evidence that humanitarian concerns are likewise shaping the response to the infectious disease threat in all its dimensions.

NOTE

REFERENCES

1.   Lederberg J, Shope RE, Oaks SC Jr, editors. *Emerging infections: microbial threats to health in the United States.* Washington: National Academy Press; 1992.

2.   Rodier GR, Ryan MJ, Heymann DL. Global epidemiology of infectious diseases. In: Strickland GT, editor. *Hunter's tropical medicine and emerging infectious diseases.* 8th ed. Philadelphia: WB Saunders Company; 2000.

3.   Heymann DL, Rodier GR. Hot spots in a wired world. *Lancet Infectious Diseases* 2001;1:345–53.

4.   Woolhouse MEJ, Dye C, editors. Population biology of emerging and re-emerging pathogens. *Philosophical Transactions of the Royal Society for Biological Sciences* 2001;356:981–2.

5.   Tauxe RV, Mintz ED, Quick RE. Epidemic cholera in the New World: translating field epidemiology into new prevention strategies. *Emerging Infectious Diseases* 1995;1:141–6.

6.   World Health Organization. *Global defence against the infectious disease threat.* Geneva: World Health Organization; 2003.

7.   Weekly Epidemiological Record. Yellow fever, Senegal (update). *Weekly Epidemiological Record* 2002;77:373–4.

8.   World Health Organization. *Dengue prevention and control.* Report by the Secretariat; World Health Assembly Document A55/19. Geneva: World Health Organization; 2002.

9.   Weekly Epidemiological Record. Urgent call for action on meningitis in Africa: vaccine price and shortage are major obstacles. *Weekly Epidemiological Record* 2002;77:330–1.

10. Tauxe RV. Emerging foodborne diseases: an evolving public health challenge. *Emerging Infectious Diseases* 1997;3:425–34.

11. World Health Organization. *The increasing incidence of human campylobacteriosis.* Report and proceedings of a WHO consultation of experts; Document No. WHO/CDS/CSR/APH 2001.7. Geneva: World Health Organization; 2001.

12. World Health Organization. *Emerging foodborne diseases.* WHO Fact Sheet 124. Geneva: World Health Organization; 2002.

13. World Health Organization. *Understanding the BSE threat.* WHO Document No. WHO/CDS/CSR/EPH/2002.6. Geneva: World Health Organization; 2002.

14. Bonn D. Spared an influenza pandemic for another year? *The Lancet* 1997;349:36.

15. Gubler DJ. Human arbovirus infections worldwide. *Annals of the New York Academy of Sciences* 2001;951:13–24.

16. Molyneux DH. Vector-borne infections in the tropics and health policy issues in the twenty-first century. *Transactions of the Royal Society for Tropical Medicines and Hygiene* 2001;95:235–8.

17. Centers for Disease Control and Prevention. *West Nile virus update: current case count*; 2003. Available from: URL: http://www.cdc.gov/ncidod/dvbid/westnile/surv&controlCaseCount03.htm, accessed on 2003 Sep 16.

18. World Health Organization. *WHO global strategy for containment of antimicrobial resistance.* Document No. WHO/CDS/CSR/DRS/ 2001.2. Geneva: World Health Organization; 2001.

19. Heymann DL. The fall and rise of infectious diseases. *Georgetown Journal of International Affairs* 2001;11:7–14.

20. Cash RA, Narasimham V. Impediments to global surveillance of infectious diseases: consequences of open reporting in a global economy. *Bulletin of the World Health Organization* 2002;78:1353–67.

21. Kassalow JS. *Why health is important to U.S. foreign policy.* New York: Council on Foreign Relations and Milbank Memorial Fund; 2001.

22. World Health Organization. *Macroeconomics and health: investing in health for economic development.* Report of the Commission on Macroeconomics and Health by Sachs JD, chairman. Geneva: World Health Organization; 2001.

23. UNAIDS. *Report on the global HIV/AIDS epidemic.* Geneva: UNAIDS; 2002 Jul.

24. Price-Smith AT. *Pretoria's shadow: the HIV/AIDS pandemic and national security in South Africa.* CBACI Health and Security Series, Special Report 4. Washington: Chemical and Biological Arms Control Institute; 2002.

25. Eberstadt N. The future of AIDS: grim toll in India, China, and Russia. *Foreign Affairs* 2002;81:22–45.

26. Elbe S. HIV/AIDS and the changing landscape of war in Africa. *International Security* 2002;27:1150–77.

27. Ostergard RL Jr. Politics in the hot zone: AIDS and national security in Africa. *Third World Quarterly* 2002;23:333–50.

28. Morrison JS. The African pandemic hits Washington. *Washington Quarterly* 2001;24:197–209.

29. Burchill S. Realism and neo-realism. In: Burchill S, Linklater A, editors. *Theories of international relations.* London: Macmillan; 1996.

30. Center for Strategic and International Studies (CSIS). *Contagion and conflict: health as a global security challenge.* Report of the Chemical and Biological Arms Control Institute and the CSIS International Security Program. Washington: Center for Strategic and International Studies; 2000.

31. Ban J. *Health, security, and U.S. global leadership.* CBACI Health and Security Series, Special Report 2. Washington: Chemical and Biological Arms Control Institute; 2001.

32. Weiner M. Security, stability, and international migration. *International Security* 1992;17:91–126.

33. Kelley PW. Transnational contagion and global security. *Military Review* 2000;May–June:59–64.

34. Nichiporuk B. *The security dynamics of demographic factors.* Santa Monica (CA): RAND; 2000.

35. Tickner JA. Re-visioning security. In: Booth K, Smith S, editors. *International Relations Theory Today.* University Park (PA): Pennsylvania State University Press; 1995.

36. Cooper R. *The post-modern state and the world order.* Los Angeles: Demos; 1996.

37. Fidler DP. Public health and national security in the global age: infectious diseases, bioterrorism, and *Realpolitik. George Washington International Law Review*;27. In press 2003.

38. Holsti KJ. *The state, war, and the state of war.* Cambridge (UK): Cambridge University Press; 1996.

39. Homer-Dixon T. Now comes the real danger. *Toronto Globe and Mail* 2001 Sep 12.

40. National Intelligence Council. *The global infectious disease threat and its implications for the United States*; 2000. Available from: URL: http://www.cia.gov/nic/graphics/infectiousdiseases.pdf–17d.html", accessed on 2003 Sep 16.

41. CISET. *Infectious diseases: a global health threat.* U.S. National Science and Technology Council Committee on International Science, Engineering, and Technology (CISET) Working Group on Emerging and Re-emerging Infectious Diseases. Washington: CISET; 1995.

42. DoD-GEIS. U.S. Department of Defense Global Emerging Infections Surveillance and Response System; 2003. Available from: URL: http://www.geis.ha.osd.mil/aboutGEIS.asp, accessed on 2003 Sep 16.

43. UN Security Council. UN Security Council Resolution 1308(2000) on the responsibility of the Security Council in the maintenance of international peace and security: HIV/AIDS and international peacekeeping operations. Adopted by the Security Council at its 4172nd meeting; 2000 Jul 17. Available from: URL: http://www.reliefweb.int/w/rwb.nsf/0/d1261fd7ea89821c85256 b8000774bfb?OpenDocument, accessed on 2003 Sep 16.

44. Feachem RGA. AIDS hasn't peaked yet — and that's not the worst of it. *The Washington Post* 2003; Jan 12.

45. World Health Organization. *Preparedness for the deliberate use of biological agents: a rational approach to the unthinkable.* Document No. WHO/CDS/CSR/EPH/2002.16. Geneva: World Health Organization; 2002.

46. Heymann DL. *Strengthening global preparedness for defense against infectious disease threats.* Statement for the Committee on Foreign Relations hearing on the threat of bioterrorism and the spread of infectious diseases. Washington: United States Senate; 2001 Sep 5. Available from: URL: http://www.who.int/emc/pdfs/Senate_hearing.pdf, accessed on 2003 Sep 16.

47. Howard-Jones N. *The scientific background of the international sanitary conferences, 1851–1938.* Geneva: World Health Organization; 1975.

48. World Health Organization. *Global health security: epidemic alert and response.* World Health Assembly Resolution WHA54.14. Geneva: World Health Organization; 2001.

49. World Health Organization. *International health regulations (1969).* Geneva: World Health Organization; 1983.

50. World Health Organization. *Revision and updating of the international health regulations.* World Health Assembly Resolution WHA48.7. Geneva: World Health Organization; 1995.

51. World Health Organization. *Communicable disease prevention and control: new, emerging, and re-emerging infectious diseases.* World Health Assembly Resolution WHA48.13. Geneva: World Health Organization; 1995.

52. World Health Organization. *Revision of the international health regulations: progress report.* Report by the Director General; World Health Assembly Document A51/8. Geneva: World Health Organization; 1998.

53. World Health Organization. *Public health response to biological and chemical weapons.* Geneva: World Health Organization; 2001. Available from: URL: http://www.who.int/csr/delibepidemics/biochemguide/en/index.html, accessed on 2003 Sep 16.

54. Knobler SL, Mahmoud AAF, Pray LA, editors. *Biological threats and terrorism: assessing the science and response capabilities.* Washington: National Academy Press; 2002.

55. Health Canada. *How Canadian initiatives are changing the face of health care.* Ottawa: Health Canada; 2002. Available from: URL: http://www.hc-sc.gc.ca/ohih-bsi/pubs/succ/national_e.html, accessed on 2003 Sep 16.

56. Chyba CF. Toward biological security. *Foreign Affairs* 2002;81:122–36.

57. G7 Health Ministers. *Ottawa plan for improving health security.* Statement of G7 Health Ministers' Meeting; 2001 Nov 7; Ottawa, Ontario, Canada. Available from: URL: http://www.g7.utoronto.ca/g7/health/ottawa2001.html, accessed on 2003 Sep 16.

58. U.S. Senate. *Global pathogen surveillance act of 2003, S871* (introduced in Senate). Available from: URL: http://capwiz.com/vvaf/webreturn/?url=http://thomas.loc.gov/cgi-bin/query/z?c108:S.871:, accessed on 2003 Sep 16.

59. United Nations. *United Nations millennium development goals.* New York: United Nations; 2000. Available from: URL: http://www.un.org/ millenniumgoals/, accessed on 2003 Sep 16.

60. Global Fund to Fight AIDS, Tuberculosis and Malaria. Available from: URL: http://www.globalfundatm.org/, accessed on 2003 Sep 16.

CHAPTER 8

HIV/AIDS: THE SECURITY ISSUE OF A LIFETIME

ALEX DE WAAL

"We spend our years as a tale that is told. The days of our years are threescore years and ten."

— Psalm 90: 9–10

INTRODUCTION

The HIV/AIDS epidemic threatens something unprecedented in modern history: namely, a protracted reduction in adult longevity for a general population. In sub-Saharan Africa, adult lifetimes have been reduced by up to two decades. We do not know what this change will entail, beyond that it is a critical and pervasive threat to human security, like no other. It is virgin territory for demographers and social scientists, though parallels with the calamitous 14th century (1) and the sequence of disasters that overwhelmed the colonized world in the last years of the 19th century (2) are suggestive. Our models for social and economic development rest on unexamined assumptions — including a 'normal' adult lifespan and the expectation of a gradient of progress in human affairs — that need to be called into question by the advent of generalized HIV/AIDS epidemics. Moreover, our demographic and epidemiological models for the course of HIV/AIDS largely fail to take into account the systemic and structural threat posed by the collapse in adult longevity. We can say with certainty that a calamity of unparalleled proportions is unfolding, but our experience and expertise does not enable us to describe the dimensions of that calamity.

This chapter focuses on sub-Saharan Africa, where the HIV/AIDS epidemic has advanced furthest and fastest, but it has implications also for other parts of the world, which are at the threshold of potentially generalized epidemics (3, 4).

Approximately 30 million people in Africa are living with HIV and AIDS. There are between four and five million new infections every year, and currently between two and three million people die every year from AIDS and related causes. Yet less than 0.2% of Africans are currently on a prescribed course of anti-retroviral treatment. Even if one million people in Africa begin anti-retroviral treatment every year for the next five years, the number of people living with untreated HIV and AIDS in the continent will continue to rise. Moreover, the nature of the epidemic means that the worst is yet to come. The time lag between HIV infection and death from AIDS is estimated at about nine years in Africa (somewhat shorter than in Europe and North America). Given the recency of the HIV epidemic, notably in South Africa, the vast majority of AIDS mortality remains in the future. The level of deaths we are witnessing now reflects infections that occurred on average nine years ago; today's HIV prevalence indicates a substantially higher number of deaths nine years hence. Figure 1 illustrates the dual nature of the HIV/AIDS epidemic.

The direct impact of HIV — namely, the deaths of tens of millions of human beings from AIDS — is the greatest threat to human life in the coming century. We are only at the beginning of the global HIV/AIDS pandemic. To appreciate what this entails for human security, we must stretch our imaginations.

Figure I.   HIV and AIDS[1]

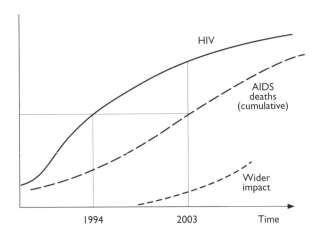

[1] Source: Adapted from Tony Barnett and Alan Whiteside, *AIDS in the 21st century: disease and globalisation;* London: Macmillan Palgrave; 2002.

Life expectancies

What is a lifetime? Let us begin by examining our statistical measures. We are accustomed to using measures of life expectancy at birth (LEB), which ranges from the upper thirties in Sierra Leone to well over eighty in Japan, as proxies for a key part of human well-being. But these figures require scrutiny. LEB figures are strongly influenced by infant and child mortality levels, and do not reflect the expected longevity of an older child or young adult. Adult deaths can be modeled by several measures, among them life expectancy on attaining adulthood (defined herein as age 20) and the chance of a 15-year-old dying before reaching age 60.

The following table matches countries with contrasting and similar LEBs. Japan has the world's highest life expectancy at 80 years, a level that is expected to increase by about 6.5 years by 2050 (5), and perhaps substantially more if gene therapy and other technologies are developed. Brazil and Bangladesh are included as a comparison for what South Africa might have expected in the absence of a generalized AIDS epidemic, and Sierra Leone is included as the country with the world's lowest LEB, absent a generalized AIDS epidemic. The figures for AIDS-impacted countries are in bold. Note that these figures are indicative only: HIV/AIDS brings added indeterminacy to Africa's already unreliable statistics. For example, current estimates for LEB in Botswana vary by up to 20 years.

Heavily AIDS-impacted countries have lost up to 15 years of LEB. This statistic actually underestimates the implications for adults: for a given level of LEB, AIDS-impacted countries have between five and 11 years *lower* adult life expectancy than countries without a generalized HIV/AIDS epidemic.

If we rank countries by child mortality rates, South Africa and Botswana are comparable to Bangladesh. If we rank by *adult* life expectancies, South Africa ranks just above Sierra Leone, while other AIDS-impacted countries are below it. According to the Zambian census data between 1980 and 2000, life expectancy at age 20 fell 11 years for men and 17 years for women. In 1990, the chance of a 15-year-old dying before reaching age 60 was 0.22 for South African women and 0.38 for men (male death rates were heightened by the violence of the time); demographers predict that by 2010 the figures will be 0.70 and 0.81, respectively (6). Three quarters of adolescents will not complete their 'normal' adult life spans. This statistic is significantly worse than Sierra Leone and Malawi today, and comparable to the historic crises in Asia in the late 19th century. Moreover, in contrast to historical crises, HIV/AIDS massively impairs a population's capacity for demographic recovery.

HIV/AIDS not only shortens lives, it reduces the quality of life. Dying of AIDS is peculiarly painful, traumatic, and expensive, for both the stricken individual and her or his family and caregivers. The psychological legacy

Table 1.   Life expectancy, related measures, and HIV prevalence for selected countries, 2000[1]

Country	Life expectancy at birth e0	Adult HIV rate 2002 (%)	Under 5 mortality 5q0	% of total deaths under 5 years	% of total deaths attributed to AIDS[2]	Adult life expectancy e20	Adult deaths 45q15 (women)	Adult deaths 45q15 (men)
Japan	80.2	<0.1	0.005	0.6	0.04	61.7	0.07	0.15
United States	76.7	0.6	0.008	1.4	0.61	57.7	0.13	0.21
Brazil	68.2	0.7	0.046	13	0.78	52.0	0.14	0.26
Bangladesh	60.6	<0.1	0.092	32	0.05	48.1	0.21	0.26
Mauritania	52.6	0.5	0.171	52	NA	45.1	0.39	0.46
South Africa	50.4	20.1	0.084	15	57	36.6	0.50	0.57
Chad	49.3	3.6	0.182	51	11	42.0	0.37	0.45
Botswana	44.5	38.8	0.084	16	99	29.8	0.67	0.70
Mali	43.7	1.7	0.226	49	4.4	38.8	0.45	0.52
Niger	43.3	3.3	0.254	65	NA	39.2	0.41	0.47
Zambia	39.4	21.5	0.164	32	53	28.6	0.69	0.72
Sierra Leone	37.9	7.0	0.278	53	10	35.6	0.53	0.59
Malawi	37.5	15.0	0.224	38	29	30.1	0.70	0.65

Legend:
e0 is life expectancy at birth (LEB)
5q0 is under 5 mortality
e20 is life expectancy at 20
45q15 is the probability of dying between ages 15 and 60

[1] WHO life tables, at www3.who.int/whosis/life/life_tables, accessed 2003 Mar 31; UNAIDS HIV prevalence figures for 2002, at www.unaids.org/hivaidsinfo/statistics, accessed 2003 Apr 18.
[2] AIDS deaths from UNAIDS, for 2001; total deaths from WHO life tables, for 2000. These data are derived by widely differing methods and have wide margins for error, as illustrated by the figure for Botswana.

Sources: WHO life tables; UNAIDS HIV prevalence figures for 2002.

inherited by millions of young Africans who have watched their parents die of AIDS is unknowable.

Losing our hold on the future

What is a lifetime? We are socialized into a subjective anticipation of longevity, which in turn determines our life choices. This is a complicated area, underresearched by social scientists. The biblical "threescore years and ten" is part of the cultural archive of the Judeo-Christian tradition. In the late Middle Ages, amidst massive waves of mortality that cut both adult and child life expectancy, 'normality' was still defined at the biblical level. "According to an anonymous poem of the mid-14th century, life's span was 72 years, consisting of twelve ages corresponding to the months of the year (7)." In Islam, only God knows the time of one's death, and so the idea of an untimely death is, strictly speaking, absurd. Nonetheless, modern Muslim societies have adopted the principle of a retirement age, usually sixty, which in turn implies a concept of a normal working life.[1]

For well over a century, life expectancies have been steadily rising in the industrialized world, so that most people can aspire to five decades of adult life (8). Until very recently, this was increasingly a statistical as well as a normative expectation in the rest of the world. Today, across sub-Saharan Africa, children are being socialized into a world filled with the premature deaths of adults. What does it mean to live in a society with a falling life expectancy? In countries with HIV prevalence above 30%, the lifetime probabilities of contracting HIV are in excess of 70%. What does it mean when the overwhelming majority of adults will not live to age 60? The minority that lives to retirement age can expect to outlast most of their peers and probably their children, too. Will they enjoy their old age?

A generalized HIV/AIDS epidemic is a societal shock that has unknowable consequences and profound implications for the worldview of the people in affected societies. Communities undergoing trauma have a tendency toward introversion and conservatism, clinging to the familiar and seeking ways to deny the reality of their trauma. In the case of HIV/AIDS, we witness a double denial: of the infection itself and of the reality of its impact. Too often, this denial begins with the political leadership, whose attempts to cling to the past and to normalcy serve as a role model for denial by their citizens.

Projecting likely trends into the future is a hazardous business, especially in the case of shocks like the HIV/AIDS pandemic. But it is precisely because the future will not resemble the past, and because the one thing we know for certain is that the HIV/AIDS epidemic is a long-wave event that is only now beginning to unfold, that it is imperative to go beyond existing data. We need to exercise our imaginations and examine the possible trajectories of social and economic processes, and the extent to which social and economic development rests upon hitherto unexamined assumptions about the length of an adult lifetime.

AIDS-RELATED POVERTY

Most current macroeconomic models for the impacts of HIV/AIDS estimate that an HIV prevalence rate of 10% will cut 0.4% off GDP growth (9, 10). There are reasons to believe that these models both underestimate and misrepresent the effects of the pandemic. The first reason is that the models assume that as the labor force size declines, the investment in both human and physical capital increases. This assumption is questionable.

A truncated lifespan will entail lower returns to investment in education and training (11) because of the reduced length of time that, on average, each individual will have to reap the benefits of time and money spent in education. We are already witnessing the phenomenon of companies in South Africa hiring two or even three skilled workers for every place they need to fill, in anticipation of AIDS mortality.

Another result of reduced longevity is lower savings rates. Expenditure on health care and treatment increases, while the incentive to save is reduced. Mortgage and life insurance companies increase their rates. Mobilizing domestic finance to meet the Millennium Development Goal of reducing poverty by half thus becomes more difficult to achieve. Investment in physical capital is also likely to be lower because of the global mobility of capital. The HIV/AIDS epidemic acts as a form of workforce employment tax, insofar as it reduces productivity through absenteeism, increases staff turnover, and increases benefits payments (12). In turn, transnational corporations have greater incentives to move their manufacturing operations to localities that are less impacted.

Given Africa's dire economic performance prior to the HIV/AIDS epidemic, the limited success of development strategies based upon the 'filling the finance gap' approach, and the continuing cascade of other insults to Africa's economies, the macroeconomic effects of the pandemic may not be separately discernible. Rather than an economic disaster in and of itself, the HIV/AIDS pandemic is primarily an intensification of existing difficulties, and an impediment to Africa's ability to find a path to recovery and development. More significant than the downturn is the erosion of the capability to withstand the shock of that downturn. Africans' ability to cope with extreme adversity and find creative solutions to the most dire circumstances has increasingly been recognized (13). This ability accounts for the flourishing of the informal economy, which in countries such as Somalia and the Congos has become the lifeline for the afflicted populace. Doubtless this resilience will find new wellsprings under the onslaught of HIV/AIDS and its attendant ills. However, we must not be too sanguine, given the way in which the epidemic undermines precisely those coping capacities.

Another way of envisioning the economic impact of HIV is to consider it an increase in the cost of staying alive. An individual living with HIV requires better nutrition to stay healthy (14); the burden of illness entails greater spending on medical treatment. Meanwhile, working adults need to support more dependents, including children orphaned by AIDS and chronically sick adults. There is controversy among demographers as to whether the HIV/AIDS epidemic will cause an overall shift in dependency ratios. It appears that the deaths of adults will be approximately matched by fewer children, due to lower fertility and higher child mortality (15). This finding is counterintuitive in light of the exceptionally high levels of adult mortality caused by AIDS. The paradox can be resolved by noting the change in the age and gender structure within the adult population. AIDS causes most losses among precisely those groups that contribute most to supporting dependents, namely women of all ages and men in their thirties and forties. The implication is that the absolute poverty level in a society relates to the specific nutritional, health care, and dependent support requirements of that society; in an AIDS-affected population, this level is higher than otherwise. The point at which an individual or family is considered to be in absolute poverty needs to be revised upwards.

Good data for accurately modeling the economic implications of HIV/AIDS are scarce. There is evidence, however, that one of the pandemic's effects is to increase inequality, through the failure of AIDS-affected households to recover and the intergenerational transmission of poverty (16). There is a curious but persistent discrepancy between a growing number of household-level studies of the impact of AIDS-related morbidity and mortality on poverty (17, 18, 19), and the relative insensitivity of aggregate indicators such as GDP and national food production to levels of HIV and AIDS.

The inequality effect of HIV/AIDS has not yet been studied in a rigorous quantitative manner. However, it is probable that the epidemic exacerbates inequalities, as affected households descend into poverty, while others that are less affected may even gain. The way in which AIDS clusters at the level of households (if one family member is infected with HIV, it is likely that her or his partner is infected as well, and there are high rates of mother-to-child transmission), combined with the sheer level of HIV prevalence in a generalized epidemic, means that the number of households on a downward economic trajectory will far exceed those that are climbing out of poverty.[2] Compared to other causes of poverty, with AIDS the way out is exceptionally difficult. As inequality increases, the headcount of the poor increases, too.

These are nonlinear effects, akin to a process of developmental regression that has been compared to "running Adam Smith in reverse" (20). In extreme circumstances, we may witness the long-term descent of societies into a situation characterized by chronic starvation among the poor, a state that I have described elsewhere as "new variant famine" (21). Such crises are not caused solely, or even principally, by HIV/AIDS: Africa is already subject to such extreme poverty and adverse global conditions, that the effect of the AIDS pandemic is to exacerbate existing economic difficulties and make them more intractable. There is no apparent reason to suppose that the global market, as it operates today, will necessarily provide Africa's poorest with a wage or livelihood sufficient to sustain life and health in the era of HIV/AIDS. The challenge is to ensure that globalization can deliver tangible benefits to the poorest, including those whose capabilities are severely constrained by HIV/AIDS.

PARALYSIS OF GOVERNANCE?

The creation and functioning of complex institutions depends upon long career trajectories. Institutions such as government ministries, large corporations, armies, and universities all depend upon the skills, experience, and networks built up by their senior staff over many years. Institutions that rely on short career paths — for example, student unions — have very different organizational models, with a flatter hierarchy and mobilization based more upon charismatic leadership than on bureaucratic process. As working lives shorten, it follows that levels of institutional complexity will shrink as well.

Variants of this phenomenon have been witnessed in a number of formal and less formal institutions. In parts of eastern and southern Africa, education and health systems have become semiparalyzed through the shortages of trained staff. These problems have been accentuated by the interconnectedness of the labor market. Thus, the private sector in South Africa hires teachers to replace skilled technicians lost to AIDS. The South African health service loses thousands of health professionals every year to industrialized countries. Doctors, nurses, and technicians leave partly because of better pay, partly because they become demoralized with the monumental demands of caring for patients with AIDS, and their incapacity to respond effectively. As a reaction, South Africa hires health workers from other African countries that have no options for replacing those who are lost.

In many countries, soldiers suffer substantially higher rates of HIV infection than the general population (22). Hard data are scarce, as are frank studies of the impact of HIV/AIDS on the effectiveness, discipline, and morale of armed forces. However, Africa's most thoughtful military commanders recognize the severe threat that HIV/AIDS poses to the integrity of armed forces (23). The impairment of military capacity has implications in turn for regional peace and security (24). Police forces and judiciaries face similar stresses, coincident with an impending increase in crime associated with the changing demographic composition of the population and possibly lower levels of schooling and socialization resulting from the growing numbers of children orphaned by AIDS (25).

These observations underlie the recognition by the U.S. National Intelligence Council and the U.N. Security Council that the HIV/AIDS pandemic represents a threat to global security (26, 27). When a country loses up to 30% of its workforce and witnesses its population's life expectancy cut by a third, a fundamental challenge arises to the legitimacy of those who preside over such a calamity. Society as a whole experiences a similarly destabilizing reversal. However, while we can speculate about the possible causal paths leading to a collapse of national security and even build plausible scenarios, there is thus far neither data nor models that could allow us to analyze with accuracy how these linkages may materialize (28). We have sufficient cause to be alarmed, but cannot yet specify exactly why.

The same phenomenon of institutional erosion afflicts political parties and civil society. There is anecdotal evidence about the decline in the quality of middle-ranking political leadership in several ruling parties in the continent. The voluntary sector is also seriously affected: small organizations risk collapse if they lose key individuals and feel pressure to shift the focus of their activities from community development and human rights toward the urgent demand of AIDS care (29).

Taken overall, the implications of shorted adult longevity on institutions and the structures of governance may be akin to "running Max Weber in reverse" (30). We should note, however, that there is already such a high level of institutional dysfunction in many parts of Africa that many of the effects will be masked by preexisting difficulties. There will be no single trajectory for how the impacts of the epidemic play out in severely affected countries. In some, we may see progress in economic development and the stalling of governance. In those already beset by crisis, decline may accelerate. Because HIV/AIDS acts as a systemic shock, interacting with other problems such as food insecurity and the outmigration of skilled labor, we may be unable to disentangle the many causative factors in a disaster. At the minimum, the impacts of the pandemic may be less the deterioration of existing systems than the incapacity to build better and more capable institutions in place of those that are currently failing. The HIV/AIDS pandemic is rendering the continent more vulnerable to reverses, and less resilient when those reverses occur.

A crisis of social reproduction?

Perhaps the most significant implication of the HIV/AIDS epidemic is the possibility of a crisis of social reproduction. It is widely noted that the greater burden of the epidemic falls upon women. Women are infected on average six to eight years younger than men, and fall sick and die at younger ages. In Malawi in 2000, the chance of a woman dying between the ages of 15 and 44 was 49% (31). This statistic is rising. Women also bear the multiple additional burdens of supporting children orphaned by

AIDS, caring for the sick, and maintaining households. Women's work is famously unmeasured in formal indexes of economic activity, and for this reason the potentially unendurable burden on Africa's women remains largely unrecognized among policymakers.

Two important secondary effects of the HIV/AIDS epidemic are the decreased fertility among women living with HIV and the imminent gender imbalance among adults due to the relatively greater and younger mortality of women. The implications of these effects are not yet understood.

The AIDS-related subsistence crisis is contributing to social fragmentation. As resources become scarce, there is a retraction of the ambit of social reciprocity — what anthropologists of disaster have called the 'accordion effect' (32). We see augurs of this in southern Africa. Reportedly, one of the reasons for the rapid increase in the planting of root crops such as cassava (the production of which doubled in the 1990s, reversing earlier trends towards growing more nutritious crops) is that it is a 'selfish crop.' A farmer who harvests maize is subjected to demands for a share from relatives; by keeping her cassava in the ground, she is freed from these demands.[3] The civil society sector, while often responding vigorously and even heroically to the challenges of HIV/AIDS, is itself weakening. The reciprocities that sustain social life are under strain. An escalating number of orphans is thrust upon the dwindling generosity of society. The crisis of social reproduction is seen most clearly in those children orphaned by AIDS that are not cared for by an extended family.

To this disturbing scenario we must add the certainty of secondary demographic insults. History teaches: "the most telling and most perverse characteristic of societies exposed to crises is that they experience them in a recurrent fashion" (33). One demographic insult predisposes to another, to the extent that students of India's population history have diagnosed the phenomenon of 'bang bang famines' (34). In the case of HIV/AIDS, we already know that there is an associated pandemic of tuberculosis and increased non-AIDS child mortality. The latter is probably associated with neglect of child care by women overburdened by the demands of sustaining a household stricken by AIDS, or ill themselves, as well as higher death rates among orphans. It is also likely that as girls are withdrawn from school to assist with domestic work and care for the sick, their lower educational achievement will contribute to higher child mortality in the succeeding generation (35).

In line with the 'new variant famine' hypothesis, we may also see new patterns of mortality associated with AIDS-related destitution and hunger. Malnourished adults living with HIV are likely to progress more rapidly toward AIDS morbidity and mortality. Already in 2002–2003, surveys in southern Africa revealed that a majority of people in AIDS-affected households regularly skips meals, to the extent of going without food for entire days (36). Therefore, AIDS cases may rise more sharply. Also, the impoverishment and social disruption caused by AIDS will cause migration to towns and the entry of many young men and women into the lowest stratum of urban society. People in this group, especially commercial sex workers, are at higher risk of HIV; thus, HIV incidence is likely to increase. Malnutrition may also contribute to an increase in mother-to-child transmission of HIV (37).

Meanwhile, a variant famine may increase tuberculosis, other infectious diseases, and malnutrition. Note, however, that the AIDS-affected households are likely to have few young children (due to lower fertility), so that in contrast to traditional famines, child malnutrition and mortality are unlikely to register as an early and sensitive indicator of crisis.

Figure 2 indicates the possible nature of vicious interactions between HIV/AIDS and its secondary effects. The scale of the increases in HIV incidence, AIDS deaths, and deaths from other causes is speculative. The key point is less the short-term scale of these increases than the negative nonlinearity, which may threaten a long-term failure to overcome the pandemic and associated demographic and socioeconomic difficulties. We are obliged to question current epidemiological models for the course of the HIV/AIDS pandemic. Although already grim, these models overlook the possibility of higher 'background' mortality associated with the pandemic's impacts, and the likelihood that these impacts will impede the prospects for reducing HIV transmission.

Unlike the economic and governance problems brought about or made worse by HIV/AIDS, the potential crisis of social reproduction is almost exclusively the product of the pandemic. It is truly a shock like no other (38), representing a reversal of recent progress in social development.

Figure 2. HIV, AIDS, and impacts: how they may interact

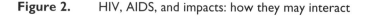

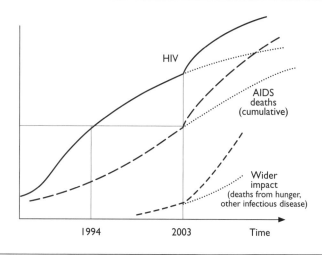

The motor of this change is the pressure on women's time. Africa's women struggle to care for and socialize the next generation. Their burdens are great, their time limited, and their lives shortened. Can social reproduction be secure when half of all adult women die before age 40? Unfortunately, over the coming decades, we are likely to observe the answer to this question.

CONCLUSION: A DISASTER WITH NO NAME

The above analysis indicates that the HIV/AIDS pandemic in sub-Saharan Africa threatens human security in many respects. The different elements of threat — demographic, economic, governance, and social reproductive — may interact in peculiarly dangerous and unforeseen ways. The coming disaster has no name and no place in today's social imagination. Is it an AIDS-related national crisis (ARNC) (39)? Such an ungainly acronym bespeaks the discourse of international institutions, remote from popular consciousness. Is it a new version of failed or collapsed states, which have figured in the political science literature of the last decade? Is it a 'low-level equilibrium trap'? Is it a crisis of social reproduction — a more precise but similarly arcane form of words? Is it new variant famine — a subsistence crisis that does not resemble a familiar drought famine? The virtue of using 'famine' is that the word has deep resonance in all cultures. The drawback is not that it is alarmist or an exaggeration; on the contrary, the most extreme word in our lexicon of disaster does not do justice to the novel enormity of what we may be about to encounter.

At the core of the threat that HIV/AIDS poses to human security is the question of ensuring lifetimes for all. Can economic development and sustainable livelihoods, the functioning of institutions and the maintenance of social structures, and the very fabric of social reproduction, be sustained with dramatically foreshortened adult longevity? At a time when children born in the richest industrialized countries can expect to live for 75 to 80 years and life spans are increasing, hundreds of millions of people in sub-Saharan Africa face lifetimes that are a fraction of that length, and much shorter than their parents' and grandparents'. It is an existential global inequality and as such, a denial of rights and a critical, pervasive, and long lasting threat to human security. Even in the unlikely event of a biomedical 'magic bullet,' the effects of the HIV/AIDS pandemic are with us for a generation at least. The challenge will not be overcome in the lifetime of most Africans alive today. But we can make a start.

NOTES

[1]   I am indebted to A.H. Abdelsalam for this point.

2 A methodological problem arises because of the tendency of AIDS-affected households to dissolve on the death of one or both adult heads, and thus disappear from a household survey-based data set.

3 I owe this observation to Tony Barnett.

REFERENCES

1. Tuchman B. *A distant mirror: the calamitous fourteenth century.* Harmondsworth: Penguin; 1978.

2. Davis M. *Late-Victorian holocausts: El Nino famines and the making of the Third World.* London: Verso; 2001.

3. U.S. National Intelligence Council. The next wave of HIV/AIDS: Nigeria, Ethiopia, Russia, India, and China. Intelligence Community Assessment 2002–04-D. 2002 Sep; Washington.

4. Eberstadt N. The future of AIDS. *Foreign Affairs* 2002 Nov–Dec:22–42.

5. United Nations Population Division. *World population prospects: the 2002 revision: Highlights.* Department of Economic and Social Affairs; UN ESA/P/WP 180. New York: United Nations; 2003. p. 71.

6. Dorrington R, Bradshaw D, Budlender D. *HIV/AIDS profile in the provinces of South Africa: data for 2002.* Cape Town: Centre for Actuarial Research, University of Cape Town; 2002. p. 28.

7. Tuchman. p. 569.

8. Riley J. *Rising life expectancy: a global history.* Cambridge: Cambridge University Press; 2001.

9. World Bank. *Confronting AIDS: public priorities in a global epidemic.* Washington: World Bank; 1999. p. 32.

10. Bureau of Economic Research. The Macro-economic impact of HIV/AIDS in South Africa. Economic research note No. 10. Matieland, South Africa: University of Stellenbosch; 2001 Sep.

11. McPherson M, Hoover D, Snodgrass D. The impact on economic growth in Africa of rising costs and labor productivity losses associated with HIV/AIDS. Cambridge (MA): JFK School of Government, Harvard University; 2000 Aug.

12. Rosen S, Simon J. Shifting the burden of HIV/AIDS. Boston: Center for International Health, Boston University; 2002 Feb.

13. Davies S. *Adaptable livelihoods: coping with food insecurity in the Malian Sahel.* London: Macmillan Palgrave; 1995.

14. Semba RD, Tang AM. Micronutrients and the pathogenesis of human immunodeficiency virus infection. *British Journal of Nutrition* 1999;81:181–9.

15. Stanecki K, Heaton L. A descriptive analysis of dependency ratios and other demographic indicators in populations affected by HIV/AIDS. Paper presented as empirical evidence for the demographic and socioeconomic impact of AIDS meeting; 2003 Mar; Durban, South Africa.

16. Lehutso-Phooko M, Naidoo R. Income inequality prospects with HIV/AIDS — a social dimension. *Labour Markets and Social Frontiers* 2002;2:11–6.

17. Barnett and Whiteside. *AIDS in the 21st century: disease and globalisation.* London: Macmillan Palgrave; 2002.

18. Kwaramba P. The Socio–economic impact of HIV/AIDS on communal agricultural production systems in Zimbabwe. Working paper 19, Economic Advisory Project. Harare: Friedrich Ebert Stiftung; 1998.

19. Rugalema G. Coping or struggling? A journey into the impact of HIV/AIDS in southern Africa. *Review of African Political Economy* 2000;26(86):537–45.

20. McPherson M, Goldsmith A. Africa: on the move? *SAIS Review* 1998;28:153–67.

21. de Waal A, Whiteside A. "New variant famine": AIDS and food crisis in southern Africa. *The Lancet.* In press 2003 Sep.

22. Yeager R, Hendrix C, Kingma S. International military human immunodeficiency virus/acquired immunodeficiency syndrome policies and programs: strengths and limitations in current practice. *Military Medicine* 2000;165:87–92.

23. Gebre-Tinsae T. HIV/AIDS in the Ethiopian military: perceptions, strategies, and impacts. Paper for Center for Strategic and International Studies (CSIS). Washington: CSIS; 2002.

24. Heinecken L. HIV/AIDS, the military, and the impact on national and international security. *Society in Transition* 2001;32(1):120–47.

25. Schönteich M. AIDS and age: SA's crime time bomb. *AIDS Analysis Africa* 1999;10:2.

26. National Intelligence Council. The global infectious disease threat and its implications for the United States. Washington: U.S. National Intelligence Council; 2000 Jan.

27. UN Security Council. Resolution 1308 (2000), on the responsibility of the Security Council in the maintenance of international peace and security: HIV/AIDS and international peacekeeping operations. Adopted 2000 Jul 17.

28. Gebre-Tinsae T, de Waal A. HIV/AIDS and conflict in Africa. London: UK Department for International Development; 2003 Feb.

29. Manning R. Is HIV/AIDS a threat to local-level (grassroots) democracy? An exploration of the impact on civil society and local government in KwaZulu-Natal, South Africa. Natal (SA): Health Economics and AIDS Research Division, University of Natal; 2002.

30. de Waal A. How will HIV/AIDS transform African governance? *African Affairs* 2003;102(2003):1–24.

31. World Health Organization. WHO life tables, 2000. Geneva: World Health Organization; 2000.

32. Laughlin CD, Brady IA. Introduction: diaphasis and change in human populations. In: Laughlin CD, Brady IA, editors. *Extinction and survival in human populations.* New York: University of Columbia Press; 1978.

33. Palloni A. Comment: on the role of crises in historical perspective. *Population and Development Review* 1998;14:145–58. p. 148.

34. Dyson T. Famine in Berar, 1896–7 and 1899–1900: echoes and chain reactions. In: Dyson T, Gráda CÓ, editors. *Famine demography: perspectives from the past and present.* Oxford: Oxford University Press; 2002.

35. Whiteside A, Barnett T, George G, van Niekerk A. Through a glass darkly: data and uncertainty in the AIDS debate. *Developing World Bioethics* 2003;3(1): 49–76.

36. Southern African Development Community (SADC), Vulnerability Assessment Committee (VAC). Towards identifying impacts of HIV/AIDS on acute food insecurity in southern Africa and implications for responses in 2003–04. Harare, Zimbabwe: SADC VAC; 2003 Apr.

37. Semba RD, Miotti PG, Chipangwi JD, et al. Maternal vitamin A deficiency and mother-to-child transmission of HIV-1. *The Lancet* 1994;343:1593–7.

38. Baylies C. The impact of AIDS on rural households in Africa: a shock like any other? *Development and Change* 2002;33:611–32.

39. de Waal A. AIDS-related national crises. Justice Africa; AIDS and Governance Discussion Paper No. 1. London; 2001 Sep.

CHAPTER 9

AIDS: A Threat to Human Security

OLIVE SHISANA, NOMPUMELELO ZUNGU-DIRWAYI, AND
WILLIAM SHISANA

*"Today marks the first time, after more than 4,000 meetings
stretching back more than half a century, that the Security Council
will discuss a health issue as a security threat. We tend to think
of a threat to security in terms of war and peace. Yet no one can
doubt that the havoc wreaked and the toll exacted by HIV/AIDS
do threaten our security. The heart of the security agenda is protecting lives — and we now know that the number of people who
will die of AIDS in the first decade of the 21st century will rival
the number that died in all the wars in all the decades of the 20th
century. When 10 people in sub-Saharan Africa are infected every minute; when 11 million children have already become orphans, and many must be raised by other children; when a single
disease threatens everything from economic strength to peacekeeping — we clearly face a security threat of the greatest magnitude."*

— U.S. Vice President Al Gore, U.N. Security Council,
January 10, 2000

INTRODUCTION

The words of former Vice President Al Gore are an important acknowledgment of history because for the first time, the United Nations Security
Council considered that a health issue constituted a security threat. We
argue that AIDS like other epidemics such as bubonic plague, smallpox,
and influenza, has the potential to annihilate human populations, destroy
communities, and stifle economic growth, especially in heavily affected
countries. Thus, it constitutes a clear threat not only to national security
or the security of states, but more importantly to human security — the

security of individuals and communities. We discuss the cumulative impact of AIDS on social, economic, political, and military sectors and suggest specific policy options aimed at reducing this threat to human security.

HIV/AIDS: THE PROBLEM

Since the beginning of the AIDS epidemic more than 20 years ago, an estimated 60 million people have been afflicted; 20 million have died from AIDS, and 40 million were living with HIV/AIDS at the end of 2001 (1). In 2001, five million people became infected, including 3.5 million in sub-Saharan Africa, with a total population of about 28.5 million people living with HIV/AIDS. This means that sub-Saharan Africa accounted for 70% of the new HIV infections globally. An estimated 9% (compared with 1.2% globally) of sub-Saharan Africans aged 15 to 49 years were living with HIV/AIDS; 58% were women (2).

Most of the infections in this part of the world are transmitted heterosexually, although new information raises the possibility of inadequate medical care as a potential source of 20 to 40% of HIV infections (3). When we consider that people with HIV/AIDS live for an average of seven to 10 years after infection, or longer if they receive highly effective antiretroviral therapies, the probability of a single individual infecting many others is great. This possibility, coupled with the high level of human movement, gives HIV/AIDS the potential to become a global pandemic.

REGIONAL DIFFERENCES

Half of all the people in sub-Saharan Africa living with HIV/AIDS reside in the Southern Africa Development Community (SADC) (Fig. 1). This region remains badly affected, with HIV rates increasing among pregnant women in countries like Botswana, Zimbabwe, and Namibia. South Africa reports a drop in HIV prevalence rates among youth but a rise in the 20 to 34 age group (4). Zimbabwe, Swaziland, and Lesotho have adult prevalence rates of more than 30%. South Africa carries the largest burden of HIV/AIDS cases and is considered home to 12.5% (5 million out of 40 million) of all people living with HIV/AIDS in the world. East African countries have made and maintained gains against the epidemic. For example, in Uganda the HIV prevalence rate among pregnant women has dropped from 29.5% in 1992 to 11.25% in 2000. Challenges remain as new infections are reported to be rising at a high rate (5).

The rise in the rate of infections has also been observed in the Asia and Pacific region, in spite of its prevention programs (6). New evidence suggests that low national prevalence figures have hidden localized problems in the region. This is said to be true in South and Southeast Asia, which have the second largest number of people living with HIV/AIDS, after sub-Saharan Africa (6).

Eastern Europe and Central Asia are currently experiencing a rapid spread of the HIV/AIDS epidemic. In this region, Russia leads in the number of people being infected with HIV/AIDS (6). Unlike in sub-Saharan Africa, here injecting drug use spreads the epidemic. In Latin America and the Caribbean region, the epidemic 'is well established' and there is a danger that it will spread rapidly in the absence of effective response (6). This region has a few countries with a high prevalence rate, making it second after sub-Saharan Africa. Haiti (6%) and Bahamas (4%) are reported to be the worst affected.

The Middle East and North Africa region also shows a trend toward increasing HIV rates, although rates are still relatively low. Here the mode of infection is predominantly sexual intercourse, with outbreaks of HIV infections among injecting drug users. Western Europe has low rates of people living with the virus, but has also experienced an increase in the number of infections (6). Due to access to resources such as AIDS drugs, this region has reduced the impact of AIDS. Here transmission is mainly via injecting drug use; heterosexual transmission remains very low.

DETERMINANTS OF HIV/AIDS

The World Health Organization (WHO) maintains that: "HIV infection thrives on poverty and marginalization. The epidemic is sustained by social disruption; by historical inequalities of wealth, gender, and race; and by migrant labor practices. HIV/AIDS thrives in unstable conditions, such as armed conflict and social and economic crises (7)." The history of Africa,

Figure 1. Prevalence of HIV/AIDS by region at the end of 2001

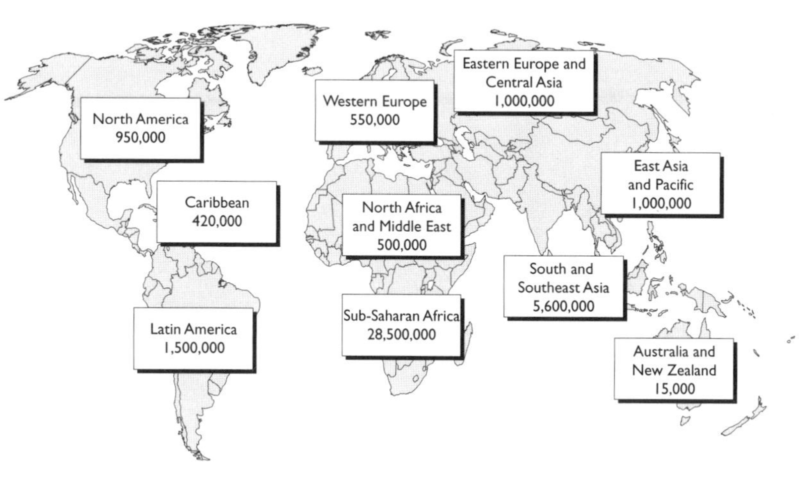

Source: UNAIDS; 2002.

and more so of southern Africa, adequately fits this description. No less than 28 of the 53 states have been involved in wars (8). War disrupts economies; diverts spending to military programs; increases violence against women, including rape; causes migration of soldiers, displacement of communities, and breakdown of social mores. It impedes the delivery of health services. War leads to preoccupation with human survival, making the HIV/AIDS messages irrelevant. Under these circumstances infections spread uncontrolled.

In Southern Africa, the migratory labor system that involved at least nine of the 14 countries in the SADC region created hospitable conditions for the spread of HIV. Many men left their families for 11 months out of a year to work in the mines of South Africa and Botswana. The majority of them lived in single-sex hostels. This isolation resulted in some of them engaging in risky sexual behavior, including interaction with sex workers. Some of the female partners left at home also engaged in sexual relationships with other men. When the migrant laborers returned home they infected or were infected by their partners, facilitating rampant spread of the disease.

Cross-national migration is not the only contributor to the spread of HIV. Economic development resulted in a need for physical infrastructure such as roads, dams, and airports. Men involved in the building of this infrastructure and the transporting of goods in the SADC region spent months away from home. Furthermore, for reasons of employment, many people moved from rural to urban areas, which contributed to the more rapid spread of the disease. Botswana and South Africa are examples of the latter. The rural areas carry a burden of AIDS because some of those incapacitated by the disease return from urban areas to their homes to die, thus depleting the limited resources in these areas.

In addition to economic migration, 11 of the 14 SADC countries were involved in wars that created refugees. In 1985, the United Nations High Commission for Refugees (UNHCR) recorded 11 million refugees worldwide. In 2001, Africa had the second largest number of refugees (6 million); the SADC region had a 7.8% increase in the number of refugees (9). This instability creates a favorable climate for the spread of communicable diseases.

Other factors that account for such high prevalence of HIV/AIDS in the SADC region include social, cultural, political, and behavioral determinants. Social and cultural factors mitigate against the use of barrier methods such as male and female condoms, leading to an increased risk of infection. Lack of financial and human resources for procuring preventive services lead to a spread of HIV, especially in the rural and poor communities. In addition, variable responses to prevention programs may account for different levels of infection rates. For example, countries like Botswana and Zimbabwe show an increase in condom use (Table 1). On the other hand, Haiti shows low levels of condom use (14%) and a high level of risky behavior (55%) in males. The figures for high-risk behavior in Zimbabwe are high although improving (42.5% for males). These figures suggest that prevention programs need to be strengthened to ensure healthy sexual practices and modified to fit local social norms. Given that knowledge is a necessary but insufficient condition for change in behavior, we need to incorporate a wide range of approaches.

Lastly, biological cofactors contribute to susceptibility to HIV infections. These include high rates of sexually transmitted infections, particularly ulcerative ones such as syphilis and herpes. People in the northern countries seem to be less susceptible than people in the tropico-equatorial areas whose immune systems are compromised by various infections (10). The high prevalence of HIV/AIDS in the SADC region suggests that the interaction of psychosocial, cultural, and economic factors with unsafe sex, coupled with biological susceptibility, puts people at even greater risk of HIV infection.

If we examine HIV/AIDS in the context of previous epidemics, we predict that its impact on some countries will be more devastating than on others.

UNDERSTANDING THE IMPACT OF AIDS ON HUMAN SECURITY

AIDS affects the security of states and the security of individuals to live in safe communities and meet their basic needs. This section explores the national and human security dimensions of AIDS. First, through a comparison with the great plague epidemic six centuries ago, we explore how AIDS affects demographics and thereby threatens the security of individuals and communities. We then consider the political dimensions of the AIDS epidemic and explore the link between the insecurity of people and the resulting insecurity of states as they struggle to respond. Finally, we examine the direct connection of AIDS to the military and national security. Taken together, these three perspectives provide a comprehensive view of AIDS' multifaceted impact on security.

EPIDEMICS, DEMOGRAPHIC SHIFTS, AND PEOPLE'S SECURITY

AIDS has changed the demographic, as well as the social and political landscape of every country it has touched. The former U.S. Surgeon General, David Satcher, stated: "While the modern epidemic affects people of all age groups, those of working age are at highest risk, posing potentially dire economic, social, and political consequences for the global community. Unfortunately, the world continues to devote greater attention and resources to traditional national security issues such as wars, postponing notice of an epidemic that, if left to spread unchecked, will kill more people than any of the terrible conflagrations that have so marked this century (11)." The Norwegian Minister of International Development, Hilde

Table I. Selected countries' behavior indicators

COUNTRY	Median age at first sex (20–24)			Reported high–risk sex for adults (15–49) in the last year (%)			Reported condom use (%)		
	Male	Female	Year	Male	Female	Year	Male	Female	Year
Botswana	–	17.4	1988	–	–	–	85.0	–	1996
South Africa	–	–	–	–	–	–	30.3	24.7	2002
Zimbabwe	19.5	18.9	1999	42.5	16.0	1999	70.2	42.0	1999
Uganda	19.4	16.7	2000	28.4	14.1	2000	58.9	37.8	2000
Japan	–	–	–	23.7	16.3	1996	–	–	–
Papua New Guinea	–	–	–	15.0	12.0	1994	38.0	12.0	1994
India	21.0	18.0	2001	11.8	2.0	2001	51.2	39.8	2001
Armenia	–	19.7	2000	18.9	0.6	2000	43.3	–	2000
France	17.9	18.4	1998	13.3	5.6	1990	64.7	50.2	1993
Portugal	17.4	19.8	1997	–	–	–	–	–	–
Sudan				3.0	1.0	1995	20.0	16.7	1995
Canada	–	17.8	mid–1990s	8.4	6.0	1997	72.3	71.9	1997
USA	–	17.2	mid–1990s	11.0	–	1997	65.0	–	1997
Haiti	–	18.2	2000	55.4	31.9	2000	25.5	14.4	2000
Mexico	–	20.7	1987	15.4	–	1997	62.8	–	1997
Peru	–	19.6	2000	13.6	1.5	1996	14.6	17.9	2000

Source: UNAIDS Global Report 2002; Nelson Mandela/HSRC Study of HIV/AIDS, 2002.

Johnson, echoed this statement by remarking, "According to some estimates, we are projected to have a hundred million HIV cases by 2005. If that happens, it will be the biggest epidemic since the Black Death (12)."

Epidemics such as bubonic plague have reversed human development and changed the structure of populations (13). HIV/AIDS threatens to reverse the development gains made over the last 30 years. We need only look at the Human Development Index (HDI) of countries affected by HIV over the last two decades to see that this reversal has already started (14). The HDI shows that in countries classified as having both middle to low human development and high rates of HIV/AIDS, there is a decline in human development. The two indicators of social and economic development — namely, child survival and adult life expectancy — have been halted or reversed.

In countries that are less developed and have high rates of HIV/AIDS, there has been an increase in the number of deaths among children under age five. In 2002, the child mortality rate in South Africa was 97 deaths per 1,000; without AIDS, this rate would have been 61 deaths per 1,000 (15). In Zimbabwe, half the child deaths are linked to AIDS. Life expectancy had been slowly rising until the emergence of AIDS in the mid-1980s, which caused a decline in life expectancy from 60 years and above to 40 years or less in many sub-Saharan countries (16). In Botswana for example, life expectancy dropped from almost 60 years before AIDS to 39 years currently, and is likely to drop further to 26.7 years by 2010 (16).

The premature death of economically active people has a negative impact on economic growth. The International Crisis Group, citing a World Bank study, showed that an adult AIDS "prevalence rate of 10% might reduce the growth of national income by up to a third. At infection levels of about 20%, studies show that a nation can expect a decline in GDP of 1% per year (17)." By killing millions of young, economically active people in a continent still trying to shake the legacy of colonialism and apartheid, AIDS threatens the economic development of Africa. It is likely to change the demographic structures of countries it heavily affects. Many diseases are fatal to infants and the elderly; AIDS targets society's young adults.

In developing countries, the population structure is generally described as a pyramid. Now AIDS has begun to introduce a completely new shape, the 'population chimney.' The implication is that large numbers of men die prematurely, and some young women die during their reproductive years, while others become infertile. For those who have babies, a third of these newborns become infected with HIV and hence die before adolescence and before they reproduce. The net result is that fewer babies are born, resulting in loss of population (18). Botswana is already experiencing a negative population growth as of 2002; its projection for 2010 is an example of a change in structure from a pyramid to a chimney (19). A country like South Africa that has the highest burden of HIV/AIDS is projected to have a population of 31 million in 2050, which is half what the population would have been without AIDS related mortality (19). According to the U.S. Census Bureau, countries like Lesotho, Mozambique, South Africa, and Swaziland in sub-Saharan Africa will experience a population decline by 2010, while in Malawi, Namibia, and Zimbabwe, the population growth is expected to halt.

POLITICS, POLITICAL ECONOMY, AND AIDS

The demographic changes highlighted above will have an impact on political structures. The heavily affected countries in the SADC region are likely to experience major political changes. HIV/AIDS threatens political stability in both developed and developing countries and also between multilateral organizations and private sectors. The governments' responses to HIV/AIDS are increasingly becoming a yardstick for the fitness of politicians to lead. At the July 2002 World AIDS conference, Dr. Piot of UNAIDS expressed this sentiment when he stated, "Let's bring forward the day when leaders who [don't] keep their promises on AIDS...lose their jobs to those who will (20)." Considering a few instances of what has happened to some political leaders, this threat should not be taken lightly.

Many leaders have been subjected to questions by the media and protest action by AIDS activists. President Mbeki was criticized on his overseas trips even when his visits were about different issues. He was perceived to deny the existence of the link between HIV and AIDS, and his government was seen as intransigent with respect to providing antiretroviral therapy. South Africa offers a good illustration of how HIV/AIDS can tear a country asunder and cause tensions between the people and the government (Sidebar 1).

Tommy Thompson, the U.S. Secretary for Health, is another leader who was targeted by activists at the recent Barcelona AIDS conference (2002). Activists drowned him out by shouting slogans and prevented the delivery of his address. He finally left the stage without the audience hearing his presentation (21). The main issue was that he represented G8 governments that have not made a significant contribution to the $10 billion needed annually for the Global Fund to Fight AIDS, Tuberculosis, and Malaria. Money is needed for the provision of antiretroviral therapies, among other things.

AIDS activists hounded former U.S. Vice President Al Gore during his presidential campaign because of his perceived support for the pharmaceutical companies that produce AIDS drugs. These companies were accused of making huge profits by pricing their drugs beyond the reach of the poor. When Gore announced his presidential candidacy in Carthage, Tennessee on 16 June 1999, protestors disrupted him. They alleged that he had "threatened severe international trade sanctions against South Africa if it allows production of generic drugs (22)." On 30 April, Gore had authorized a review of South African policies on compulsory licensing and set a 30 September deadline for South Africa to comply or suffer sanctions (23). Wherever he spoke, activists stalked him until he changed his position and became a strong supporter of AIDS programs. He later took the issue of AIDS to the U.N. Security Council.

AIDS has the potential to cause tensions between various sectors of society and between nations in a complex way. For example, in South Africa the issue of access to drugs pits activists and government against pharmaceutical companies on the one hand, and government against civil society on the other. In 1997, the South African government introduced a bill in parliament to amend its Medicines and Related Substance Use Act. The amendment made provision for doctors to substitute patented drugs with generic ones, and for parallel importation and compulsory licensing, so that South Africa could buy medicines from the least expensive source.

Advocacy and militancy are increasing due to the lack of access to drugs by the most affected regions. As Dr Gro Harlem Brundtland told the Executive Board of WHO, "The drugs are in the North and the disease is in the South (24)." This kind of inequity cannot continue. Indeed, the realization of inequity is galvanizing activists. The formation of the Pan-African HIV/AIDS Treatment Access Movement (PHATAM) illustrates the escalating tensions surrounding HIV/AIDS.

Seventy AIDS activists from 21 African countries met in Cape Town in August 2002 to form the PHATAM. The convenor, Mill Katana, articulated the rationale for the group when he stated that, "We know ARV [anti-retroviral] treatment is feasible in our countries and are launching a movement to demand ARV treatment and we won't take 'no' for an answer (25)." The impatience reflected in this statement was echoed by Dr. Eric Goemaere, Head of Mission for Médecins Sans Frontières (MSF) in South Africa, who said, "The time to scale-up is long overdue and this will only be possible with political action at the national and international level. This community-based movement must provoke the necessary political response (25)." Presumably, this statement targets those governments that have no political will to implement full-scale treatment programs and those that do not contribute financially to the Global Fund to Fight AIDS, Tuberculosis, and Malaria.

The militancy and frustration is not limited to activists but includes some professional associations. The South African Medical Association (SAMA), representing 70% of South African doctors, has taken a strong position regarding the provision of treatment for HIV/AIDS. Its President, Dr. Kgosi Letlape, declared that doctors could no longer be part of a system "that commits genocide (26)." To equate the South African government's approach to HIV/AIDS with genocide is a serious charge that reflects the potential for HIV/AIDS to unleash conflict between the government and the governed. The statement is also indicative of the internal conflict that health care professionals experience when national policies restrict them from doing what they were trained to do — namely, save lives.

HIV/AIDS AND THE MILITARY

It has been estimated that there are high rates of HIV infection among the armed forces in Africa. Statistics vary: the World Bank, UNAIDS, and the Economic Commission on Africa estimate HIV prevalence rates in the military of African nations at 10 to 50%. According to the International Crisis Group, in many African nations the rate of infection among military personnel is as much as five times that of the civilian population. Other figures suggest that the rates are as high as 80% in countries where the virus has been present for more than 10 years (27). Armed forces are made up of young, sexually active males who are at great risk of being infected with HIV. With many of them involved in peacekeeping missions, it is easy for them to spread the disease. Table 2 shows the different rates of infection for Southern Africa.

Estimates as high as 80% clearly have negative implications for the ability of armed forces to defend their countries and serve on peacekeeping missions. The possibility that countries will be unable to defend themselves due to HIV/AIDS is an important concern. As Fourie and Schönteich point out, "Armed forces form the basis of a country's defense and constitute the underpinning of stability both within states and between them.

Table 2.   Estimated HIV/AIDS infection by country. Prevalence within national armed forces and percentage Gross Domestic Product (GDP) for southern Africa.

Country	Size of population, 2001	HIV/AIDS %, 1999	Size of forces, 2001	HIV prevalence in armed forces (%) for year indicated	Defense budget as % of GDP
Angola	10,860,000	2.78	113,000	50 (1999)	16.5
Botswana	1,450,000	35.80	7,800	33 (1999)	5.2
DRC	50,340,000	6.43	31,100	50 (1999)	7.8
Lesotho	20,090,000	23.57	2,050	40 (1999)	4.2
Malawi	9,840,000	15.96	10,800	50 (1999)	1.8
Mozambique	16,700,000	13.22	6,100	Not available	4.1
Namibia	1,880,000	19.54	8,100	16 (1996)	4.4
South Africa	42,830,000	19.94	90,500	15–20 (2000)	1.3
Swaziland	970,000	25.25	3,000	48 (1997)	2.5
Zambia	10,240,000	19.95	21,500	60 (1998)	2.5
Zimbabwe	12,290,000	25.06	36,000	55 (1999)	6.1

Sources: UNAIDS and WHO, 1999; Du Plessis, 2001.

If they become debilitated by disease, national security is compromised (28)."

The countries that are most vulnerable in terms of HIV/AIDS are in the region that has been experiencing military conflict. Conflicts such as those in the Democratic Republic of Congo do not necessarily remain internal, but attract defense forces from other nations as different countries take sides. Unlike U.N. peacekeepers, the deployment of military personnel is at the discretion of countries or formations. These various forces do not have a uniform HIV/AIDS protocol to prevent the infected from being sent to the theater of conflict. Developed countries such as the USA have already indicated their reluctance to send their personnel on peacekeeping missions unless all countries involved adopt a uniform HIV/AIDS protocol (29). This concern is justified because in a situation of military conflict there is a higher probability of soldiers coming into contact with blood.

The risk of contracting HIV is not unidirectional. Beyond the risk of contracting HIV in the course of duties, military personnel may transmit or contract HIV through sexual contact with the locals involving lovers, sex workers, and most disturbing, rape. There are cases of women and girls being raped, sometimes gang-raped, in front of their families. Soldiers — in some cases, young child soldiers — have been forced to rape women as punishment (30). Rape is used as a weapon to humiliate and terrorize the community; when the perpetrator is HIV positive, this act becomes a lethal weapon capable of mass destruction. Due to dysfunctional health services associated with military conflicts, the survivors have no access to prophylactic treatment and other necessary care. Survivors live with great emotional fear, not knowing whether they are infected and if they are, facing the reality of a slow death without health care. Thus, the physically and psychologically debilitative effect of conflict and AIDS weakens communities, thereby reducing their productive capacities and ability to defend themselves.

The fight for access to AIDS drugs has not been limited to pharmaceutical companies only. Recently activists have begun targeting multinational conglomerates like Anglo and Coca-Cola to provide AIDS drugs to their employees living with HIV/AIDS.

GOVERNMENTS' RESPONSES AND LESSONS FROM AFRICA

There are encouraging cases of countries grappling with HIV/AIDS in a decisive manner. The first case of HIV/AIDS was discovered in 1982, and within 10 years Uganda had the highest HIV prevalence and incidence. The country put HIV/AIDS high on the agenda and took drastic measures to deal with it on a sustainable basis. The President of Uganda, Yoweri Museveni, mobilized the international community to support his country's effort to fight the epidemic. He dealt effectively with the stigma against the disease. The commitment paid off and the epidemic was turned around.

Sidebar 1.   An example of AIDS-related political tensions: The case of South Africa

In South Africa, the issue of HIV/AIDS has united people from a wide spectrum. People living with the disease and those affected are uniting across political parties and across religious, socioeconomic, and labor lines, bringing with them activists, scientists, and the media to exert pressure on the state to deal with HIV/AIDS effectively. The Treatment Action Campaign (TAC) has played an important role in setting the agenda and fighting for the rights of those infected and affected in South Africa.

The TAC, medical practitioners, and the Children's Rights Center tried in vain to influence the government to make accessible to ordinary HIV positive pregnant women the program to prevent transmission of HIV from mother to child (PMTCT). These groups resorted to intensifying their campaign and took the government to court (31). Eminent people such as former South African President, Nelson Mandela; former Anglican Bishop, Desmond Tutu; labor union officials of the Congress of South African Trade Unions; opposition party leaders such as the United Democratic Movement, Democratic Alliance, Inkatha Freedom Party, and the Secretary of the ANC Health Committee; and the former President of the Medical Research Council, to name a few, joined the call for PMTCT.

The state lost the case and appealed all the way to the Constitutional Court. Activists took to the street demonstrating against the continued refusal of the Ministers of Health to supply Nevirapine in health facilities where there was capacity to do so. The Constitutional court ordered the government to take steps to remove obstacles and make Nevirapine and voluntary counseling and testing available for PMTCT at public hospitals outside of the pilot sites.

This conflict takes on a much more serious dimension in the context of Mark Heywood's statement: "In a democracy such as South Africa's, the pressure of the electorate and our rights to freedom of expression are a vital duty that we must exercise to remind government of its priorities and duties. At times like these, we need organizations like the National Association of People Living with HIV/AIDS (NAPWA) to stand up and shout. Engage in civil disobedience: occupy government offices. Let the voices of poor and marginalized people whose decision-making powers the government has falsely appropriated under the rubric of poverty, be heard (32)." Moreover, during this conflict over the provision of Nevirapine, calls were made from different quarters for the removal of the Minister of Health from her position. This situation illustrates how tensions related to HIV/AIDS can be used to evaluate leaders' fitness for political positions.

Main points:

■ HIV/AIDS has the potential to cause conflict between government and civil society.

■ Civil organizations and society are setting the HIV/AIDS agenda.

■ HIV/AIDS can cause people to engage in civil disobedience against the government.

Uganda reduced HIV/AIDS prevalence from 8% in 1999 to 5% in 2000, making it the first country to register a fall in new HIV cases in Africa, giving hope to sub-Saharan Africa. Museveni demonstrated that with leadership commitment backed by action on the ground, it is possible to reverse the high rates of HIV within a reasonable period of time (33). However, there are concerns that this reduction may not be sustainable. The AIDS Information Center (AIC) has registered an increase in new HIV infections in Uganda and indicates prevalence at 22% (34). This means that a more concerted effort is needed.

Other examples of leadership commitment are found in Botswana and Senegal. Botswana President Festus Mogae acted decisively when he realized the potential of HIV/AIDS to annihilate his small country of 1.5 million people. He mobilized national and international resources in the form of experts, pharmaceutical companies, donors, and the public to support his plan to make drugs accessible to his people. His intervention was prudent, as the latest HIV/AIDS statistics show that 38% of the adult population in Botswana is living with HIV/AIDS. Senegal also shows that through commitment there is the potential to control the spread of HIV. Here, equally strong measures were put in place and consequently, this country has managed to keep the prevalence rate below 2%, and it is falling.

The hope offered by the countries above is no reason for complacency. The most important lesson we can take from Uganda is that it is possible to turn the epidemic around; however, prevention messages alone are not enough, because some people continue to be infected in the midst of wide public campaigns. For prevention to be a success, other methods are needed such as vaccines, which historically have been used to combat infectious diseases.

The development of a cost-effective and affordable vaccine is still underway in Africa. Lack of funding, poor infrastructure, lack of experienced research teams, sociocultural and political considerations are slowing progress. Moreover, vaccine development takes time. Uganda has been involved in vaccine development since the late 1980s. In 1991, a phase 1, randomized, placebo-controlled trial evaluating the safety of a vaccine was initiated (35). Other countries in Africa have followed suit, including Kenya and South Africa, which are undertaking HIV vaccine trials.

Reducing new HIV infection requires interventions beyond those discussed above. These include the PMTCT program that has shown success in Uganda in reducing vertical transmission of HIV from mother to child using ARVs. Many countries have replicated the PMTCT program; this bodes well for Africa. Educating the sexually active to either abstain or practice safer sex using barrier methods such as male and female condoms is also necessary. Other prevention methods that must be encouraged are: reduction of multiple concurrent as well as serial partners, treatment of sexually transmitted infections, and use of voluntary counseling and testing services.

The development of microbicides must be supported to empower women with a prevention method they can control.

Dealing effectively with HIV/AIDS requires that prevention programs be complemented by universal access to ARVs. Africa is showing progress in this area, too. Several southern African countries such as Zimbabwe, Mozambique, and Zambia are indicating their desire to make ARVs available to their people within their limited budgets (36, 37). Botswana already provides ARVs universally to its citizens. Ironically, pressure forced South Africa (Sidebar 1), a country that fought national and international battles to gain access to affordable medicines, to contemplate some movement in this direction. On April 17, 2002, the South African cabinet announced that ARV drugs could improve the quality of life of people living with HIV/AIDS "if administered at certain stages...in the progression of the condition, in accordance with international standards (38)."

There is hope for South Africa when taking the latter pronouncement in conjunction with President Mbeki's address to Parliament in February 2002. He said that the government was committed to "intensifying its comprehensive program against AIDS" and had "initiated discussions with some of [the pharmaceutical companies] to examine new ways of making drugs more affordable and to strengthen our health infrastructure (38)." However, the slow pace from pronouncement of intentions to implementation is a matter of concern. Already the TAC is increasing its campaign against the South African government to speed up the process of making drugs available.

CONCLUSION

In summary, we have presented information that supports the arguments that HIV/AIDS creates political tensions, reverses human development gains, affects the economy, and reduces the ability of the military to undertake its duties, including peace keeping operations. We have drawn from historical evidence to show that epidemics pose a danger to society. We have also demonstrated that some political leaders are aware of the impending disaster, and that efforts are being made to tackle the problem of HIV/AIDS. From this brief presentation, it is clear that AIDS is a threat to human security and may lead to the annihilation of some populations. It is therefore fitting that the United Nations Security Council consider HIV/AIDS a human security issue. We believe that AIDS must be included in the report of the Commission on Human Security.

In treating AIDS as a threat to human security, we need to take the following steps.

Implementation of 10 key prevention strategies

- Encourage abstinence
- Discourage multiple sexual partners
- Increase accessibility of condoms
- Identify and treat STIs early
- Encourage voluntary counseling and testing
- Encourage late sexual initiation by teens
- End the migratory labor system
- Do away with single sex hostels
- End wars that lead to displacement of people
- Keep peace keeping forces and soldiers based near home

Broad recommendations

- Countries with HIV/AIDS prevalence of 10% or more should declare AIDS an emergency and take urgent steps to reorient their budget from unnecessary military spending to programs that tackle HIV/AIDS, poverty, and food security in order to save the lives of their citizens.

- It is urgent that the G8 countries contribute the necessary resources to the Global Fund to Fight AIDS, Tuberculosis, and Malaria.

- Developing countries may follow the example of Zimbabwe and introduce a levy to finance HIV/AIDS programs.

- The affected countries, with the assistance of the international civil society, should raise funds to establish voluntary counseling and testing services that will be incorporated into primary health care.

- Although anti-retroviral drugs are not a cure for AIDS, they do prolong life. Therefore, countries should ensure accessibility to this treatment by, among other things, using generic drugs and negotiating with pharmaceutical companies to put public interest over profits.

- To reduce political tensions, governments must include all stakeholders and act decisively to combat HIV/AIDS.

References

1. UNAIDS. Report on the global HIV/AIDS epidemic. UNAIDS/02.26E. Geneva: UNAIDS; 2002. p. 22.

2. UNAIDS, WHO. Regional HIV/AIDS statistics and features. Geneva: UNAIDS; 2001.

3. Gisselquest D, Rothenberg R, Potterat J, Drucker E. HIV infections in the sub-Saharan Africa not explained by sexual or vertical transmission. *International Journal of STD & AIDS* 2002;13:657–66.

4. UNAIDS. Report on the global HIV/AIDS epidemic. UNAIDS/02.26E. Geneva: UNAIDS; 2002. p. 25.

5. UNAIDS. Report on the global HIV/AIDS epidemic. p. 23.

6. UNAIDS. Report on the global HIV/AIDS epidemic.

7. Brundtland GH. AIDS and global security. Speech delivered at Nobel Centenary Roundtable by Dr. David Nabarro on behalf of Dr. Gro Harlem Brundtland; 25 Jan 2002; Paris, France.

8. Buve A, Bishikwabo-Nsarhaza K, Mutangandura G. The spread and effect of HIV-1 infection in sub-Saharan Africa. *The Lancet* 2002 Jun 8;(359):2011–7. Available from: URL: http://www.thelancet.com, accessed on 2002 Sep 9.

9. United Nations High Commissioner for Refugees (UNHCR). Refugees by numbers: 2002 edition. 2002 Aug 8. Available from: URL: http://www.unhcr.ch/cgi-bin/texis/vtx/home?page=search, accessed on 2002 Sep 9.

10. Montagnier L. The future of AIDS research: what to do. In: Lanza R, editor. *One world: the health and survival of the human species in the 21st century.* Santa Fe (NM): Health Press; 1996.

11. Satcher D. The global HIV/AIDS epidemic. *Journal of the American Medical Association* 1999 Apr 8;281(16).

12. Johnson HF. Speech at seminar on AIDS and global security; 2002 Jan 25; Paris, France.

13. South African History Online. Chronology: 1700–1799; 1713. Available at: URL: http://www.sahistory.org.za/pages/chronology/thisday/pages/1713-02-13.htm, accessed on 2002 Sep 12.

14. United Nations Development Program. *Human development global report 2002: HDI index 1975–2001.* New York: Oxford University Press; 2002.

15. Stanecki K. The AIDS pandemic in the 21st century. Draft report presented at XIV International Conference on AIDS; 2002 Jul; Barcelona, Spain. Available at: URL: www.usaid.gov/pop_health/aids/Publications/docs/aidsdemoimpact.pdf, accessed on 2002 Sep 3.

16. Lamptey P, Wigley M, Carr D, Collymore Y. Facing the HIV/AIDS pandemic. *Population Bulletin* 2002;57(3),1–38.

17. International Crisis Group. HIV/AIDS as a security issue. Washington/Brussels; 2001 Jun 19. Available at: URL: www.crisisweb.org/projects/issues/hiv_aids/reports/A400321_19062001.pdf, accessed on 2002 Aug 15.

18. UNAIDS. AIDS and population fact sheet. Available at: URL: http://www.unAIDS.org/fact_sheets/files/Demographic_Eng.html, accessed on 2002 Sep 3.

19. U.S. Census Bureau. Demographic estimates and projection (2002). In: Lamptey P, Wigley M, Carr D, Collymore Y. Facing the HIV/AIDS pandemic. *Population Bulletin* 2002;57(3),1–38.

20. BBC News. UNAIDS warning to world leaders. Sunday, 2002 Jul 7, 20:27 GMT.

21. Litte J. U.S. rep hooted off AIDS stage. Med-Tech Center; Today's headlines. 2002 Jul 9; Barcelona, Spain. Available at: URL: http://www.wired.com/news/medtech/0,1286,53728,00.html, accessed on 2002 Sep 3.

22. McLarty S. Gore, AIDS drugs, and South Africa. *Z Magazine.* Available at: URL: www.zmag.org/ZMag/articles/mcclarty.htm, accessed on 2002 Aug 8.

23. Gore A. Letter to James E. Clyburn, endorsing the use of compulsory licensing and parallel imports of pharmaceutical drugs in South Africa; 1999 Jun 25.

24. Brundtland GH. Epidemiology: WHO outlines three-pronged attack against AIDS epidemic. *AIDSWEEKLY Plus* 2000 Feb 7. Available at: URL: http://www.aegis.com/pubs/aidswkly/2000/AW000201.html, accessed on 2002 Aug 12.

25. Pan-African HIV/AIDS Treatment Access Movement. Declaration of action: plan of action. 2002 Aug 22. Available at: URL:http://www.globaltreatment access.org/content/press_releases/02/082202_PTM_ PP_PLAN_ACT.htm, accessed on 2002 Sep 9.

26. Jordan B. Doctor calls AIDS policy "genocide." *Sunday Times* 2002 Jul 28; p. 7.

27. Heinecken L. HIV/AIDS, the military, and impact on national and international security. *Society in Transition* 2001:32(1),120–7.

28. Fourier P, Schönteich M. Africa's new security threat: HIV/AIDS and human security in Southern Africa. *African Security Review* 2001;10(4). Available at: URL: http://www.iss.co.za/Pubs/ASR/10No4/Content.html, accessed on 2002 Sep 9.

29. U.N. Security Council. Security council meets on HIV/AIDS and peacekeeping operations, hears from peacekeeping under-secretary-general, UNAIDS. Security Council 4,259th meeting; 2001 Jan 19; New York, NY. Available at: URL: http://www.un.org/News/Press/docs/2001/sc6992.doc.htm, accessed on 2001 Jul 01.

30. UNICEF Adult wars, child soldiers: Voices of children involved in armed conflict in the East Asia and Pacific region. Available at: URL: http://www.unicef.org/media/publications/adultwarschildsoldiers.pdf, accessed on 2002 Sep 12.

31. Treatment Action Campaign. Demonstration and new court hearing on access to Nevirapine. Pretoria High Court; 2002 Mar 1; Pretoria, South Africa.

32. Heywood M. Something missing in the debate about mother-to-child transmission. South African Medical Research Council: *AIDS Bulletin* 2000;9(4),10–1.

33. Mbulaiteye SM, et al. Declining HIV-1 incidence and associated prevalence over 10 years in a rural population in Southwest Uganda: a cohort study. *The Lancet* 2002;360:41–6.

34. Kisambira E. HIV/AIDS infections on the increase. AIC: the new vision. 2002 Sep 21. Available at: URL: http://www.newvision.co.ug/detail.php?main NewsCategoryId=8&newsCategoryId=13, accessed on 2002 Sep 23.

35. Mugyeni PN. HIV vaccine: the Uganda experience. Vaccine 20, 1905–1908. 2002.

36. Parirenyatwa D. Financing HIV/AIDS: responses using the AIDS levy in Zimbabwe. Paper presented at the Social Aspects of HIV/AIDS Research Alliance. 2002 Sep 1–4; Pretoria, South Africa.

37. Mocumbi P. HIV/AIDS in Southern Africa: what are the challenges? Paper presented at the Social Aspects of HIV/AIDS Research Alliance. 2002 Sep 1–4; Pretoria, South Africa.

38. Mbeki T. Address to parliament on 2002 Feb 17; Cape Town, South Africa.

SECTION III

VIOLENCE AND RISKS

Violence and Human Security: Policy Linkages[1]

David R. Meddings, Douglas W. Bettcher, and Roya Ghafele

Introduction

The World Health Organization defines violence (1) as:

> "The intentional use of physical force or power, threatened or actual, against oneself, another person, or against a group or community, that either results in or has a high likelihood of resulting in injury, death, psychological harm, maldevelopment, or deprivation."

Figure 1 provides a typology that allows one to consider different types of violence according to the characteristics of those committing the violent act. Thus, self-directed violence refers to violence inflicted upon oneself, interpersonal violence refers to violence inflicted by another individual or a small group of individuals, and collective violence refers to violence inflicted by larger groups such as states or organized political and military groups.

This chapter discusses some of the health linkages of human security that are mediated through violence. It develops and supports five assertions:

- Violence is a central threat to human security under all widely prevailing conceptions of human security

- The types of violence constituting this threat include both collective violence and interpersonal violence

- These types of violence share determinants that are inextricably linked with some of the major issues underlying the increased attention that human security has received over the last decade

- Coherent policy recommendations to prevent violence would have cross-cutting benefits in terms of reducing a number of threats to human security

Figure I.   A typology of violence (1)

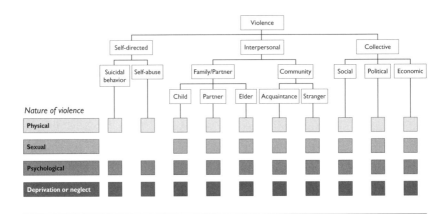

Violence, as a human security threat, constitutes a core public health issue

Finally, in an era of globalized threats requiring international cooperation, the discussion focuses on the interstate spillover effects of violence, or in other words, the transnational dimensions of the problem. These arguments are linked to the notion of security as a 'contested concept' in the 21st century; in particular our analysis focuses on the implications of the violence case study for conceptualizing sovereignty, the core concept underpinning international relations.

Violence as a health problem

Before developing discussion around these five points, some attention should be given to the attributes and effects of violence that may make it difficult for some to perceive violence as a health problem. On its face, some may feel such discussion unnecessary. After all, one need only consider a physical assault requiring medical attention to make the point that health effects can and do arise following perpetration of violence.

However, even though there are obvious health effects that result from violence, these effects arise in a much more manifest way from the interaction of a person with his or her external environment than most other communicable or noncommunicable health conditions. With infectious disease, while the external environment is exceedingly important in providing suitable conditions for infectious agents and their various vectors, one tends to consider the 'illness' within the context of the physiological processes that begin following the entry of an infectious agent into a human host. Similarly, the 'illness' aspects of noncommunicable conditions such as cardiovascular diseases or malignant processes tend to be considered in terms of physiological changes occurring within a person.

In contrast, the health effects arising from perpetration of violence clearly involve an interaction between a victim and a perpetrator. Whether the mechanism by which violence is inflicted involves forcible restraint or threat of lethal injury during rape or a speeding bullet, there can be no denying that this use of force, essential to the definition of violence, occurs external to the body.

While the intentional use of physical force or power against a person is characteristic of violence, and requires that the health effects of violence are mediated through one's external environment, this feature is by no means unique among the various processes that lead to health outcomes. Although one may focus more easily on the internal physiological changes such as fever and convulsions in a child with malaria, the fact remains that the malaria parasite (or any other infectious agent) has entered that child through an interaction with the child's external environment. Similarly, with many noncommunicable diseases, well prior to a cancerous change within a cell or the deposition of fatty material within a blood vessel, an interaction has taken place with one's external environment.

On reflection therefore, the external environment is an important consideration for many health outcomes. A major and striking difference with violence, however, is that the time lag between an interaction with one's environment and the health effects produced tends to be very short. While there are certainly long-term health effects arising from exposure to violence, the immediate health effects — the fractured bones, the collapse in blood volume — appear without an incubation or latency period to temporally separate the connection between these effects and the contributory role of one's environment.

Whether this clear and immediate connection with the external environment causes people to view violence more as a criminal justice issue; whether since violence so frequently involves an interaction between individuals, some see it from a sociological perspective; or whether it is so patently obvious that health effects arise from violence that people overlook the health connection in order to establish more meaningful connections; some need to be reminded that violence is, among other things, a health issue.

Indeed, it is not merely because violence gives rise to health effects that it is important and useful to consider violence from a public health perspective. Those with an interest in the health of populations have always attempted to understand interactions between humans and their environment, and determine how this relates to health problems. Deeper consideration of violence reveals many attributes shared with other health problems — the most important being that violence is not a random event.

Age is one of the more striking associations: violence disproportionately affects individuals during their most productive years. In 1998, interpersonal violence, collective violence, and self-directed violence accounted for three of the top six causes of death for individuals of either sex aged 15 to 44 in low- and middle-income countries (2). Interpersonal and self-directed violence were the second and third leading causes of death for the same age group in high-income countries (2). In 2002, the World Health Organization released the *World Report on Violence and Health,* which estimates that 1.6 million people worldwide lost their lives to violence during 2000 (1). Apart from the associations with age, the *Report* also draws attention to a number of the gender dimensions of violence, with males being victims in over three quarters of homicides and females overwhelmingly represented as victims of forms of interpersonal violence such as intimate partner and sexual violence.

Over and above the age and gender associations, country income is a potent predictor of violence rates. Violent death rates for low- to middle-income countries are more than twice those of high-income countries, and over 90% of violent deaths occur in low- and middle-income countries (1). As will be developed later in this paper, socioeconomic gradients at more localized levels also correlate closely with rates of violence.

Thus, not only is violence a significant contributor to global morbidity and mortality, its occurrence is far from random. Violence is poorly explained as a criminal act committed by isolated individuals, and much more usefully understood as a behavior determined by economic and social development fault lines at the transnational and societal levels, interacting with individual-, familial-, and community-level factors. In sum, violence is a global public health problem that requires a multisectoral approach. On reflection, something which is not so very different from the large-scale drainage projects in southern Europe to eradicate malaria, or combined efforts of government and industry to control and reduce exposure to lead.

VIOLENCE IS A THREAT TO HUMAN SECURITY

So it seems both useful and eminently appropriate to consider violence as a global public health problem, but is it a threat to human security? A brief look at any of the widely prevailing conceptions of human security leaves little doubt that violence is indeed a threat to human security.

A characteristic of the human security perspective is that the individual, rather than the state, is the referent object of concern; the value base of human security is squarely people-centered. However, when it comes to defining how broadly or narrowly one should consider threats to the individual, opinions diverge.

Those who consider a broad range of threats typically have a development-oriented view of human security. In 1994, the *Human Development Report* from the United Nations Development Program (UNDP) articulates a widely cited conception of human security:

"Human security encompasses economic security, food security, health security, environmental security, personal security, community security, and political security" (3).

Under this conception, human security includes threats arising, *inter alia,* from poverty, hunger and famine, health outcomes, violence, political repression, and environmental degradation. In discussing the threat of violence the report elaborates:

"Perhaps no other aspect of human security is so vital for people as their security from physical violence. In poor nations and rich, human life is increasingly threatened by sudden, unpredictable violence" (3).

Those who view threats to human security more narrowly tend to emphasize those issues posing a direct threat to the personal safety and well being of the individual. The Canadian government is one of the more readily identified proponents of a narrower range of threats (4, 5).

A criticism of the broad conception of human security has been that it conflates a broad range of threats to the individual under the banner of 'insecurity.' While this heading may offer advantages of advocacy and mobilizing diverse constituencies, it has been argued that it does so at the cost of undermining the descriptive power of the concept of human security. On the other hand, the broader conception of threats better reflects the values underlying concern for the well-being of individuals, and is less concerned with analytical methods to support it.

This chapter does not advocate either a broad or narrow conception of threats. Of far greater relevance is that violence remains a central concern to either viewpoint. Indeed, as Kanti Bajpai points out, violence figures prominently in the overlap between the two threat agendas:

"Most of the threats listed by both the UNDP and Canadian government papers relate to personal safety and well being. Both identify indirect and direct threats. Amongst the direct threats, they both list everyday violent crime, child abuse, and abuse of women. Much higher up the ladder towards more organized direct violence, they both list government repression, terrorism, and genocide. Canada lists, in addition, various other kinds of direct violence — call it societal violence — that endanger personal safety including the existence of private security forces, banditry, warlordism, internal war, and ethnic violence. The Canadian writings in particular include organized violence that is more familiar in security thinking — transnational violence and international/global violence" (6).

Clearly, the threat of violence to the individual remains a central preoccupation, whether one's conception of human security focuses on a narrow range of threats or a broader one. Violence — whether interpersonal or collective — has been a central and consistently articulated concern for many scholars and political figures who have sought to define human security from either a broad or a narrow perspective.[2, 3, 4, 5] Moreover, both of these perspectives contend that the traditional concept of security that dominated the Cold War era, focusing on the threat of military aggression across borders and the military means to face such threats, is not sufficient to conceptualize the international security challenges that have emerged in the post Cold War era. While the end of the Cold War does not mean that these traditional security issues are no longer relevant, there are mounting demands that the security agenda should provide space for the threats to human life and collective security, often nonmilitary in origin, such as interpersonal and ethnic violence, organized crime, and economic instability (7).

More recent developments in refining the concept of human security also keep violence squarely anchored within the human security discourse. Through a variety of meetings and consultations since its inception, the Commission on Human Security has elaborated a working definition of human security that advocates the objective of human security is to safeguard the vital core of all human lives from critical and pervasive threats (8). The term 'vital core' includes elements such as the rights and freedoms allowing survival, livelihood, and basic dignity. The two essential attributes of the term 'critical and pervasive threats' are that these threats affect core activities of human lives and do so on a large scale and/or in a nonanomalous manner (8). Clearly violence in many forms has direct negative impacts on survival, livelihood, and basic dignity. The large scale and nonanomalous aspects of violence will be covered in the next section, which develops a profile of the forms of violence that constitute critical and pervasive threats to populations around the globe.

VIOLENCE AS A CRITICAL AND PERVASIVE THREAT: A GLOBAL OVERVIEW

Table 1 provides estimated deaths due to collective violence from the 16th through the 20th centuries. Despite the large degree of uncertainty surrounding these estimates, the rise in death rates, particularly pronounced in the 20th century, is nevertheless striking.

According to the *World Health Report 2001*, an estimated 310,000 people lost their lives as a direct result of collective violence during 2000, with over half of these deaths occurring in sub-Saharan Africa, and men aged 15 to 44 accounting for well over a third of mortality (9). Estimating nonfatal outcomes is difficult; however, the numbers are likely to be substantial given that the ratio of injured to killed among military personnel across a wide range of conflict settings, derived by dividing the number

Table 1.   Estimated historical deaths and annual rates of death due to collective violence, 16th to 20th centuries

Century	Estimated deaths during century (millions) (1)	Estimated mid-century population (millions) (54)	Estimated annual death rate per 100,000
16th	1.6	500	3.2
17th	6.1	545	11.2
18th	7.0	790	8.9
19th	19.4	1,260	15.4
20th	109.7	2,520	43.5

of combatants wounded to those killed, has been reported to range from 1.9 to 13.0, with an average around 3.0 (10).

A wide variety of indirect effects on health arise from the disruptive social changes that accompany collective violence. Collective violence typically creates population displacement and a substantial degradation of social infrastructure, such as health care systems and food production and distribution networks (11, 12). Not infrequently, life-sustaining civilian infrastructure is specifically targeted in conflicts through acts such as the destruction of food and water distribution complexes and the execution of health care workers (13, 14). Research in these settings has shown a significant reduction in indicators such as vaccination status that accompany collective violence (15). Furthermore, many efforts to control or eradicate disease that have been dramatically successful elsewhere founder in settings where collective violence is occurring.

While it is difficult to estimate with precision the burden of health effects that are attributable to these changes, evidence suggests it is substantial. Crude mortality rates in displaced populations fleeing collective violence have been reported at five to 12 times the baseline rates (16), and were substantially higher among those fleeing the Rwandan genocide who arrived in Goma (17). The primary causes of death in these circumstances are communicable diseases and malnutrition, and the incidence of AIDS in Africa is thought to have increased considerably as a direct result of civil wars (18, 19). Beyond the morbidity and mortality related to communicable disease and malnutrition, a broad range of health outcomes has been documented in populations exposed to collective violence, including disability and psychosocial and reproductive health sequelae (17).

Furthermore, due to the nature of collective violence, it seems reasonable to expect that these indirect health effects would not be limited to the time period during which the violence occurs. A recent statistical assessment using cross sectional data indicates that the total disability adjusted life years (DALYs) lost in 1999 due to the indirect effects of collective violence from 1991 to 1997, was about the same as the number lost through direct effects of collective violence in 1999 (16).

There seems to be little doubt that collective violence constitutes a 'critical and pervasive threat' to the vital core of human well-being in regions where it is occurring. Indeed, most people who think of violence in relation to human security probably consider war as the primary violence-mediated human security threat. The Rwandan genocide and ethnic cleansing in the former Federal Republic of Yugoslavia are rightly viewed as watershed events in the development of the human security discourse, not least for the catastrophic loss of life that accompanied this collective violence, but also for the dilemma these events posed to an international community struggling to value state sovereignty and human security simultaneously.

But what about interpersonal violence? Are there settings in which interpersonal violence constitutes a critical and pervasive threat? The *World Report on Violence and Health* estimates that in the year 2000, interpersonal violence accounted for almost twice as many deaths as collective violence (1). There is an obvious difference in terms of public visibility — collective violence tends to be heavily mediatized while interpersonal violence in many forms tends to be concealed. For example, Brazil is not a country at war. Largely because of this, few people would be aware that in addition to the 467 Israeli or Palestinian minors killed due to conflict from 1987 to 2001, a staggering 3,937 children under the age of eighteen were murdered by firearms in the municipality of Rio de Janeiro alone — an eightfold difference (20).

Across Latin and Central America, particularly in urban areas, violence is a daily threat. The ACTIVA project was a multicenter study coordinated by the Pan American Health Organization to assess violence and related norms and attitudes in selected cities in Latin and Central America as well as Madrid (21). Almost 11,000 interviews were conducted among a sample that stratified population groups according to socioeconomic level and population density within the eight cities involved. The sample represented the relevant urban populations from ages 18 to 70, and was of sufficient size to permit estimates with 95% reliability. The proportion of respondents indicating that they had been victims of violence (armed robbery, extortion by a public authority, physical assault, or knife or bullet wounds) during the prior 12 months ranged from 10.6% in Santiago, Chile, to 38.5% in San Salvador, El Salvador.

Urban violence has begun to attract an increasing amount of research attention; some aspects will be discussed in the subsequent section. It should be noted however that while the largest cities were located in high-income countries until the 1960s, this is no longer the case. Today some of the world's largest cities, and the megacities of the future, are found in the developing world (22). It has been estimated that every five years, 60%

of inhabitants of cities with populations of 100,000 or more become victims of violence (22).

The Banshbari slum is located in the midwestern part of Dhaka, Bangladesh. Although throughout the 1970s it was a rapidly growing urban slum, its residential population has decreased during the 1990s, due to newly established housing societies, to around 2000. Those who remain are both politically and economically marginalized. Participatory rural appraisal methods have been used to probe residents' perceptions of violence and insecurity (23). Those interviewed report that the occurrence of firearm-related violence has increased steadily since the mid-1990s through to the time of the appraisal, that essential tasks such as gathering firewood are fraught with insecurity, and that residents do not go outside after nightfall. There are frequent references to the deliberate targeting of women for abduction, rape, and trafficking, with one woman reporting:

> "I wish I could run and escape from them because anything can happen to me. I can be raped by a number of them....They can traffic me out of the country or sell me to a brothel; they can keep me in captivity and use me as a prostitute for life. Even if I come back from them somehow, the society will not accept me; they will think I am spoilt and nobody will marry me. My family will lose face in the society."

A central problem in shedding light on the nature of the threat of interpersonal violence in settings where it is pervasive is the absence of reliable data. South Africa has made considerable inroads in addressing this issue by establishing the National Injury Mortality Surveillance System (NIMSS) (24). NIMSS is a mortuary-based surveillance system that captures key information on fatal injuries. As of 2001, the system provides descriptive data from 32 mortuaries in six provinces and is estimated to provide this information for just over a third of externally caused deaths within South Africa. The data are biased towards urban areas, although 14 of the mortuaries serve largely rural areas. Homicide was the leading cause of death and accounted for 44% of the 25,361 fatal injuries recorded in 2001, with over half of these inflicted by firearms.

The United States, long cited as the setting with the highest firearm homicide rates among high-income countries, experienced what has been described as an epidemic of firearm-related violence from the mid-1980s to 1993 (25). During the peak of the epidemic, firearm-related homicide rates reached almost seven per 100,000 for the American population as a whole. However, this aggregate figure disguises the fact that rates among age and ethnic groups were much higher. In fact, in many American cities a black male who turned 18 in 1989 had roughly a one in 20 chance of being murdered by 1995 (26). While the ability to disaggregate data to these finer levels makes such analyses possible, it is sobering to reflect that while rates of firearm-related violence in the United States are definitely high relative to other high-income settings, they pale in comparison to rates observed in many low- and middle-income settings. Indeed, firearm homicide rates of 40 and 50 per 100,000 — roughly sixfold higher than the peak of the U.S. epidemic — have been reported to the WHO for Brazil and Colombia respectively (27).

SHARED DETERMINANTS: IMPLICATIONS FOR THE HUMAN SECURITY POLICY AGENDA

Despite the readily discernible difference in public visibility, there are a number of notable similarities between collective and interpersonal forms of violence. Most important for the human security discourse and its policy implications is that both forms share a number of determinants and the capacity to be self-perpetuating. Indeed, if a central challenge for those engaged in furthering the human security discourse is to propose integrated responses to approaching human security threats, then discussion of these issues is highly relevant.

The vulnerability of populations to either interpersonal or collective violence is influenced by a variety of factors in the political, economic, and social spheres. These include:

1. Weak economic development at the country level
2. Inequalities in access to economic, political, and social resources at the societal level
3. Weak forms of governance and forms that are not socially redistributive
4. A number of factors linked to globalization, including:
   - Abrupt changes in political and social structures
   - Aspects of globalization linked to financial movements and opportunities
   - Transnational flows of weapons, particularly small arms

PER CAPITA GDP

A striking association with both rates of interpersonal violence and the occurrence of collective violence is low per capita gross domestic product (GDP) at the country level. Over the years, a number of studies have demonstrated the relationship between country level GDP per capita and homicide rates (28, 29), and Figure 2 shows geographical distribution of estimated rates of youth homicide for 2000.

Analysts who have studied causes of civil war tend to agree that per capita GDP is an important predictor of the risk of armed conflict, although there is disagreement on the nature of this relationship. Some stress the importance of incomes that rely on primary commodity exports (30), while others offer evidence to contradict this view. Others still posit that

Figure 2.   Estimated homicide rates[a] among youth aged 10–29 years, 2000 (1)

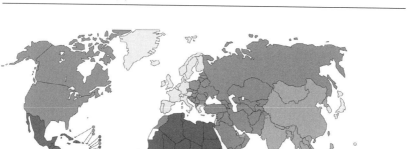

[a] Rates were calculated by WHO region and country income level and then grouped according to magnitude.

Source: WHO Global Burden of Disease project for 2000, Version 1 (see statistical annex).

economic growth generates political instability and potentially fuels collective violence in poor economies, while offering a protective effect in richer countries (31).

Horizontal inequalities

Disparities in access to economic, political, and social resources at the societal level also have been demonstrated to correlate with both interpersonal and collective violence. Increasing inequalities in income distribution as measured by indicators such as the Gini coefficient correlate with rising homicide rates; this relationship persists despite statistical control for a variety of national characteristics and appears repeatedly across a number of study settings (32). Similarly, a number of analysts have argued that in addition to inequalities in income distribution, unequal access to political and social resources, or predominance of one ethnic community over another, are powerful drivers of political instability and collective violence (31, 33).

Quality of governance

Given that the vast majority of conflicts occur within states, it is perhaps not surprising that a number of scholars cite real or perceived failures of governance — whether related to the provision of services and redistribution of social goods, the degree of political inclusiveness, or other aspects of perceived quality of governance — as an important determinant of conflict (33, 34). In this respect, Axworthy observes that:

> "The meaning of security is being transformed. Security traditionally has focused on the state because its fundamental purpose is to protect its citizens. Hobbled by economic adversity, outrun by globalization, and undermined from within by bad governance, the capacity of some states to provide this protection has increasingly come into question" (35).

Notwithstanding the logic of this viewpoint, it is important to note that there are a number of areas where consensus is lacking on fundamental issues such as the importance of inclusive democracies as a form of governance, and the causal relationship between grievances related to governance and civil conflict. These and a host of other issues related to policymaking in relation to collective violence have recently received a thorough review (36).

Forms of governance that provide social redistribution of collective goods and social protection correlate with lower rates of interpersonal violence. For example, homicide arrest rates have been found to be negatively associated with homicide rates, suggesting that modes of governance that actively support the rule of law help to deter further violence (37). Various forms of collective social protection, and forms of redistribution such as welfare expenditures, have also been shown in association with lower rates of interpersonal violence (38, 39).

Effects of Globalization

Globalization has been defined as a set of processes that intensify human interaction by eroding boundaries of time, space, and ideas that have historically separated people and nations in a number of spheres of action, including economic, health and environmental, social and cultural, knowledge and technology, and political and institutional (40). While globalization is not a new phenomenon, the manner in which the world has become increasingly interdependent in recent times has created the conditions under which populations experience rapid and fundamental social, political, and economic changes; globalization in recent times has assumed a magnitude — and taken on patterns — unprecedented in world history (41). The interaction of the processes of globalization and the international system is changing the face of the security discourse.

Health development in the 21st century must take advantage of the opportunities afforded by global change and at the same time, minimize the risks and threats associated with globalization, such as the negative effects of violence. In this way, the dramatic improvements in the health of the world's population achieved in the 20th century can be maintained in the

21st century (41). Negative changes are associated with both collective and interpersonal violence and exemplify a downside human security risk that may be substantially greater in population impact than would have been observed in a less globalized world.

The end of the Cold War era brought relatively abrupt and far-reaching consequences to the political and social structures of the former Soviet bloc, as well as radical changes affecting livelihood strategies. Comparison of regional trends in youth homicide between western Europe and some countries of the former Soviet bloc between from 1985 to 1995 illustrates some of the associated changes in interpersonal violence that were observed during this period of transition. Homicide rates in the 10 to 24 age bracket increased by over 150% from 1985 to 1994 in the Russian Federation, and by 125% over the same period in Latvia (1). In both settings the proportion of homicides attributable to firearms more than doubled. By contrast, homicide rates and the proportion attributable to firearms within western Europe remained generally low and stable.

There is general consensus that political instability is a predictor of collective violence (31, 36). Furthermore, it has been argued that transitional states are particularly at risk for civil war, whereas either repressive autocracies or inclusive democracies tend to have low levels of civil violence (42).

Financial factors related to globalization may also contribute to changes in violence. A recent study of predictors of foreign direct investment indicates that poor rule of law and corruption are most detrimental for investment (43). Since forms of governance that support respect for the law are associated with lower rates of interpersonal violence, countries with high or increasing rates of interpersonal violence would appear to be at risk for reduced investment or capital flight, potentially aggravating socioeconomic inequities with the possibility for further increased rates of interpersonal violence (7).

With respect to collective violence, there is little doubt that economic motivations have played a major role in initiating conflicts, and that the access to global markets and trade in commodities from conflict areas has played a substantial role in maintaining the ability of parties to the conflict to continue their struggle. The aspects of globalization that permit easily concealed payments and expedite exchanges of assets greatly facilitate this economic activity. A wide variety of economic networks have been used to conduct transborder trade and exploit the global economic system in order to support war economies (44).

TRANSNATIONAL SPILLOVER EFFECTS

The impact of interpersonal violence on the international system, in particular the transnational spillover effects, has yet to be fully studied. However, the global epidemiology of interpersonal violence, which clearly demonstrates a world dividing into clusters of high-violence and low-violence societies, does not bode well for the future stability of the international system. As noted above, these clusters of violence coincide, for the most part, with the division between low-to-middle income and high-income countries. To the extent that interpersonal violence leaches a society's economic growth potential, it is reasonable to conclude that interpersonal violence is widening the gap between the rich and poor.

Such disparities and the emergence of clusters of intense violence within nations enhance the probability of state collapse and disintegration, and the emergence of failed states. It may be argued that the contemporary international system already contains states and quasi-states, a different situation from a world containing only states (45). Such quasi-states have a greater probability of becoming failed states, which may be defined as:

> "A situation where the structure, authority (legitimate power), social, and political order of a state have fallen apart. This is accompanied by social violence and the privatization of security" (46).

Collapsed or quasi-states often pose a direct threat to their citizens or fail to protect them. Failed states and the ensuing seemingly random violence, both local and transnational, that results from such collapse set off waves of domestic and transnational catastrophes such as migration, epidemics of communicable diseases, undernutrition and malnutrition, and rape or unsafe sex. Such environments also become prime breeding grounds for organized crime and terrorism. These few examples show how the root causes of violence are intimately linked and have the potential to propagate other public health problems, such as infectious disease epidemics. The uneven and contradictory characteristics of our emergent global society are accompanied by global social movements, both positive and negative, and the fragmentation of many nation-states.

Therefore, from an international perspective, violence has the capacity to seriously weaken worldwide stability. People flee from violence. According to UNHCR, "armed conflict is now the driving force behind most refugee flows" (47). In other words, in a globalized world one cannot be secure if one's neighbor, even a distant neighbor, is not secure. Violence has significant spillover effects. In Austria, for instance, the refugee flows from the Balkans led to an anti-foreigner referendum, and most likely contributed to the success of the extreme right party in the elections of 1999.

Another aspect of globalization that is associated with both collective and interpersonal violence is the issue of transnational flows of weapons, particularly small arms. The movement of these weapons over porous borders following conflicts and in the wake of organized crime and the drug trade has attracted increasing international concern and attention in recent years. Both collective violence, through perpetuation of conflicts and exacerbation of regional instabilities, and interpersonal violence, through noncombat-related assaults, have been linked to the uncontrolled and widespread availability of these weapons (48).

Given these shared determinants, it should come as no surprise that collective violence and interpersonal violence are interrelated, and that the effects of interpersonal violence in an interconnected world are not hermetically contained within state boundaries, or for that matter within nonexistent failed state borders. Collective violence is associated with an increase in homicide and other crimes, both during the phase of violence and thereafter, and also has been shown to lead to increased suicide rates in settings bordering civil wars (16). The experience of international war has been reported to make the use of violence within states more common (49, 50). Moreover, the spillover effects of violence and political disintegration are waves of other public health problems such as communicable disease epidemics, rape, the rampant spread of sexually transmitted diseases, and mass migration. Thus, interpersonal violence and the concomitant political instability it brings represent serious transnational challenges to both the international system and global public health.

SECURITY AS A CONTESTED CONCEPT

In the emerging international relations discourse of the 21st century, many writers agree that security is a contested concept. While there is general agreement that security implies freedom from threats to core values (for both individuals and groups), there are diverging views whether the main focus of the emerging security discourse should be on individual, national, or international security (51). Traditionalists argue that security issues are within the realm of domestic and not international responsibility. However, this realist approach is unable to deal with threats that states bring upon their citizens or violent threats that arise within the state; realism conceptualizes a historic and abstract international system where anarchy and power dominate the relations between states. The concept of state sovereignty dominates this view of international relations and is rooted in the origins of the modern international system traced back to the Treaty of Westphalia in 1648.

This chapter argues that the security discourse must go beyond a tightly defined realist perspective focusing on interstate military force to include emerging threats, especially violence and the determinants of interpersonal violence, as integral human security concerns. In an increasingly globalized world, security threats stem from complex systems, both natural (e.g., the ecosystem) and human made (the global economy and interpersonal violence), in which individuals, states, and the system all play a part, and in which economic, societal, and environmental factors are as important as political and military ones (52). In this regard, challenges to the international system such as interpersonal violence require a rethinking of state sovereignty that includes global attention to the subnational and transnational dimensions of interpersonal violence as both a human security and public health priority. A sole emphasis on the state, state sovereignty, interstate relations, and interstate security — the traditional security paradigm — cannot address the security issues outlined in our analysis.

The human security issues enumerated in this chapter provide other dimensions to the emerging global security agenda that characterizes the post-Cold War era. A security paradigm for the 21st century must include space for individual, state, and transnational problems, such as the proliferation of interpersonal violence in many areas of the world. In other words, it requires a rethinking of conventional notions of world politics and international relations. No country alone can address the security challenges of this new era in world affairs. In this respect, we believe that contesting traditional concepts of security is a positive development, and one that can only lead to more effective ways of addressing serious human security challenges such as interpersonal violence.

Conclusion

Consideration of these shared determinants for interpersonal and collective violence should bring to mind some areas of policy action that would advance the human security agenda. Viewed broadly, the intent of these policies should be to address the transnational- and societal-level determinants of these forms of violence. Strengthening mechanisms may be used to reduce inequalities, promote effective and inclusive forms of governance, and protect individuals and populations from the downside risks of globalization through better control and transparency of certain international markets. Efforts in these areas would have cross-cutting benefits for a number of other health and nonhealth threats to human security as well.

On its face, advancing such an agenda may seem problematic to differences in North-South priorities. However, the North has a rational interest in preventing violence in the South — not least because it effectively bankrolls the costs of this violence through collapsed development initiatives, humanitarian aid, and peacekeeping. Illegal migration arising from this violence is a volatile political issue for the North (34).

Interpersonal violence and collective violence exemplify threats to human security, and a policy agenda responding to their fundamental determinants would have benefits for a number of other human security threats. In addition, interpersonal violence and collective violence are important global public health problems; in fact, a particularly apt description of *ill* health was provided by Thomas Hobbes in the seventeenth century in describing life without security:

> "In such condition there is no place for industry...no arts; no letters; no society; and which is worst of all, continual fear, and danger of violent death; and the life of man, solitary, poor, nasty, brutish, and short (53)."

We therefore contend that if international society ignores the threats to human security and public health posed by interpersonal violence, it does so at its peril.

NOTES

[1] © Copyright World Health Organization 2003. All rights reserved. The World Health Organization has granted the publisher permission for the reproduction of this article.

[2] "Once synonymous with the defense of territory from external attack, the requirements of security today have come to embrace the protection of communities and individuals from internal violence." Kofi Annan Millennium Report, Chapter 3, p. 43-44.

[3] "Several key elements make up human security. A first essential element is the possibility for all citizens to live in peace and security within their own borders. This implies the capacity of states and citizens to prevent and resolve conflicts through peaceful and nonviolent means and, after the conflict is over, the ability to effectively carry out reconciliation efforts." Sadako Ogata, Asian Development Bank Seminar, 27 April 1998.

[4] "What do we mean by human security? We mean, in its most simple expression, all those things that men and women anywhere in the world cherish most: enough food for the family; adequate shelter; good health; schooling for the children; protection from violence whether inflicted by man or by nature; and a State which does not oppress its citizens but rules with their consent." United Nations Deputy Secretary-General Louise Frechette, Vienna International Center, 9 October 1999.

[5] "Human security relates to the protection of the individual's personal safety and freedom from direct and indirect threats of violence." Kanti Bajpai, Joan B. Kroc Institute Report, No. 19. Fall 2000, p. 48.

REFERENCES

1. Krug EG et al., editors. *World report on violence and health*. Geneva: World Health Organization; 2002.

2. Krug EG, Sharma GK, Lozano R. The global burden of injuries. *American Journal of Public Health* 2000 April;90(4):523–6.

3. United Nations Development Programme. *Human development report 1994*. New York: Oxford University Press; 1994.

4. Axworthy L. Canada and human security: the need for leadership. *International Journal* 1997;52:183–96.

5. Department of Foreign Affairs and International Trade (DFAIT), Government of Canada. Human security: safety for people in a changing world. 1999. Available from DFAIT website: URL: http://www.dfait.maeci.gc.ca/foreignp/HumanSecurity/secur-e.htm, accessed on 2003 February 15.

6. Bajpai K. Human Security: Concept and measurement. Occasional Paper 19:OP:1. Notre Dame (IN): The Joan B. Kroc Institute for International Peace Studies. 2000 Aug. p. 25–6.

7. Wipfli H, Bettcher D, Ouseph R, Monteiro M, Butchart A, Cosivi O, et al. Health security issues. In: *Encyclopedia of life support systems*. In press 2003.

8. Alkire W. Conceptual framework for human security. 2002 Feb 16. Available from: URL: http://www.humansecurity-chs.org/doc/frame.html, accessed on 2003 February 15.

9. World Health Organization (WHO). *World health report 2001*. Geneva: WHO; 2001.

10. Coupland RM, Meddings DR. Mortality associated with use of weapons in armed conflicts, wartime atrocities, and civilian mass shootings: literature review. *British Medical Journal* 1999;319:407–10.

11. Collier P. On the economic consequences of civil war. *Oxford Economic Papers* 1999;51:168–83.

12. Stewart F. War and underdevelopment: can economic analysis help reduce the costs? *Journal of International Development* 1993;5(4):357–80.

13. Fitzsimmons DW, Whiteside AW. Conflict, war, and public health. Conflict Studies 276. London: Research Institute for the Study of Conflict and Terrorism; 1994.

14. Toole MJ. Displaced persons and war. In Levy BS, Sidel VW, editors. *War and public health*. Updated edition. Washington: American Public Health Association; 2000.

15. Garfield RM, Frieden T, Vermund SH. Health-related outcomes of war in Nicaragua. *American Journal of Public Health* 1987;77:615–8.

16. Ghobarah H, Huth P, Russett B. Civil wars kill and maim people long after the shooting stops. *American Political Science Review*. In press 2003.

17. Meddings DR. Civilians and War: A review and historical overview of the involvement of non-combatant populations in conflict situations. *Medicine, Conflict and Survival* 2001;17:6–16.

18. Reid E. A future, if one is still alive: the challenge of the HIV epidemic. In: Moore J, editor. *Hard choices: moral dilemmas in humanitarian intervention*. Lanham (MD): Rowman & Littlefield; 1998. p. 269–86.

19. Epstein H. AIDS: The lesson of Uganda. *New York Review of Books* 2001;48(11):18–23.

20. Dowdney L. Child combatants in organised armed violence: a study of children and adolescents involved in territorial drug faction disputes in Rio de Janeiro. First edition for presentation at the Seminar on Children Affected by Organised Armed Violence; 2002 Sep 9–13; Rio de Janeiro, Brazil. p. 125.

21. Cruz JM. Victimization from urban violence: levels and related factors in selected cities of Latin America and Spain. Research in Public Health Technical Papers Project Activa 4. Washington: Pan American Health Organization; 1999 Jan.

22. Cornelius-Taylor B, Handajani YS, Jordan S, Köhler G, Korff R, Laaser U, et al. Urbanization and public health — a review of the scientific literature. In: Strohmeier KP, Köhler G, Laaser U, editors. *Pilot research project on urban violence and health: Determinants and management; a study in Jakarta, Karachi and conurbation Ruhrgebiet.* Lage: Jacobs; 2002. p. 31–77.

23. Regional Centre for Strategic Studies. Small arms and human insecurity. Colombo: Regional Centre for Strategic Studies; 2002.

24. Matzopoulos R. A profile of fatal injuries in South Africa. Third annual report of the National Injury Mortality Surveillance System. Johannesburg: Medical Research Council of South Africa, University of South Africa; 2002 Dec.

25. Wintemute G. Guns and gun violence. In: Blumstein A, Wallman J, editors. *The crime drop in America.* Cambridge: Cambridge University Press; 2000. p. 45–96.

26. Cook PJ, Laub JH. The unprecedented epidemic in youth violence. In: Moore MH, Tonry M, editors. *Crime and justice: a review of research.* Chicago: University of Chicago Press; 1998. p. 101–38.

27. Department of Injuries and Violence Prevention, World Health Organization. *Small arms and global health.* Geneva: World Health Organization; 2001.

28. Rahav G, Jaamdar S. Development and crime: a cross-national study. *Development and Change* 1982; 13(4):447–62.

29. Krahn H, Harnagel TF, Gartrell JW. Income inequality and homicide rates: cross-national data and criminological theories. *Criminology* 1986;24:269–95.

30. Collier P, Hoeffler A. Greed and grievance in civil war. Manuscript. World Bank; 2001. Available from: URL: http://econ.worldbank.org/files/12205_greedgrievance_23oct.pdf, accessed on February 15, 2003

31. Gates S. Empirically assessing the causes of war. Paper presented to the 43rd Annual Convention of the International Studies Association; 2002 Mar 24–27; New Orleans, USA.

32. Messner F. Economic discrimination and societal homicide rates: further evidence of the cost of inequality. *American Sociological Review* 1989;54:597–611.

33. Stewart F. Root causes of violent conflict in developing countries. *British Medical Journal* 2002 Feb 9;324:342–345.

34. Gurr TR. *Minorities at risk: a global view of ethnopolitical conflicts.* Washington: Institute of Peace Press; 1993.

35. Axworthy L. Human security and global governance: putting people first. *Global Governance* 2001;7(1):19.

36. Mack A. Civil war: academic research and the policy community. *Journal of Peace Research* 2002;39(5):515–25.

37. World Bank Latin American and Caribbean Studies. Viewpoint Series. *Determinants of crime rates in Latin America and the world.* Washington: World Bank; 1998.

38. Pampel FC, Gartner R. Age structure, socio-political institutions, and national homicide rates. *European Sociologic Review* 1995;11(3):243–60.

39. Messner SF, Rosenfeld R. Political restraint of the market and levels of criminal homicide: a cross-national application of institutional-anomie theory. *Social Forces* 1997;75(4):1393–1416.

40. Lee K, Dodgson R. Globalization and cholera: implications for global governance. *Global Governance* 2000;6(2):213–36.

41. Yach D, Bettcher D. The globalization of public health I: threats and opportunities. *American Journal of Public Health* 1998;88(5):735.

42. Hegre H, Ellingsen T, Gates S, Gleditsch NP. Towards a democratic civil peace? Democracy, political change, and civil war. *American Political Science Review* 2001;95(1):33–48.

43. International Finance Corporation. Investment and uncertainty, a comparative study of different uncertainty measures. Technical Paper 4. Washington: International Finance Corporation; 1997.

44. Duffield M. Globalization, transborder trade, and war economies. In: Berdal M, Malone D, editors. *Greed and grievance: Economic agendas in civil wars.* Boulder:Lynne Rienner; 2000. p. 69–90.

45. Jackson R. *Quasi-states: sovereignty, international relations and the Third World.* Cambridge (UK): Cambridge University Press; 1990.

46. Zartmann W. *Collapsed states: the disintegration and restoration of legitimate authority.* Boulder (CO): Lynne Rienner; 1995. 1: 1–320.

47. UNHCR. *Human rights and small arms: the human rights impact of small arms and light weapons.* Geneva: UNHCR; 2001. 283: 1–320.

48. Meddings DR. Weapons injuries during and after periods of conflict: retrospective analysis. *British Medical Journal* 1997 Nov 29;315:1417–20.

49. Stein AA. *The nation at war.* Baltimore (MD): Johns Hopkins University Press; 1980.

50. Archer D, Gartner R. Violent acts and violent times: a comparative approach to postwar homicide rates. *American Sociological Review* 1976; 41(4):937–63.

51. Baylis J. What is meant by the concept of security? In: *The globalization of world politics.* Baylis J and Smith S, editors. Oxford: Oxford University Press; 1997. p. 194.

52. Buzan B, *Peoples, states and fear: an agenda for international security studies in the post-Cold War era.* Hemel Hempstead: Harvester Wheatsheaf; 1991.

53. Hobbes T, *Leviathan.* Everyman's Library. New York: Dutton; 1950. p. 103–4.

54. United Nations Population Division. *The world at six billion.* New York: United Nations; 1999.

CHAPTER II

Gender, Health, and Security[1]

Sonali Johnson and Claudia García-Moreno

Introduction

There are different perspectives on the meaning of human security. For some, human security refers to freedom from fear and freedom from want (1). Others define it as a broad 'spider web' concept, encompassing a variety of issues that affect human experience. These issues are often interrelated and include, according to the UNDP definition: economic security, personal security, health security, environmental security, political security, food security, and community security (2). By incorporating different discourses into its analytical framework (e.g., development, human rights, legal, political), human security has the potential to address a wide range of social issues and conceptualize their impact upon individuals and collective societies.

Whichever definition is used, gender inequality is central to the human security framework. Access to and experience of basic security needs outlined above — such as economic opportunity, food, good health, natural resources, and so on — are all subject to socially defined gender norms and, particularly, to the unequal balance of power between women and men. Thus, human security is a gendered phenomenon.

Gender, broadly defined as the array of societal beliefs, norms, customs, and practices that define masculine and feminine attributes and behaviors, often acts as a filter leading to patterns of inclusion or exclusion in access to basic needs and services, including those related to health (3, 4, 5). It also affects the ability to protect oneself from disease, violence, and fear, and to exercise one's rights, resulting in different health and human security outcomes for women and men. Consequently, women and men often experience different sources of insecurity during the course of their lives. Women's insecurity in particular is often a direct result of societal gender norms, values, and expectations, hence the proposal to use the term *gender insecurity*. If half of the population is vulnerable to gender insecurity, the achievement of human security is clearly at stake.

This chapter discusses gender insecurity in the context of health. Health is an important marker of human security since it is a primary indicator of the welfare and subsequent survival of the individual, and a necessary condition for security. Health is often the area in which economic, personal, environmental, and other forms of insecurity interact, since insecurities or 'fear factors' experienced by individuals in a society often manifest in their mental or physical health. Understanding gender norms and values, and gender discrimination in particular, is crucial to public health since gender roles and unequal gender relations interact with other social and economic variables to produce different and often inequitable patterns of exposure to health risks as well as health outcomes. Gender is a factor in differential access to and utilization of health information, care, and services, where these differences have a clear impact on health outcomes. Gender also leads to different social and economic consequences of disease for women and men (6, 7).

The first part of this chapter discusses the influence of gender norms on the framework of most societies and its impact on health and human security, especially that of women. The gendered nature of the public and private spheres is highlighted, including the influence of inequality in power relations between women and men, particularly in negotiating access to resources. This section also reviews the impact of gender inequality on public health, including health seeking behavior and access to health care services.

The second part of the chapter focuses on two important public health issues: HIV/AIDS and gender-based violence. Both are closely related to gender inequality and impact profoundly on health and human security. Poverty, discrimination, and power inequalities facilitate the transmission and impact of HIV/AIDS with particularly severe consequences for women. There are also gender dimensions to the social and economic consequences of HIV/AIDS, including the responses to the epidemic at the household, community, and national levels.

Violence is also gendered, manifesting itself in different forms and with different consequences for men and women. Violence against women, in all its forms, is an extreme example of gender insecurity. It is part of the daily lives of many women and girls worldwide and is a major risk factor for their ill health. The causes of violence are complex and symptomatic of a number of inequalities associated with age, gender, socioeconomic, and cultural background. Violence against women, particularly that perpetrated by partners, underpins the lack of human security and health for many women. If women cannot be free from fear within their own homes, their overall health and well-being, as well as their sense of security and ability to pursue social opportunities and fulfill their potential, are deeply affected. There are also links between HIV/AIDS and gender-based violence that will be discussed in the section on gender-based violence.

The final section of the chapter outlines some action points and recommendations for addressing gender insecurity in health. In discussing gender-related insecurity, the purpose of this chapter is not to expose women as victims or men as perpetrators. It recognizes the agency of both men and women in dealing with the multitude of insecurities that may affect them during the course of their lives. The objective of the chapter, however, is to highlight general societal trends and inequities that are created or shaped by gender norms and values, and result in increased risk of insecurity and ill health for women.

GENDER INSECURITY IN THE PUBLIC AND PRIVATE DOMAINS

In order to understand gender insecurity in the context of public health it is necessary to discuss the significance of gender to the structure of society. To do this, it is important to make the critical distinction between sex and gender since the two are often erroneously used as interchangeable.

An individual's sex refers to those characteristics that are biologically determined. Gender however, is a social construct produced by learned behavior. This behavior is informed by social emphasis on biological difference that assigns diverse value and roles to women and men. One is born male or female but learns to be a man or a woman (8). Gender is not a fixed category but evolves over time and manifests differently in a variety of settings. However, gender is a fundamental thread in the social fabric, shaping women's and men's sense of identity and participation in society as a whole, as well as their differential access to and control over power, influence, and resources.

The sexual division of labor is apparent in both the public and private domains[2] and has been shaped by the understandings and expectations of what it means to be a man or woman (i.e., gender). Access to and involvement in the public and private spheres is greatly influenced by gender norms and stereotypes that discriminate against women, leading to inequity and insecurity. Historically and across most societies, women have been associated with the private sphere — that of the family and home. The public sphere, particularly the formal work place, has traditionally been the domain where men engage in their role as breadwinners. Women's household and childcare work are viewed as an extension of their physiology; their productive labor has been largely ignored by neoclassical economics (9). Women's contribution to family income tends to be overlooked because most of it is unpaid or takes the form of repetitive services rather than products that can be counted as contribution made (10). Although this situation is changing in many societies, gender norms and values that influence the types of jobs women and men typically occupy in the public sector, as well as the division of labor within the home environment, evolve much more slowly. Inequality is also demonstrated by the fact that women worldwide still earn far less than men for the same jobs (11).

Amartya Sen's model of *cooperative conflicts* illustrates the significance of the sexual division of labor as a social arrangement that affects inter-household allocation of resources (12). Sen argues that households face two types of problems simultaneously in securing the prosperity of the household. The first involves cooperation, where members contribute to total household capability, and the second involves conflict, where re-sources are divided among members of the household. Social arrangements regarding who does what, who consumes what, and who makes what decisions, are outcomes of what Sen refers to as the combined problem of cooperation and conflict. These decisions are arrived at through inter-household bargaining, where notions of hierarchy and authority, per-ceived[3] interest and perceived contribution to the household, come into play. Gender power relations are a factor in all of the above and conse-quently, inter-household allocation of resources often privileges men's interests over women's, especially where resources are scarce. Sen extends his argument even further to consider the outcome when the cooperative conflict union fails and terms this *the breakdown position* (12).

Gender inequalities are present in many societies, resulting in a higher rate of illiteracy and less access to education and economic opportunity for women, thus making their breakdown position worse than that of men. Women's fear of this position therefore affects their bargaining power in households where there is a greater likelihood of 'settling' and cooperat-ing with the social arrangement despite an unfavorable outcome relative to men. Fear of the breakdown position may also be a factor preventing women from leaving violent relationships. Therefore, intrafamily decisions involving significant inequalities in the allotment of food, money, and health care have important implications for the welfare, health, and se-curity of women (12).

GENDER INSECURITY AND HEALTH

According to a 1999 WHO report providing life tables for 191 countries, although sex differentials in life expectancy of three years and more in favor of women were observed in most countries (especially in more de-veloped countries), the differential was only half a year or less in coun-tries such as Nepal, Uganda, Turkey, and Djibouti, with male life expectancy exceeding that of females in a handful of countries including Zimbabwe, the Maldives, Namibia, and Botswana (13).

Women's longer life expectancy, compared to men's, is often used to imply that gender inequity with regard to health works in favor of women. However, data from the 2001 WHO World Health Report listing 2000 estimates of healthy life expectancy (HALE)[4] in all WHO member states shows that in every country, expectation of healthy years lost at birth for females is higher than males (14). Similarly, the percentage of total healthy life expectancy lost is consistently higher for females than for males. These data essentially show that although the probability of mortality may be higher in males than females, the probability of life with illness or disability is higher in females than males. In addition, in many countries women suffer from avoidable mortality, such as that related to pregnancy and childbirth (15).

In societies with son preference (mainly in South and Southeast Asia), gender discrimination may be experienced at birth through the practice of infanticide, and even pre-birth through sex-selective abortion (16, 17). The phenomenon of 'missing women' in India and China is a direct example of the impact of gender discrimination on the health and human security of millions of women.[5] Evidence of health and gender related insecurity for girls and women is also apparent in sex-selective nutrition and medical care for illness in certain countries (19).

The model of cooperative conflict, therefore, applies in childhood as well as adulthood. Since men are viewed as bringing home higher returns than women (especially in economic terms), more family resources may be spent on boys than on their sisters, particularly where resources are scarce and gender norms strongly favor males. A study conducted in Papua New Guinea on treatment seeking patterns for malaria, for example, found that mothers not only take their male infants more frequently to primary health clinics, but they also walk further with them in search of care (20).

In adulthood, access to and utilization of health services is also influenced by gender-related factors in many settings. Health service issues such as cost, distance, and opening hours may affect men and women differently, particularly where women have restricted mobility or less access to resources.

Two significant factors tend to delay women's decisions to seek treatment when ill: their workload in the home, and their care giving roles with small children or other family members who are sick (21, 22, 23). Other factors that affect women's access to health services include the need for permission from husbands or senior members of the household to seek treatment, and restrictions upon physical mobility outside the home (15, 20). Little data is available on the gender dimensions of the burden of cost for treatment. However, as stated earlier, in situations where resources are scarce, women may have less control over those resources and consequently may be less likely to seek treatment, especially for conditions that are not viewed as serious (22, 23) (Figure 1).

In addition, gender differences in decision-making may also affect access to health facilities. For example, a study conducted in Tanzania found that while men made independent decisions to seek voluntary counseling and testing (VCT) services for HIV/AIDS, women felt compelled to discuss

Figure 1.   Reasons for women's lack of access to health care

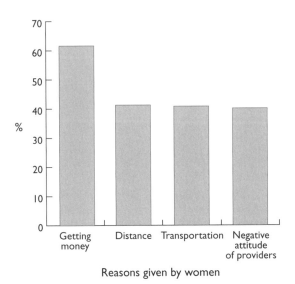

Source: Uganda Demographic Health Survey, 2000–2001.

testing with their partners before accessing the service (24). In some societies cultural taboos against consulting male practitioners may discourage women from visiting health facilities if they perceive these facilities to consist almost exclusively of male staff. In a study in Uganda, women reported that since most health workers are men, they could not discuss intimate problems such as STDs and HIV/AIDS with them (25). Similarly, many men may not seek services if they perceive these services to be directed exclusively at women, such as antenatal or family planning services.

It is well known that poverty is closely linked to increased risk of disease and ill health (for example, tuberculosis, malaria, HIV/AIDS, reproductive ill health, and malnutrition) as well as violence (26). While poverty affects the health and well-being of both men and women, as stated earlier, gender inequality often means that women are at a greater disadvantage in protecting their health in resource poor settings, since they may be less able to access prevention and treatment. For example, a study in Benin showed that since women were financially dependent on their husbands, they were unable to purchase insecticide treated nets (ITNs) for prevention of malaria without their husband's permission (27).

The intersections between poverty, gender inequality, and vulnerability to two major public health issues, HIV/AIDS and violence, will be discussed respectively in the next section.

GENDER INSECURITY AND HIV/AIDS

The HIV/AIDS pandemic continues to disrupt and destroy the fabric of families, communities, and societies around the world. According to current global estimates, the number of people living with HIV/AIDS is now 42 million (28), which is significantly higher than the 2000 estimates of 36.1 million (28). HIV/AIDS is a critical human security issue as it is a threat to socioeconomic development as well as to human survival (29).

In the early stages of the HIV/AIDS epidemic, infection was predominantly among men. However, as of the end of 2002, 50% of all new infections were occurring in women. Women constitute 19.2 million of the 38.6 million adults living with HIV/AIDS (28). Estimates from 2001, showed that in North Africa and the Middle East, women constituted 40% of HIV infected adults (30). Data from 2002 reveals that women now make up 55% of adults infected with HIV. In sub-Saharan Africa, 58% of HIV infected adults are women (28). The latest estimates show a higher prevalence rate for young women aged 15 to 24 years compared to young men of the same age (28) (Figure 2). Most men are infected 10 years later, between the ages of 25 and 35 (31).

Figure 2.   Sex distribution of young people (aged 15–24) living with HIV/AIDS, 2002

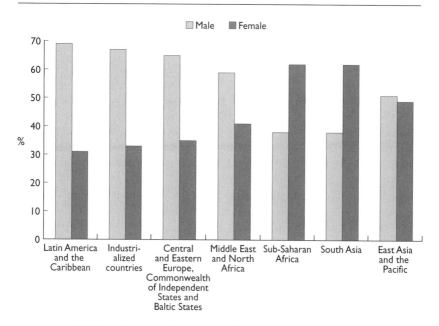

Source: UNAIDS/UNICEF 2001 in Young People and HIV/AIDS: Opportunity in Crisis; produced by UNICEF, UNAIDS, and WHO, 2002.

Evidence from some studies indicates that women may have higher biological vulnerability to HIV infection than men, since the odds of male to female transmission are significantly higher than those of female to male (32, 33). Although gender norms and values create pathways of vulnerability to HIV/AIDS for both men and women, a number of social factors, shaped by gender norms that reflect inequality, significantly increase vulnerability to HIV/AIDS for women, especially young women. Gender inequality is also apparent in the negative social and economic consequences of HIV/AIDS and determines the level and quality of care, treatment, and support received. Consequently, HIV/AIDS is a critical issue of gender insecurity.

Masculinity, femininity, and gender insecurity for HIV/AIDS

Attitudes towards sex, informed by gender norms and expectations, are an important factor in the increasing vulnerability to HIV infection for both men and women. However, the unequal power between girls and boys and women and men (i.e., gender inequality) means it is often more difficult for girls/women to protect themselves, as they cannot control where and when sex takes place as much as boys/men, nor can they enforce the use of condoms.

Notions of masculinity and femininity contain an inherent double standard in the accepted sexual behavior of men and women. In many societies, a culture of silence surrounding sexual issues and an emphasis on the virginity of unmarried women has resulted in shame, embarrassment, guilt, and consequently the reluctance of women to discuss their sexual health (3, 31). Studies report that many young women are afraid to seek information on contraception and sexually transmitted infections (STIs) since this may label them as sexually active regardless of the true extent of their sexual experience (31). Research also shows that young men do not seek information on STIs or HIV since ignorance about matters pertaining to sex may be viewed as a sign of weakness (34). A UNAIDS report on sexual behavior among young people, compiling research conducted in seven countries (Cambodia, Cameroon, Chile, Costa Rica, Papua New Guinea, the Philippines, and Zimbabwe), reveals that there is a marked perception that young men are sexual beings, while young women must retain their purity (35). In Cambodia, young men view the 'deflowering' of young women as the ultimate sport; however, a high value is placed on virgin brides. As the report states, "That they cannot see the paradox in the position in which they place young women, and find themselves, remains one of the great conundrums in sexual culture" (35).

Condoms and prevention of HIV/AIDS

The promotion and distribution of condoms is a major component of HIV/AIDS prevention programs. However, condom use is heavily influenced by notions of femininity and masculinity. In contexts where virility is seen as an integral part of masculinity and sexual innocence a marker of femininity, many young, sexually active women hesitate to insist on condom use for fear that they will be seen as promiscuous. Research conducted in Thailand as part of a Women and AIDS Research Program found that both young men and women interviewed felt that a girl who requests condom use would be perceived as 'bad,' 'unclean,' 'promiscuous,' or 'easy' (36).

Research carried out in several countries shows that communication between adults on sexual behavior and condom use is also problematic (37, 38). Many adult married women are unable to request that their partner wear a condom for fear of being accused of infidelity, abandonment, or violence (36). In response to the power issues surrounding male condoms, female condoms, which are used by women, have been heralded as an effective empowering alternative (39). Although female condoms have been well received by a number of women, their cost (often between four and ten times the price of male condoms) and usage difficulties may discourage many women from buying or using them. Other women still require the permission of their husbands (39).

Monogamy is often cited as a means to protect against HIV, yet marriage is often the context in which many women are exposed to HIV infection. The double standards of social norms, referred to above, often accept men having extramarital and premarital relationships as normal. Women's inability to negotiate safer sex, even when they suspect their partner may be infected with HIV, makes HIV infection a risk even among women with only one partner.

Men and women often have different levels of knowledge regarding HIV/AIDS. A recent analysis of levels of knowledge of HIV prevention in 23 developing countries found that on average, 75% of men had accurate knowledge about HIV/AIDS transmission and prevention, compared to 65% of women (40).

In most contexts, appropriate sexual behavior for men means heterosexual behavior, often with different female partners. These norms can render men who have sex with men particularly vulnerable since in many countries sex between men is highly stigmatized or illegal. This stigma acts as an important deterrent for men who have sex with men to obtain information on safe sex practices or to seek treatment when ill. Adolescent men may have sex with other males of their age group as well as older men. Younger-older male-to-male sexual relationships occur in many settings, and sex may be consensual or coercive (41). In either case, the young men concerned are vulnerable, especially if they are uninformed about the risks of acquiring HIV and are having sex with an older, more experienced partner. Men who have sex with men also may have sex with women. A study in India reveals that 90% of male clients of male sex workers are married (31). As a result, their wives are also exposed to potential infection.

POVERTY, GENDER INSECURITY, AND HIV/AIDS RISK

Economic dependence, lack of education, the inability to negotiate safe sex, as well as the need to resort to sex for a living contribute to the vulnerability of women and adolescent girls to HIV/AIDS. A study conducted in South Africa between 1992 and 1999 on women's awareness and responses to HIV/AIDS reveals that the lack of economic opportunity is viewed by many women as significantly increasing their risk of exposure to HIV. Many women were explicit about their economic needs, stating, "Poverty makes prostitutes of us." When asked who was most at risk, they immediately replied that women are, due to their economic dependency and knowing their partners have intercourse with other women. Women across the study sites experienced great difficulties in asking their partner to wear a condom, even when they were aware of their risk, for fear this could be viewed as challenging his authority (37).

The exchange of sex for money or food in situations of poverty has been reported in a variety of settings. Studies reveal that adolescent girls often engage in sex with older men for cash, while others are trafficked into the sex industry (31, 42). A study in Malawi found that two-thirds of the 168 female adolescents who reported having sexual intercourse acknowledged accepting money or gifts for sex (43). Many of these encounters involve coercion or violence.

In many societies, cultural norms support the early marriage of girls, often to older men (44). Anecdotal evidence reveals that in parts of Africa, men may seek younger partners for sex or marriage in the belief that they are 'safe' (45). Again, evidence suggests that in many instances, these encounters are not consensual but take place through force (46). In addition, older men typically have more sexual experience than adolescent girls and therefore are more likely to have been exposed to sexually transmitted infections, including HIV.

In addition to economic factors, gender inequality in the political and legal domains, as well as some cultural practices,[6] also have implications for women's health and human security. Lack of political representation may limit the number and quality of policies that address women's needs in health and other areas. In many countries women experience substantial discrimination in their legal status and treatment under the law compared to men. They may have only limited rights to hold, inherit, or dispose of property, or to make decisions about education, marriage, or the education of their children (47). These factors may put women at risk by increasing their poverty and making it more difficult for many to make independent decisions regarding their health and welfare.

STIGMA AND DISCRIMINATION

Stigma and discrimination may be seen as risk factors and outcomes of HIV/AIDS. Fear of stigma and discrimination may prevent men and women, and particularly adolescents, from seeking information about

HIV. Stigma attached to HIV/AIDS has resulted in segregation of HIV positive men and women in schools and hospitals, refusal and termination of employment, the denial of the right to marry, expulsion from communities and violence (48). However, HIV related stigma does not manifest equally among men and women. For instance, the previously mentioned UNAIDS study on sex and youth across seven sites found that in each study site, men with HIV were barely questioned about how they became infected and were generally treated well. Women, on the other hand, were often accused of having had extramarital sex (whether or not this was the case) and received lower levels of support (35).

Health workers usually share the gender norms and values of the wider society; these views are likely to be reflected in their attitudes towards patients. For instance, in Brazil, despite a policy of free and universal access to antiretroviral drugs for AIDS, women are often diagnosed at later stages of infection than men (3). Data suggests that women's lack of use of services could be the result, among other things, of the discrimination they face by health workers (3).

In addition to stigma and discrimination, the threat of violence may affect women's decisions to seek testing and counseling. In a recent review of studies of disclosure of HIV status, fear of abandonment (closely tied to fear of loss of economic support from their partner), fear of violence, and fear of rejection or discrimination were the most often mentioned barriers to disclosure (49). Disclosure-related violence ranged from 0.4% to 4% in U.S.A. and 3.5% to 14.6% in sub-Saharan Africa (49). The intersections between gender-based violence and HIV/AIDS are of increasing concern and will be discussed further in the next section.

Women bear the greatest burden of HIV/AIDS since they provide the majority of care and support to those affected by the disease. Their quality of life, economic situation, and security are therefore directly affected by this burden. AIDS widows often experience a severe decline in food security and in many cases face destitution and abandonment by relatives (25). Even in countries where both men and women engage in crop production, the death of a male household head can have a significant impact on food security for the family. A study of farming households in Kenya found that the decline in the total value of output was much more significant after the death of a male household head, compared to the death of other household members, including the death of a female spouse (50). The relative poverty of many female headed households compared to male headed households may make it more difficult for women to purchase treatment for a variety of health conditions including HIV/AIDS, and may severely affect their health and human security and that of their family.

To conclude, the evidence is overwhelming that gender norms, values, and relations impact on the HIV/AIDS epidemic. Therefore, it is critical that the norms and values that shape masculinity and femininity, and in particular gender inequality, be addressed by policies and programs aimed to control HIV/AIDS. Although gender inequality has been addressed in international policy recommendations such as the United Nations General Assembly Special Session on HIV/AIDS (UNGASS) Declaration of Commitment, it is urgent that national governments translate these commitments into concrete actions. Furthermore, it is necessary to implement measures that will elevate the status of women in general, address their specific needs, and reduce their vulnerability to HIV/AIDS.

GENDER-BASED VIOLENCE, HEALTH, AND HUMAN SECURITY

Violence is a pervasive public health problem that affects all aspects — mental, physical, and spiritual — of the health of individuals, as well as impacting on families and communities. Violence also violates human rights and as such, is a major contributor to human insecurity, especially with regard to personal safety. While the human security discourse has highlighted the impact of collective violence, particularly armed conflict, it is interpersonal violence that generates insecurity in the daily lives of many people globally (51).

Although both men and women experience violence, gender leads to different vulnerabilities to specific types of violence. The forms of violence experienced by women and men and their effects are therefore different. For instance, most of the violence that men encounter, such as homicide, criminal assault, drug-related crime, and violence in war, occurs in the public space. Women also encounter violence as a result of conflict and other social upheavals, and are exposed to violence in public spaces such as the work place and community. However, violence against women and girls occurs most frequently in the private sphere, by partners, other family members, or acquaintances. Thus, many women and girls live their daily lives in fear and insecurity, even in the spaces where they are meant to be 'secure.'

Significantly, most of the violence that women experience, whether in public or private, is directed against them by men and is often the result of unequal gender power in relationships. Consequently, violence against women is also referred to as *gender-based violence*. According to the United Nations Declaration on the Elimination of Violence Against Women, violence against women and girls is defined as "any form of gender-based violence that results in, or is likely to result in, physical, sexual, or psychological harm or suffering to women, including threats of such acts, coercion, or arbitrary deprivation of liberty, whether occurring in public or private life" (52).

Violence against women takes many forms, including physical, sexual, and psychological abuse, and can be perpetrated and/or condoned by the family, the community, and the state (53). Some forms of violence are linked to particular cultural or traditional practices of various countries, such as female genital mutilation, child marriage, murders in the name of honor ('honor killings')[7] or dowry-related abuse. Other forms of violence, such as trafficking of women and forced prostitution, are often linked to situations of extreme poverty, where gender roles and power relations within families and communities increase women's vulnerability.

Male dominance in the gender hierarchy does not by itself fully account for gender-based violence since it does not explain why some men indulge in violence and others do not. The ecological framework proposed by Heise et al. for violence against women (54) is a useful tool for understanding the multidimensional nature of gender-based violence. It consists of four levels of causative factors, many of which have been alluded to in the previous discussion on gender insecurity in the public and private domains.

All of the levels of the ecological framework include some dimension of gender inequality and discriminatory norms. The initial level refers to an individual and includes personal factors such as witnessing violence as a child. The second level is related to the immediate context (the family or relationship) within which abuse takes place and includes factors such as male dominance in the family, male control of household resources, and marital or verbal conflict. The third, or community, level refers to external structural inequalities that give women a subordinate status in the community and home environment. These include low socioeconomic status, unemployment, and social exclusion. The fourth societal level, or the *macrosystem*, is where the factors in all other levels are legitimized through societal acceptance of gender norms and values, including notions of masculinity linked to aggression and dominance (54). This framework is a useful way of understanding the multiple factors associated with violence and, in particular, the interaction across these factors in culturally diverse settings.

The social acceptance of gender inequality and discrimination is influenced by, and in turn reinforces, inequalities at the family and community levels, and therefore can lead to violence against women. Thus, changing the underlying gender norms is an important prerequisite for reducing violence against women and for achieving health and human security.

PARTNER VIOLENCE AND SEXUAL VIOLENCE

There are a growing number of studies documenting the prevalence of physical and sexual violence against women, particularly by partners and ex-partners. This data highlights partner violence as a major public and women's health problem worldwide (16). A review of a number of well designed, population-based surveys on partner violence indicates that between 10% to over 50% of women report having been abused physically by a male partner at least once in their lives (54, 51) (Table 1). This violence often persists and may even start during pregnancy. A review of

Table 1.   Prevalence of physical violence against women by an intimate male partner

Country	Coverage	Year of study	Sample size	Percentage of adult women who have been physically assaulted by an intimate partner		
				In past 12 months	In current relationship	Ever (in any relationship)
Australia (56)	Metro Melbourne	1993-1994	1,494[6]	22.4[5]		
Bangladesh (57)	National (villages)	1992	1,225	19.0		47.0
Canada (58)	National	1993	12,300	3.0[3]		29.0
Canada (59)	Toronto	1991-1992	420[4]			27.4
Chile (60)	Metro Santiago and Santiago province	1993[2]	1,000		26.0	
Chile (61)	Santiago	1997	310	22.5		
Colombia (62)	National	1995	6,097[4]			19.3
Egypt (63)	National	1995-1996	7,121			34.4
Ethiopia (64)	Meskanena Woreda	1995	673	10.0[1]		45.0
India (65)	Rural areas in 2 states	1993-1994	1,842		40.0	
Kenya (66)	Kisii District	1984-1987	612		42.0	
Korea, Republic of (67)	National	1989	707	37.5[5]		
Mexico (68)	Durango City	1996	384			40.0
Mexico (69)	Metropolitan Guadalajara	1996	650	15.0		27.0
Netherlands (70)	National	1986	1,016			20.8
Nicaragua (71)	Leon	1993	360		27.0[5]	52.2
Nicaragua (72)	Managua	1997	378	30.2		
Nigeria (73)	Not stated	1993[2]	1,000			31.4
Norway (74)	Trondheim	1989[2]	111			18.0
Papua New Guinea (75)	National, rural (villages)	1982	628			67.0
Papua New Guinea (75)	National, Port Moresby (low income)	1984	298			56.1
Paraguay (76)	Western state, except Chaco region	1995-1996	6,465[4]			9.5
Peru (77)	Metropolitan Lima (middle and low income)	1997[2]	359	30.9		
Philippines (78)	National	1993	8,481			5.1
Puerto Rico (79)	National	1993-1996	7,079[4]			48.2
Switzerland (80)	National	1994-1996	1500	6.3[3]		12.6
Thailand (81)	Bangkok	1994	619		20.0	
Turkey (82)	East and Southeast Anatolia	1998	599[4]			
Uganda (83)	Lira & Masaka Districts	1995-1996	1,660		40.5	57.9
United Kingdom (84)	North London	1993[2]	430[4]	12.0		30.0
United States of America (85)	National	1998	8,000[4]	1.3		22.1
West Bank & Gaza Strip (86)	National (Palestinians)	1995	2,410	48.0		

1   In past 3 months.
2   The year of publication is listed because the research paper did not state fieldwork dates.
3   Physical or sexual contact.
4   Sample group included women who had never been in a relationship and therefore were not in exposed group.

5   Definition includes throwing objects.
6   Respondents were recruited from women visiting medical practitioners' offices or hospitals/health care centers.

Source: World Health Organization database on violence against women (as of July 1999).

studies on the prevalence of violence against pregnant women found that prevalence of physical violence ranged from 0.9% to 20.1% (55).

A multicountry study coordinated by the World Health Organization (WHO) is gathering comparable data on violence against women, by partners and ex-partners, and many other aspects of women's health and lives in seven countries (Bangladesh, Brazil, Japan, Namibia, Peru, United Republic of Tanzania, and Thailand) (87). Preliminary analysis confirms that violence against women by current and past partners is highly prevalent in all sites studies (88). For example, in Lima, Peru, 23% of women reported sexual violence while in the rural region of Cusco, Peru, 47% reported sexual assault (89).

Data on sexual violence is more limited, but in general shows that around one in five women have experienced some form of sexual violence by partners, strangers, or acquaintances (51). Sexual abuse during childhood is another form of violence that is more widespread than previously believed. A meta analysis prepared for WHO on child sexual abuse found that prevalence was 25% for females and 8% for males (90).

The high prevalence rates within the family of violence against women and abuse of children merit deep analysis by those concerned with health and human security. They impact profoundly on freedom from fear and on people's ability to exercise choice, pursue social opportunities, and plan for their futures, all considered hallmarks of human freedom and security (91). Since gender-based violence, particularly violence within the family, affects women in practically all societies and across different social classes, religions, and cultures, it is essential to address this issue in order to achieve human security for the entire population.

TRAFFICKING AND GENDER INSECURITY

Trafficking is another compelling example of human insecurity and, as it often involves women and girls, is also a form of gender-based violence. Trafficking of women and children feeds on poverty and vulnerability and commonly entails violence, deception, intimidation, and coercion of vulnerable groups. The expansion of transnational sex industries, in combination with local demand, is considered to be a major contributing factor to trafficking (92, 93). Women are most commonly affected, as trafficking most often fills a demand for jobs that require 'feminine attributes,' such as work in the 'entertainment industry,' domestic help, and the manufacturing sector (92).

Although instances of trafficking are vastly underreported due to fear or stigma, available data indicate that a vast number of women are being trafficked both within countries and internationally. In recent years, countries of the former Soviet Union and those of Eastern and Central Europe have become the main sources of trafficked women and children in Western Europe for indecent labor and commercial sexual exploitation. It is estimated that over 175,000 persons are trafficked annually from this region (94).

In 1999, U.S. governmental and nongovernmental experts estimated that 45,000 to 50,000 women and children were trafficked to the United States. The primary source countries appear to be Thailand, Vietnam, China, Mexico, Russia, Ukraine, and the Czech Republic, although women have also been trafficked to the U.S. from other countries (95). A CIA report on the problem of trafficking in the U.S. states that women are primarily trafficked into the sex industry, working in prostitution, stripping, peep and touch shows, and massage parlors that offer sexual services. Women are also trafficked into sweatshop labor, agricultural work, domestic servitude, and hotels and motels as maids. The average age of trafficked women is estimated at 20 years old, yet the report states that some women from Asia may have been trafficked at a younger age to cities such as Bangkok before being trafficked to the U.S. (95).

A variety of health problems may result from trafficking, such as mental trauma, injury, unwanted pregnancy and abortion, and sexually transmitted infections, including infection with HIV. A report on the trafficking of Burmese women and girls into brothels in Thailand found that 50 to 70% of the women and girls interviewed were HIV positive (93).

VIOLENCE AGAINST WOMEN IN ARMED CONFLICT

Armed conflict is undoubtedly a major concern when considering human security and health. Any war has a profound impact on women and men, boys and girls. Men often bear the brunt of combat as part of the warring factions, but conflicts greatly affect the human security of civilians. Human rights abuses, including rape and other forms of violence are a common occurrence in war (96). Throughout the history of conflict, in addition to injury and death, rape and other forms of sexual abuse have been inflicted upon women as weapons of war. It is estimated that between 20,000 and 50,000 women were raped as part of a deliberate strategy during the 1992–1995 conflict in Bosnia-Herzegovina (97). A mission undertaken by the Special Rapporteur on Violence against Women to Sierra Leone found that all the warring factions committed gross violations of human rights. The following is an excerpt from the report:

> "According to statistics based on 733 testimonies collected from Sierra Leonean women and girls, 72 percent of them reported having experienced human rights abuses. Over 50 percent of them reported having been subject to sexual violence; 47 percent reported having been raped; 55.7 percent reported having been gang raped; and 1.4 percent reported having been raped with a foreign object....Slightly less than half of the interviewees (41.7 percent) were abducted by the various factions. Of these interviewees, the majority (87.9 percent) reported having been raped and subjected to sexual slavery; 8.2 percent reported that they were forced to marry their abductor; 1.6 percent reported that they were forcibly conscripted" (98).

HEALTH CONSEQUENCES OF VIOLENCE

The health consequences of violence can be very serious. It increases the risk for a variety of adverse health conditions and premature death. Violence against women can affect physical, mental, and reproductive and sexual health. Survivors of abuse commonly suffer a variety of trauma-induced symptoms such as depression, alcohol abuse, obsessive-compulsive disorder, eating and sleeping disorders, and anxiety (51). In addition to injuries, intimate partner violence is often associated with chronic pain syndromes, gastrointestinal and gynecological problems, unwanted pregnancy, and sexually transmitted infections including HIV/AIDS (99, 51). Violence against women during pregnancy is associated with low birth weight, miscarriage, or perinatal death (51).

There is a growing recognition of the interactions between violence and HIV/AIDS, where violence can have both a direct and an indirect impact on women's reproductive health and their susceptibility to HIV infection (96). Sexual violence increases the risk of vaginal tearing and therefore heightens susceptibility to contracting STIs, including HIV. In a study in Rwanda, more than 3% of women had been raped, almost half of them teenagers. Of the women who had been raped, 17% tested HIV positive, compared to 11% of those who had not been raped (28).

As mentioned earlier, the threat of physical violence may deter women from asking their partner to wear a condom even when they suspect that their partner may be infected. Violence can also be an outcome of revealing a positive HIV status within households or communities. Although HIV positive men may face violence, evidence shows that women are more vulnerable to violence associated with their HIV infection than men. A study in the U.S., for example, found that 20.5% of women surveyed reported physical harm after HIV diagnosis, compared with 11.5% of men reporting sex with men and 7.5% of heterosexual men (100).

OTHER CONSEQUENCES OF VIOLENCE

Gender-based violence impacts not only women's health, but all aspects of their lives. It hinders women's productivity and ability to participate in public life, and seems to have a consistent impact on women's earnings and their ability to remain in a job (101). In addition, studies on domestic violence from Latin America by the Inter-American Development Bank find an impact on overall productivity (102).

THE RESPONSE TO PARTNER VIOLENCE

The response of women to violent situations is not uniform, but often depends upon the options available to them. Most women who experience domestic violence are not passive victims but use active strategies to maximize their safety and that of their children. These strategies include resistance, leaving the violent situation, and attempting to 'keep the peace' with their husbands (54). However, the prevalence of violence by intimate partners, especially sexual violence and psychological abuse, is vastly underreported. A variety of reasons contribute to this situation, including shame, fear of retribution, and stigma.

Data from different contexts illustrate that many women share the notion that men have the right to discipline their wives through use of force (54). For example, a study conducted in rural Egypt in 1996 found that at least 80% of women interviewed felt that beatings are justified under certain circumstances, such as when a woman refuses her husband sex. Approximately 59% of high school females in Papua New Guinea felt that violence is justified if a woman speaks disrespectfully to her husband (54).

These findings illustrate the deep-rooted nature of gender norms and the accepted behavior of men and women. Gender-based violence often occurs in an environment that accepts gender inequality as a natural occurrence. The socialization of gender inequality and internalization of gender values and norms by both women and men means that some women may feel that this is normal behavior and just 'the way things are.'

A major problem in combating gender-based violence in a number of countries is that it is considered to be a private or family affair, even by public services such as the police or health care sector. Health personnel often are not trained to deal with women suffering violence, or may feel inadequate, powerless, and isolated, especially in areas with few referral services (53). Others may feel that a woman should be able to stop the violence at any time by leaving her partner, or imply that the woman herself provoked the incident (15).

Structural factors may impede reporting, especially in instances of sexual violence. In many under resourced settings, there may be no private facilities and examination rooms. In such cases, the perpetrator of the violence may accompany a woman to an interview by medical staff, and fear of reprisal may affect the truthfulness of her account. Health services may not have the resources or staff to provide adequate treatment and care or to do a forensic examination when necessary. They also may not have the capacity to conduct proper counseling or refer women to appropriate services. Finally, in some settings health workers and providers may be unsympathetic and even abusive of women, to the point where women may be revictimized by the services. Ultimately, the health sector is often not in a position to ensure the safety and security of a woman who has come to report a violent incident and seek treatment.

CONCLUSIONS AND RECOMMENDATIONS

Gender dynamics in households, communities, and institutions affect access to food, health care, education, income, and employment — all elements of human security — usually to the disadvantage of women. Consequently, gender inequality is at the heart of human security and must be addressed in order to achieve health and human security for all humanity.

Gender issues must be addressed by programs and policies designed to create more equitable patterns of health and development. Such programs must be participatory and take into account the variety of women's needs and interests, while ensuring their security, and promoting their empowerment.

Eradicating gender-based violence is key to achieving both health and human security for women, and requires a concerted multisectoral response that has community backing and strong political commitment. Prevention strategies must include challenging gender discrimination by changing attitudes, norms, and behaviors that promote or tolerate violence against women, as well as addressing other sources of vulnerability to violence, such as poverty.

The following recommendations address gender issues in public health, including gender-based violence:

■ All data on the burden of disease and other aspects of health must be disaggregated by sex and analyzed from a gender perspective. In addition, more research is needed on the gender dimensions of health seeking behavior of women and men and on the health service response for a cross section of health conditions. Ultimately, health policies and programs need to respond more effectively to the specific needs of women and men, girls and boys.

■ Rather than use interventions based upon stereotyped notions of gender roles, it is important to design interventions to promote equitable relationships based on the reality of women's and men's lives in a particular community or setting.

■ HIV/AIDS programs and interventions must prioritize gender issues, including gender-based violence. As a minimum, programs should not foster stereotypes that are harmful to health in the long term. Services such as voluntary testing and counseling need to address the gender-related barriers to testing and disclosure.

■ HIV/AIDS Information, Education, and Communication (IEC) programs for adolescents should incorporate gender issues into their framework. Such programs should enable young men and women to have a better understanding of how norms related to masculinity and femininity increase vulnerability to HIV, and help them think about how to work towards relationships that are equitable, respectful, and responsible.

■ Health care providers and facilities must be able to identify and provide sympathetic and appropriate health care or referral to those suffering from violence and its consequences. This approach will require concerted training and support as well as structural changes to health services and close linkages with local services.

- A zero tolerance attitude towards gender violence should be promoted by the health community and integrated into interventions for a variety of health conditions. Awareness messages about how violence affects the health and lives of women, their families, and children could be promoted through the mass media and other health initiatives.

- Men must be encouraged to share in care giving responsibilities and in transforming gender norms. For example, involving men in prevention of mother to child transmission of HIV programs can increase men's awareness and sense of responsibility. Awareness programs can also inform men and women about how inequality and violence contribute to instability and disharmony within families and communities.

- Governments and others can improve the health and security of women by ensuring their access not just to health care but also to education, employment, and equal pay as men for the same job and political representation. All these factors are critical to achieve health and human security.

In the long term, public health and human security need to integrate a gender perspective more fully into their analyses and responses. These must not reinforce existing gender notions that discriminate against women, but rather promote equity in health care and overall, as well as women's empowerment. It is only when women are empowered that they can realize all of their capacities, participate fully in society, and live free from fear in their homes and communities. Women's empowerment and gender equality are therefore key foundation stones for achieving health and human security.

NOTES

[1] © Copyright World Health Organization 2003. All rights reserved. The World Health Organization has granted the publisher permission for the reproduction of this article.

[2] Although the public/private dichotomy is an artificial distinction and can be blurred, particularly in the case of some agrarian societies, it is often useful in theorizing men's and women's participation in social networks.

[3] Note that for both interest and contribution, *perceived* is distinct from *actual* interest or contribution made.

[4] Healthy life expectancy (HALE) is based on life expectancy (LEX) but includes an adjustment for time spent in poor health. HALE measures the equivalent number of years in full health that a newborn child can expect to live based on the current mortality rates and prevalence distribution of health states in the population (14).

⁵ Exact figures for the global shortfall of women vary, but some estimate that the number of missing women may exceed 100 million (18). The growing imbalance between men and women in countries such as China has created new issues in gender relations as many men are unable to find wives.

⁶ For example, 'widow cleansing' which is practiced in parts of Africa, where a widow is expected to have sex with or marry one of her dead husband's brothers.

⁷ Honor killings refers to the killing of women who have sexual activity outside marriage, including rape and forced sex, by their own male family members with the claim to protect 'family honor.'

REFERENCES

1. Annan K. Secretary-General salutes international workshop on human security in Mongolia. Press release SG/AM/7382. Two-day session in Ulaanbaatar; 2000 May 8–10.

2. UNDP. Human development report 1994. New York: Oxford University Press; 1994. p. 23.

3. WHO. Integrating gender into HIV/AIDS programmes. Review paper for Expert Consultation, WC 503.71. 2002 Jun 3–5; Geneva, Switzerland.

4. Doyal L. Gender equity in health: debates and dilemmas. *Social Science & Medicine* 2000;51:931–9.

5. Hartigan P. The importance of gender in defining and improving quality of care: some conceptual issues. *Health Policy and Planning* 2001;16(Suppl 1):7–12.

6. Vlassof C, García-Moreno C. Placing gender at the centre of health programming: challenges and limitations. *Social Science & Medicine* 2002;54:1713–23.

7. Moss N. Gender equity and socioeconomic inequality: a framework for the patterning of women's health. *Social Science & Medicine* 2002;54:649–61.

8. Butler J. *Gender trouble: feminism and the subversion of identity*. London: Routledge; 1990.

9. Mies M. *Patriarchy and accumulation on a world scale: women in the international division of labor*. London: Zed Books; 1986.

10. Elson D. *Male bias in the development process*. 2nd ed. Manchester: Manchester University Press; 1995.

11. Plantenga J, Hansen J, Heidi I, Carnoy M, Claes M, Elder S, et al. International Labour Organization. Women, gender, and work (Part II). *International Labour Review* 1999;138(4):special issue.

12. Sen AK. Cooperative conflicts. In: Tinker I, editor. *Persistent inequalities*. Oxford: Oxford University Press; 1990.

13. Lopez AD, Saloman J, Ahmad O, Murray C, Mafat D. Life tables for 191 countries: data, methods, and results. GPE discussion paper series No. 9. Geneva: World Health Organization; 1999.

14. World Health Organization. *World health report 2001*. Geneva: World Health Organization; 2001.

15. World Health Organization. Women of South-East Asia: a health profile. Delhi: WHO Regional Office for South-East Asia; 2000.

16. Watts C, Zimmerman C. Violence against women: global scope and magnitude. *The Lancet* 2002 Apr 6;359(9313):1232–7.

17. Kristof ND. China: ultrasound abuse in sex selection. *Women's Health Journal* 1993 Oct–Dec;4:16–7.

18. Sen A. Many faces of gender inequality: an essay by Amartya Sen. *Frontline* 2001;18(22):4–15.

19. Osmani S, Sen A. The hidden penalties of gender inequality: fetal origins of ill-health. *Economics and Human Biology* 2003;1:105–21.

20. Muller I, Smith T, Mellor S, Rare L, Genton B. The effect of distance from home on attendance at a small rural health centre in Papua New Guinea. *International Journal of Epidemiology* 1998;27:878–84.

21. Vlassof C, Bonilla E. Gender-related differences in the impact of tropical diseases on women: what do we know? *Journal of Biosocial Science* 1994;26:37–53.

22. Okojie CE. Gender inequalities of health in the Third World. *Social Science & Medicine* 1994;39(9):1237–47.

23. Standing H. Gender and equity in health sector reform programmes: a review. *Health Policy and Planning* 1997;12(1):1–18.

24. Maman S, Mbwambo J, Hogan NM, Kilonzo GP, Sweat M. HIV and violence: the implications for HIV voluntary counselling and testing (VCT), Dar es Salaam, Tanzania. Meeting report, WHO/FCH/GWH/01.8. In: *Violence against women and HIV/AIDS: setting the research agenda*. Geneva: World Health Organization; 2001.

25. Topouzis D. The socio-economic impact of HIV/AIDS on rural families with an emphasis on youth. Rome: Food and Agricultural Organization of the United Nations; 1994 Feb. Available from: URL: http://www.fao.org/docrep/t2942e/t2942e02.htm, accessed on 2002 Oct 15.

26. Gwatkin DR, Guillot M. The burden of disease among the global poor: current situation, future trends, and implications for strategy. Washington: The World Bank; 2000.

27. Rashed S, Johnson H, Dongier P, Moreau R, Lee C, Crépeau R, et al. Determinants of the permethrin impregnated bednets (PIB) in the Republic of Benin: the role of women in the acquisition and utilization of PIBs. *Social Science & Medicine* 1999;(49):993–1005.

28. UNAIDS. AIDS epidemic update, UNAIDS/02.46E. Geneva: Joint United Nations Programme on HIV/AIDS (UNAIDS) and World Health Organization (WHO); 2002 Dec.

29. Kristoffersson U. HIV/AIDS as a human security issue: a gender perspective. Expert group meeting on The HIV/AIDS pandemic and its gender implications; 2000 Nov 13–17; Windhoek, Namibia. Available at: URL: http://www.unorg/womenwatch/daw/csw/hivaids/kristoffersson.htm, accessed on 2002 Aug 6.

30. UNAIDS. AIDS epidemic update, UNAIDS/01.74/WHO/CDS/CSR/NCS/2001. Geneva: Joint United Nations Programme on HIV/AIDS (UNAIDS) and World Health Organization (WHO); 2001.

31. UNAIDS. Gender and HIV/AIDS: taking stock of research and programmes, UNAIDS/99.16E. Geneva: Joint United Nations Programme on HIV/AIDS; 1999.

32. Padian N, Shiboski S, Jewell N. Female-to-male transmission of human immunodeficiency virus. *Journal of the American Medical Association* 1991 Sep 25;266(12):1664–7.

33. Nicolosi A, Corrêa Leite ML, Musicco M, Arici C, Gavazzeni G, et al. The efficiency of male-to-female and female-to-male sexual transmission of the human immunodeficiency virus: a study of 730 stable couples. *Epidemiology* 1994 Nov;5(6):570–5.

34. United Nations Development Programme (UNDP). HIV/AIDS and the challenges facing men. Issues paper No.15; 2001. Available at: URL: http://www.undp.org/hiv/publications/issues/english/issue15e.htm, accessed on 2001 Jun 1.

35. UNAIDS. Sex and youth: contextual factors affecting risk for HIV/AIDS, UNAIDS/99.26E. Geneva: UNAIDS; 1999.

36. Weiss E, Rao Gupta G. Bridging the gap: addressing gender and sexuality in HIV prevention. Washington: International Center for Research on Women; 1998.

37. Susser I, Stein Z. Culture, sexuality, and women's agency in the prevention of HIV/AIDS in southern Africa. *American Journal of Public Health* 2000 Jul;90(7):1042–8.

38. Welbourn A. Gender, sex, and HIV: how to address issues that no one wants to hear about. Paper presented at "Tant qu'on a la Santé" symposium; 1999 Jan; Geneva, Switzerland.

39. Kaler A. "It's some kind of women's empowerment": the ambiguity of the female condom as a marker of female empowerment. *Social Science & Medicine* 2002 Mar;52(5):783–96.

40. Gwatkin DR, Deveshwar-Bahl G. Inequalities in knowledge of HIV/AIDS prevention: an overview of socio-economic and gender differentials in developing countries. In: Integrating gender into HIV/AIDS programmes. Review paper for expert consultation; 2002 Jun 3–5; Geneva, Switzerland. Geneva: World Health Organization; 2002.

41. UNAIDS. AIDS and men who have sex with men. UNAIDS Technical Update, May 2000. Geneva: UNAIDS; 2000.

42. Poudel P, Carryer J. Girl-trafficking, HIV/AIDS, and the position of women in Nepal. *Gender and Development* 2000 Jul;8(2):74–9.

43. Weiss E, Whelan D, Rao Gupta G. Vulnerability and opportunity: adolescents and HIV/AIDS in the developing world. Washington: International Center for Research on Women; 1996.

44. Population Council. Early marriage in a human rights context. Supporting event of the United Nations special session on children; 2002 May 8–10; New York, New York.

45. Schoepf BG. AIDS, sex, and condoms: African healers and the reinvention of tradition in Zaire. *Medical Anthropology* 1992;14:225–42.

46. Wood K, Maforah K, Jewkes R. "He forced me to love him": putting violence on adolescent sexual health agendas. *Social Science & Medicine* 1998 Jul;47(2):233–42.

47. Matlin S, Spence N. The gender aspects of the HIV/AIDS pandemic. Expert group meeting on the HIV/AIDS pandemic and its gender implications. 2000 Nov 13–17; Windhoek, Namibia.

48. UNAIDS. HIV and AIDS-related stigmatization, discrimination, and denial: forms, contexts, and determinants. Research studies from Uganda and India; UNAIDS/00.16E. Geneva: UNAIDS; 2000 Jun.

49. Maman S, Medley A. Gender dimensions of HIV status disclosure to sexual partners: rates, barriers, and outcomes. Geneva: World Health Organization. In press 2003.

50. Yamano T, Jayne TS. Measuring the impacts of prime-age adult death on rural households in Kenya. Tegemeo Working Paper 5. Tegemeo Institute of Agricultural Policy and Development; 2002 Oct; Nairobi, Kenya.

51. World Health Organization. *World report on violence and health*. Geneva: World Health Organization; 2002.

52. United Nations. Declaration on the elimination of violence against women. General Assembly. New York: United Nations; 1993.

53. García-Moreno C. Violence against women: consolidating a public health agenda. In: Sen G, George A, Ostlin P, editors. *Engendering international health: the challenge of equity*. Cambridge (MA): MIT Press; 2002.

54. Heise L, Ellsberg M, Gottemoeller M. Ending violence against women. Population reports, series L, No.11; Population Information Program. Baltimore: John Hopkins University of Public Health; 1999 Dec.

55. Gazmararian JA, Lazorick S, Spitz AM, Ballard TJ, Saltzman LE, Marks JS. Prevalence of violence against pregnant women. *Journal of the American Medical Association* 1996 Jun 26;275(24):1915–20.

56. Mazza D, et al. Physical, sexual, and emotional violence against women: a general practice-based prevalence study. *Medical Journal of Australia* 1996;164(1):14–7.

57. Schuler SR, et al. Credit programs, patriarchy and men's violence against women in rural Bangladesh. *Social Science and Medicine* 1996;43(12):1729–42.

58. Rodgers K. Wife assault: the findings of a national survey. *Juristat Service Bulletin of the Canadian Centre for Justice Statistics* 1994;14(9):1–22.

59. Randall M, et al. Sexual violence in women's lives: findings from the women's safety project, a community-based survey. *Violence Against Women* 1995,1(1):6–31.

60. Larrain-Heiremans S. Violencia familiar y la situacion de la mujer en Chile. [Domestic violence and the situation of women in Chile.] Unpublished; 1993.

61. Morrison A, et al. The socio-economic impact of domestic violence against women in Chile and Nicaragua. Washington: Inter-American Development Bank; 1997.

62. Demographic and Health Surveys (DHS). Encuesta national de demografia y salud 1995. [National Demographic and Health Survey 1995.] Colombia: Profamilia and DHS/Institute for Resource Development and Macro International; 1991.

63. Demographic and Health Surveys (DHS). Egypt demographic and health survey. Cairo, Egypt: National Population Council and Macro International; 1995.

64. Deyessa N, et al. Magnitude, type, and outcomes of physical violence against married women in Butajira, southern Ethiopia. Unpublished; 1996.

65. Jejeebhoy S, et al. State accountability for wife-beating: the Indian challenge. *The Lancet* 1997;348(Suppl):SI10–2.

66. Raikes A. Pregnancy, birthing, and family planning in Kenya: changing patterns of behaviour. A health service utilization study in Kisii District. Copenhagen, Denmark: Centre for Development Research; 1990.

67. Kim K, et al. Epidemiological survey of spousal abuse in Korea. In: Viano E, editor. *Intimate violence: interdisciplinary perspectives*. Washington: Hemisphere Publishing Corporation; 1992.

68. Alvarado-Zaldivar G, et al. Prevalencia de violencia doméstica en la ciudad de Durango. [The prevalence of domestic violence in the city of Durango.] *Salud pública de México* 1998;40(6):481–6.

69. Ramirez Rodriguez JC, et al. *Una espada de doble filo: la salud reproductiva y la violencia doméstica contra la mujer.* [A double edged sword: reproductive health and domestic violence against women.] Presentation to Seminario Salud reproductiva en América Latina y el Caribe: temas y problemas; 1996; Brazil.

70. Römkens R. Prevalence of wife abuse in the Netherlands. *Journal of Interpersonal Violence* 1997;12(1):99–125.

71. Ellsberg MC. *Candies in hell: domestic violence against women in Nicaragua.* Umea, Sweden: Department of epidemiology and public health, Umea University; 1997.

72. Morrison A, et al. *The socioeconomic impact of domestic violence against women in Chile and Nicaragua.* Washington: Inter-American Development Bank; 1997.

73. Odujinrin O. Wife battering in Nigeria. *International Journal of Gynecology and Obstetrics* 1993;41:159–64.

74. Schei B, et al. Gynaecological impact of sexual and physical abuse by spouses: a study of a random sample of Norwegian women. *British Journal of Obstetrics and Gynecology* 1989;96:1379–83.

75. Bradley C. Wife-beating in Papua New Guinea: is it a problem? *Papua New Guinea Medical Journal* 1988;31:257–68.

76. Centro Paraguaya de estudios de poblacion. Encuestra nacional de demografia y salud reproductiva, 1995–1996. [National demographic and reproductive health survey 1995–1996.] Paraguay: Centro Paraguaya de estudios de poblacion [Paraguayan center for population studies]; 1996.

77. Gonzales de Olarte E, et al. *Poverty and domestic violence against women in metropolitan Lima.* Washington: Inter-American Development Bank; 1997.

78. Demographic and Health Surveys (DHS). Domestic violence and rape. In: *National safe motherhood survey 1993.* Calverton (MD): Macro International Inc.; 1994.

79. Departmento de Salud y la Escuela de Salud Pública de la Universidad de Puerto Rico and Centers for Disease Control and Prevention Puerto Rico. Encuesto de salud reproductiva 1995–1996. [Reproductive health survey, 1995–1996, summary of findings.] *Resumen de los Hallazgos.* Puerto Rico: Universidad de Puerto Rico/CDC; 1998.

80. Gillioz L, et al. Domination masculine et violences envers les femmes dans la famille en Suisse. [Male dominance and violence against women in the family in Switzerland.] Geneva, Switzerland: Unpublished; 1996.

81. Hoffman KL, et al. Physical wife abuse in a non-western society: an integrated theoretical approach. *Journal of Marriage and the Family* 1994;56:131–46.

82. Ilkkaracan P, et al. Exploring the context of women's sexuality in eastern Turkey. *Reproductive Health Matters* 1998;6(12):66–75.

83. Blanc AK, et al. *Negotiating reproductive outcomes in Uganda.* Kampala: Institute of Statistics and Applied Economics and Macro International Inc., Makere University; 1996.

84. Mooney J. *The hidden figure: domestic violence in North London.* London: Middlesex University; 1993.

85. United States Department of Justice. *Prevalence, incidence, and consequences of violence against women: findings from the national violence against women survey.* Washington: U.S. Department of Justice; 1998.

86. Haj-Yahia MM. *The incidence of wife-abuse and battering and some sociodemographic correlates as revealed in two national surveys in Palestinian society.* The Palestinian Authority Ramallah: Besir Center for Research and Development; 1998.

87. World Health Organization. WHO multi-country study on women's health and domestic violence against women; WHO/FCH/GWH/02.2. Geneva: World Health Organization; 2002 Jun.

88. García-Moreno C. Personal communication with Sonali Johnson; 2003 Mar 18.

89. Flora Tristan Center for Peruvian Women and WHO. Violencia Sexual y Fisica contra las mujeres en el Peru. [Physical and sexual violence against women in Peru]. Lima, Peru: Cayetano Heredia Peruvian University; 2002.

90. WHO Collaborating Centre for Evidence and Health Policy in Mental Health. Comparative risk assessment: child sexual abuse. Sydney, Australia: St. Vincent's Hospital; 2001 May 4.

91. Chen LC, Narasimhan V. A human security agenda for global health. In: Chen L, Leaning J, Narasimhan V, editors. *Global Health Challenges for Human Security*. Cambridge (MA): Global Equity Initiative, Asia Center, Faculty of Arts and Sciences, Harvard University; 2003.

92. Boonchalaksi W, Guest P. Prostitution in Thailand. Phuttamonthon, Thailand: Institute for Population and Social Research, Mahidol University; 1994.

93. Asia Watch and The Women's Right Project. A modern form of slavery: trafficking of Burmese women and girls into brothels in Thailand. New York: Human Rights Watch; 1993.

94. UNFPA (United Nations Population Fund). A conceptual framework for integrating the prevention and control of trafficking in women and children in population and development programmes. New York: United Nations; 2002 Sep.

95. Richard A. International trafficking in women to the United States: a contemporary manifestation of slavery and organized crime. An intelligence monograph; DCI Exceptional Intelligence Analyst Program. Washington: Center for the Study of Intelligence; 1999 Nov.

96. García-Moreno C, Watts C. Violence against women: its importance for HIV/AIDS. *AIDS* 2000;14(Suppl 3):S253–65.

97. UNICEF (United Nations Children's Fund). Women in transition. The MONEE project CEE/CIS/Baltics regional monitoring report No.6. Florence (Italy): United Nations Children's Fund International Child Development Centre; 1999.

98. United Nations, ECOSOC. Commission on Human Rights, 58th Session. Report of the special rapporteur, Ms. Radhika Coomaraswamy, on violence against women, its causes and consequences, submitted in accordance with Commission on Human Rights, resolution 2001/49*. Mission to Sierra Leone 2001 Aug 21–29. Geneva: United Nations; 2002.

99. Campbell JC. Health consequences of intimate partner violence. *The Lancet* 2002 Apr 13;359(9314):1331–6.

100. Zierler S, Cunningham WE, Andersen R, et al. Violence victimization after HIV infection in a U.S. probability sample of adult patients in primary care. *American Journal of Public Health* 2000;90:208–15.

101. Lloyd S, Taluc N. The effects of male violence on female employment. *Violence Against Women* 1999;5(4):370–92.

102. Morrison AR, Orlando MB. Socio and economic costs of domestic violence: Chile and Nicaragua. In: Morrison AR, Biehl ML, editors. *Too close to home: domestic violence in the Americas*. Washington: Inter-American Development Bank; 1997. p. 51–80.

CHAPTER 12

HEALTH PROBLEMS AS SECURITY RISKS: GLOBAL BURDEN OF DISEASE ASSESSMENTS[1]

KENJI SHIBUYA

INTRODUCTION

HEALTH AND HUMAN SECURITY

Although it is not a new concept, human security emerged in the international policy agenda with the end of the Cold War. It is not concerned with weapons; it is concerned with human life and dignity (1, 2, 3). Creating the idea and fostering the goal of human security has also led to the intersection of the international development and national security communities; their goals are to seek freedom from both want and fear (4, 5). Human security is often considered to include a variety of issues related to the domains of human well-being (3, 6).

In the theories of human welfare, several principles are invoked to decide which components of subjective or objective states should be included in an overall conception of well-being (7, 8). For instance, some domains are intrinsically valuable, such as health, education, and freedom; others are important instruments of achieving well-being, such as income and absence of violence (9, 10). The challenge for the human security concept is to present an integrated approach to addressing the wide challenges while operationalizing the concept into practice in concrete ways (4). As a consequence, the definition, research, and policy agenda for human security have proliferated and the approaches taken by the different parties in this new paradigm vary substantially.

One conclusion in this early stage is that human security means different things to different people. For some scholars in the traditional political science field, conversations about connecting health to human security can be confusing (11). There are few, if any, who will disagree with the extension of the human-oriented concept in the field of security and development, but there are diverging opinions on its usefulness and application in practice. Despite its holistic and comprehensive approach, human security of individuals as a concept confronts the daunting challenge of dealing with all the issues that could arise to threaten various peoples or communities (4). The concept could lose its meaning in a practical sense. Given constraints in resources, it is absolutely necessary to set priorities and targets.

Although there is no easy ranking among the proposed domains of welfare (3, 6, 12), human survival and health are invariably considered to be key elements of human well-being, as demonstrated by the Human Development Index (13). Furthermore, human security can be clarified by linking it to concrete current challenges, including some specific aspects of international health. Health can add value to our understanding of the magnitude of threats to human security and how they can be alleviated. For example, when dealing with war, the health and human security linkage would enable us to analyze both direct and indirect consequences of conflict. This would change the interpretation of the security studies from a simple binary political model (a decision to war) to a continuous human one (for example, lives lost or number of disabled) (14). By linking health and human security, further attention can be drawn to the interrelationship of all of the factors involved in the cause of people's insecurity.

Health and mortality indicators can be used to map the magnitude, distribution, and time trends of human insecurity. Linking traditional health issues with the human security concept raises a number of questions. How does the linkage between health and human security alter the kinds of questions we ask about security? What are the major risks to health? How might national societal variables such as the economy or international-level factors influence health risks? Who are the most vulnerable, and from which health threats? How does a focus on human security affect public health policies? The primary purpose of this chapter is to address some of these issues based on a descriptive analysis of the best available data on the global burden of disease.

RISK ASSESSMENT

Risk assessment is one of the key elements to understanding the magnitude of health problems and implementing early warning and protective measures (11, 14). We need to understand traditional disease categorizations (such as the International Statistical Classification of Diseases and Related Health Problems) as well as the magnitude of causes of ill health, such as malnutrition, unsafe sex, and tobacco use. Such proximal determinants of health are further confounded by the root causes of human insecurity such as poverty and socioeconomic inequality within and between nations (Figure 1).

However, such information is typically limited. The lack of a reliable and comparable risk factor assessment has created an information gap that frustrates priority setting and allows various interest groups to downplay or overestimate certain risks. There is an imbalance in information about

Figure 1. A schematic illustration of proximal and distal determinants of health and their interactions

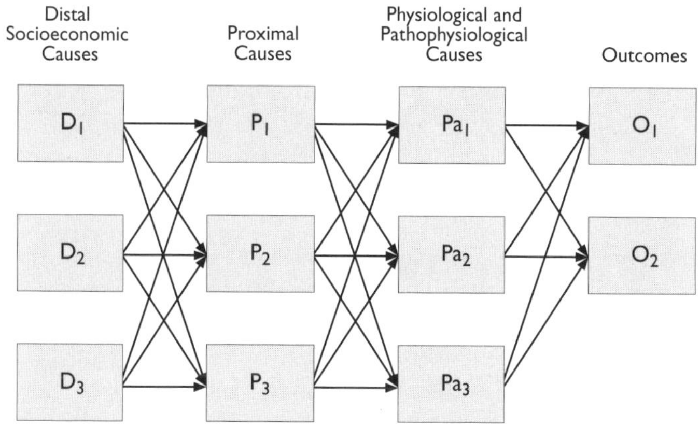

Source: World Health Organization; 2002.

risks in the press and media; typically, common, major threats to health are not considered newsworthy because they are neglected or already known, whereas rare, unusual, or catastrophic threats to health are considered highly newsworthy. As public opinion often follows the media, people tend to be more concerned with such visible risks.

Many factors are relevant in prioritizing strategies to reduce health risks: 1) the extent of various threats, 2) individual and social perceptions of risks, 3) the availability and affordability of cost-effective interventions, 4) social values and preferences against risks, and 5) community and health system characteristics (15). These factors are also key for research priorities — if major threats exist without cost-effective solutions, then these threats should be placed high on the research agenda. Governments are also likely to place particular value on ensuring their main agenda for action, which addresses the largest threats to health for their citizens. Such information can be used to reduce the unnecessary fear of future risks or risky behaviors among the public, since people tend to make choices that make them feel safer.

Quantifying the burden of disease attributable to major risk factors and the size of the potentially avoidable burden if the population distribution of risk is reduced across the board is only the first step in deciding how best to improve population health with available resources (16). The second step involves assessing the types of interventions that are available to decrease exposure to risks or to minimize the impact of exposure on health, the extent to which interventions are likely to improve population health alone and in combination, and the resources required to implement them. Cost-effectiveness analysis of interventions provides information on the priorities specific to different interventions (15, 17).

This chapter provides evidence on the causes of health risks, as well as the determinants of causes, for future implications of human health security prevention and promotion from the ongoing Global Burden of Disease 2000 (GBD 2000) project at the World Health Organization (WHO) (18). For the purpose of illustration, particular attention is paid to major proximal and distal determinants of health in developing regions.

Approaches to quantifying risks to health

The GBD 2000 method

The WHO has undertaken a fresh assessment of the Global Burden of Disease project for the year 2000 (18). The specific objectives of GBD 2000 are: 1) to quantify the burden of premature mortality and disability by age, sex, and region for 135 major causes or groups of causes; 2) to analyze the contribution to this burden of selected risk factors using a comparable framework; and 3) to develop various projection scenarios of the burden of disease over the next 30 years. The preliminary results of the first two objectives are presented here.

GBD 2000 aims to estimate global and regional mortality and morbidity based on a detailed analysis of death distributions by all causes for 191 member states of WHO. For geographic disaggregation of the GBD 2000, the six WHO regions of the world have been further divided into 14 subregions, based on mortality levels of children (under five years) and adults (15 to 59 years) (Figure 2).

The GBD 2000 study deals with the problem of systemic bias in cause-specific mortality by estimating total mortality for each country. It starts by analyzing the overall mortality upper bound for each region to ensure that the cause-specific estimates can be summed to the total all-cause mortality by age and sex. This avoids systematic over- or underestimation or double counting of deaths (19, 20). This regional cause-specific mortality envelope serves as an upper bound of mortality from a certain cause and ensures internal consistency among incidence, prevalence, and mortality rates (18).

Cause of death data were carefully analyzed to take into account incomplete coverage of vital registration in some countries and the likely differences in cause of death patterns that would be expected in the often poorer subpopulations (20). For countries lacking sufficient vital registration data, cause of death models were used first to estimate the maximum likelihood of distribution of deaths across the broad categories of communicable disease, noncommunicable disease, and injuries, based on estimated total mortality rates and income (21). A regional model pattern of specific causes of death was then constructed based on local vital registration and verbal autopsy data, and this proportionate distribution was then applied to each broad cause group. Finally, the resulting estimates were then adjusted based on epidemiological evidence from specific disease

Figure 2. Subregions of the World Health Organization based on the levels of child and adult mortality

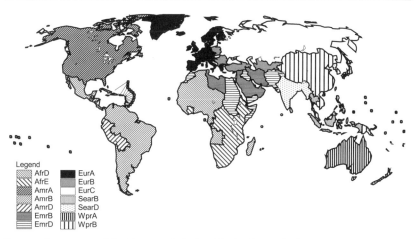

Five mortality strata were defined in terms of quintiles of the distribution of 5q0 and 45q15 (both sexes combined). Countries with low child mortality (mostly developed and middle-income countries) were split into three: A = very low child mortality, B = low child mortality and low adult mortality, and C = low child mortality but high adult mortality. Adult mortality 45q15 was regressed on 5q0 and the regression line used to divide countries with high child mortality into high adult mortality (stratum D) and very high adult mortality (stratum E). Stratum E includes the countries in sub-Saharan Africa where HIV/AIDS has had a very substantial impact.

Source: World Health Organization; 2002.

studies. Methods used to estimate global all-cause and cause-specific mortality and the incidence of these data are described elsewhere (18). The resulting estimates of incidence, duration, and age of onset yielded the disability-adjusted life years (DALYs). DALYs measure a health gap and combine information on the impact of premature death, disability, and other nonfatal health outcomes (22).

COMPARATIVE RISK ANALYSIS

The second phase of the GBD 2000 is to analyze the contribution to the burden of selected risk factors using a comparable framework. More specifically, the aims are to estimate by age, sex, and region the selected risk factors attributable to the burden of disease and injury for 2000, compared to the theoretical minimum levels of each risk factor (15, 16). For each possible risk factor-burden relationship, a systematic and documented assessment of causality was performed. The clusters of risks to health used in the GBD 2000 were as follows: risks to health and socioeconomic status, risks to the environment, addictive substances, childhood and maternal undernutrition, other diet-related risks and physical inactivity, unsafe sex, unsafe health practices, and other causes of disease and injury.

Risk factor levels in the population were the first data input in estimating potential impact fractions. For all risk factors there was a requirement to extrapolate data to some age, sex, and country groups for which direct information was not available. Wherever possible this extrapolation was based on generalizing from a particular subgroup that had similar health, demographic, socioeconomic, or other relevant indicators. The second data input into potential impact fractions was information on amounts of burden in the population by age, sex, and region. Current and future disease and injury burden was estimated as part of the GBD 2000 (18). The third data input into potential impact fractions were estimates of risk factor-burden relationships by age, sex, and region (16).

REDUCING RISKS TO DISEASE

Cost-effectiveness analysis can be undertaken in many ways and there have been several attempts to standardize methods to make results comparable, most of which have relied on the average or incremental cost-effectiveness analysis. This type of analysis may be appropriate to local decision making when policymakers are constrained to keep the current interventions and can consider only marginal improvements. However, it does not allow reevaluation of existing interventions and is not transferable across settings. WHO has developed a standardized set of methods and tools that can be used to analyze the costs and population health impact of current and possible new interventions at the same time (17). These tools and methods have been used to analyze a range of interventions that address some of the leading risks identified above. To answer key policy questions on tackling risks to health, it is necessary to compare the costs and effectiveness of interventions to the situation that would exist if they were not done (i.e., counterfactual scenario).

The analysis is used to identify interventions that are very cost-effective and those that are not cost-effective in different settings. It illustrates how, armed with information about which interventions have the potential to yield substantial improvements in population health with available resources, decision makers can begin the policy debate on prioritizing health resource allocation.

MAJOR FINDINGS

MORTALITY AND DISEASE BY CAUSE

The GBD 2000 classifies the cause of deaths into three broad categories: communicable disease, noncommunicable disease, and injuries. In 2000, approximately 56 million deaths occurred worldwide; noncommunicable disease accounted for 58% of the total number of deaths, followed by communicable disease (33%) and injuries (9%) (Figure 3). Approximately 85% of all deaths occurred in developing regions (Table 1), nearly 70% of which occurred in high mortality developing regions (AfrD, AfrE, AmrD, EmrD, and SearD).

Figure 3.   All cause mortality in world regions

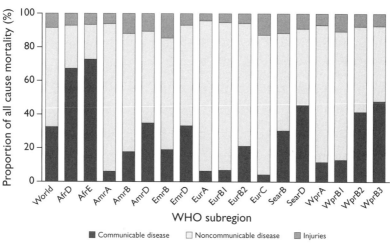

Source: World Health Organization; 2002.

In 2000 cardiovascular disease was the leading cause of mortality in the world (29% of total deaths), followed by infectious and parasitic diseases (19%), and cancers (13%). Cardiovascular disease and cancers are already major causes of deaths in absolute numbers, even in many developing countries. Both are due to accumulated risks related to aging and risky behaviors, and they are often invisible. It should also be noted that mortality risks from noncommunicable disease are generally much higher in developing regions, when comparison was made based on age-standardized mortality rates.

Whereas in middle-income regions the pace of health transition is faster and the relative importance of noncommunicable disease is increasing, in high mortality developing regions the risk of deaths from infectious disease remains quite high. The magnitude of mortality risk in terms of age-standardized mortality rate ratios is much higher from infectious disease than from other causes of deaths. Infectious disease is a typical immediate and large-scale threat. It also imposes externalities (i.e., an action or behavior of one person affects others in a society) and is particularly confounded by socioeconomic status and the availability of appropriate care, which are essential to alleviating human health insecurity. In such regions, the age-standardized mortality rate ratios of intentional injuries also tend to be high; the risks are often immediate and localized.

These overall mortality results may disguise several important patterns of attributable burden, both in different major world regions and as a result of the loss of healthy life years (Table 2). In particular, mental illness

Table 1. Global and regional number of deaths, age-standardized mortality rate, and mortality rate ratios by cause, 2000

	World	AfrD	AfrE	AmrA	AmrB	AmrD	EmrB	EmrD	EurA	EurB	EurC	SearB	SearD	WprA	WprB
Number of deaths (000s)															
All causes	54,613	4,259	6,097	1,571	2,579	528	696	3,356	4,081	1,950	3,604	2,193	12,122	1,134	10,443
1. Communicable	18,097	2,883	4,411	173	480	184	129	1,652	238	200	154	652	5,193	133	1,614
Infectious and parasitic	10,656	1,967	3,320	66	195	102	57	912	48	66	83	377	2,737	23	702
HIV/AIDS	2,571	367	1,631	15	34	24	0	49	7	1	14	46	342	0	40
2. Noncommunicable	32,541	1,070	1,233	2,387	1,778	286	464	1,420	3,643	1,636	2,986	1,251	5,748	917	7,722
Malignancies	7,022	236	296	642	385	73	78	197	1,062	289	504	229	858	337	1,837
Cardiovascular disease	16,257	469	489	1,098	758	99	272	733	1,757	1,090	2,125	556	3,126	384	3,303
3. Injuries	5,012	306	453	49	321	58	103	284	200	114	464	290	1,180	84	1,107
Intentional injuries	1,601	91	206	49	150	14	17	79	57	34	171	68	279	36	349
War and violence	720	79	189	0	124	11	6	48	5	11	73	31	73	1	66
Age-standardized mortality rate (per 100,000)															
All causes	904.3	1,659.9	2,085.8	265.6	690.7	462.3	774.7	1,208.7	446.1	801.0	673.8	915.6	1,157.1	337.6	738.1
1. Communicable	299.7	847.6	1,226.1	34.1	118.6	123.4	101.0	416.6	27.8	102.5	41.2	250.0	427.3	36.7	120.7
Infectious and parasitic	176.5	579.2	944.1	13.2	48.0	81.4	45.2	233.5	6.6	33.0	28.9	138.7	228.1	7.4	49.2
HIV/AIDS	42.6	143.4	547.8	3.9	7.9	27.0	0.2	15.4	1.5	0.6	6.3	14.8	28.0	0.1	2.5
2. Noncommunicable	538.9	694.5	707.2	399.2	496.5	273.9	585.9	697.0	384.4	648.5	454.2	561.8	625.1	264.0	545.2
Malignancies	116.3	152.9	170.1	118.8	106.5	74.5	91.6	92.9	124.9	114.0	89.9	95.6	92.3	103.4	121.2
Cardiovascular disease	269.2	330.3	309.2	170.5	216.0	96.3	366.2	389.4	169.1	429.0	289.2	259.0	352.0	101.8	236.3
3. Injuries	85.1	117.8	152.5	45.5	75.6	65.0	87.8	95.1	33.9	50.1	178.5	103.7	104.8	36.9	72.2
Intentional injuries	26.5	38.2	75.2	14.2	34.4	17.6	13.4	27.4	10.8	15.0	66.6	23.3	24.2	17.5	22.0
War and violence	12.2	32.9	68.4	6.2	28.3	13.9	5.1	16.6	1.2	5.0	30.0	10.6	6.6	0.7	4.1
Age-standardized mortality rate ratio *															
All causes	3.4	6.3	7.9	1.0	2.6	1.7	2.9	4.6	1.7	3.0	2.5	3.4	4.4	1.3	2.8
1. Communicable	8.8	24.8	35.9	1.0	3.5	3.6	3.0	12.2	0.8	3.0	1.2	7.3	12.5	1.1	3.5
Infectious and parasitic	13.3	43.7	71.3	1.0	3.6	6.1	3.4	17.6	0.5	2.5	2.2	10.5	17.2	0.6	3.7
HIV/AIDS	11.0	37.2	142.2	1.0	2.0	7.0	0.1	4.0	0.4	0.2	1.6	3.8	7.3	0.0	0.6
2. Noncommunicable	1.3	1.7	1.8	1.0	1.2	0.7	1.5	1.7	1.0	1.6	1.1	1.4	1.6	0.7	1.4
Malignancies	1.0	1.3	1.4	1.0	0.9	0.6	0.8	0.8	1.1	1.0	0.8	0.8	0.8	0.9	1.0
Cardiovascular disease	1.6	1.9	1.8	1.0	1.3	0.6	2.1	2.3	1.0	2.5	1.7	1.5	2.1	0.6	1.4
3. Injuries	1.9	2.6	3.3	1.0	1.7	1.4	1.9	2.1	0.7	1.1	3.9	2.3	2.3	0.8	1.6
Intentional injuries	1.9	2.7	5.3	1.0	2.4	1.2	0.9	1.9	0.8	1.1	4.7	1.6	1.7	1.2	1.5
War and violence	2.0	5.3	11.1	1.0	4.6	2.2	0.8	2.7	0.2	0.8	4.9	1.7	1.1	0.1	0.7

* The reference region is AmrA.

Source: World Health Organization. 2002.

Table 2. Global and regional number of disease burden (DALYs), age-standardized rate, and rate ratio by cause, 2000

	World	AfrD	AfrE	AmrA	AmrB	AmrD	EmrB	EmrD	EurA	EurB	EurC	SearB	SearD	WprA	WprB
Number of DALYs (000s)															
All causes	1,453,617	144,442	203,380	46,284	80,425	17,050	22,721	110,583	53,330	38,992	59,348	61,924	355,959	16,371	242,806
1. Communicable	609,028	102,250	150,230	3,302	17,111	6,427	5,775	59,861	2,635	7,319	4,988	20,833	169,207	1,061	58,029
Infectious and parasitic	352,111	69,215	111,144	1,443	7,425	3,332	2,314	31,095	976	2,489	2,479	11,255	84,635	358	23,951
HIV/AIDS	79,992	11,454	50,349	485	1,150	720	9	1,489	218	43	542	1,453	10,465	8	1,608
2. Non-communicable	664,880	29,295	35,322	38,380	49,572	8,383	13,018	38,631	46,378	27,196	41,939	31,552	141,885	13,646	149,684
Malignancies	189,029	2,912	3,803	5,534	4,435	883	1,068	2,842	8,623	3,299	5,434	3,049	10,424	2,731	21,064
Cardiovascular disease	142,054	5,256	5,857	6,916	7,052	1,006	2,868	8,589	9,219	8,365	16,246	5,980	34,519	2,365	27,818
3. Injuries	179,709	12,898	17,828	4,603	13,742	2,239	3,928	12,091	4,317	4,477	12,421	9,539	44,867	1,665	35,094
Intentional injuries	49,145	3,698	7,132	1,525	6,437	551	653	2,721	1,135	1,092	4,565	2,232	8,280	662	8,460
War and violence	28,571	3,418	6,679	694	5,775	452	356	1,873	162	561	2,465	1,315	2,328	35	2,458
Age-standardized DALYs rate (per 100,000)															
All causes	12,602.3	22,325.5	28,123.5	6,795.5	10,665.2	8,742.8	9,857.5	15,354.5	5,556.2	9,653.4	13,712.1	11,466.1	14,418.5	4,630.2	8,808.0
1. Communicable	4,980.0	13,154.9	17,910.0	553.4	2,008.4	2,112.0	1,752.5	6,361.3	344.5	1,964.2	1,147.9	3,857.2	6,313.3	324.0	2,142.7
Infectious and parasitic	2,998.1	9,526.4	14,310.9	228.9	932.1	1,671.2	747.2	3,576.0	132.7	638.9	756.0	2,278.0	3,511.5	120.6	922.3
HIV/AIDS	677.2	1,959.3	7,420.4	107.2	193.7	619.3	5.9	220.4	41.5	13.9	219.0	337.7	615.4	4.4	74.1
2. Non-communicable	5,664.4	6,275.7	6,608.2	5,176.4	6,110.1	4,492.5	6,002.3	6,723.9	4,432.3	6,110.7	7,256.6	5,629.6	6,157.2	3,552.9	5,217.1
Malignancies	1,531.0	756.5	888.4	617.5	540.6	402.5	527.3	554.1	708.7	765.7	725.5	538.4	469.2	590.6	774.0
Cardiovascular disease	1,253.6	1,223.3	1,222.5	847.5	1,021.9	534.0	1,789.2	1,829.3	730.0	1,872.4	2,048.1	1,156.9	1,757.5	544.6	959.9
3. Injuries	1,958.0	2,894.9	3,605.2	1,065.6	2,546.7	2,138.3	2,102.8	2,269.4	779.4	1,578.5	5,307.6	1,979.3	1,948.0	753.3	1,448.3
Intentional injuries	583.5	1,032.0	1,838.6	386.6	1,282.8	616.3	343.1	615.4	199.8	388.5	1,932.3	474.7	383.3	285.5	297.8
War and violence	383.3	946.7	1,732.7	185.4	1,166.0	540.7	217.7	465.5	30.9	210.2	1,036.5	318.4	131.4	17.9	125.3
Age-standardized DALYs rate ratio *															
All causes	1.9	3.3	4.1	1.0	1.6	1.3	1.5	2.3	0.8	1.4	2.0	1.7	2.1	0.7	1.3
1. Communicable	9.0	23.8	32.4	1.0	3.6	3.8	3.2	11.5	0.6	3.5	2.1	7.0	11.4	0.6	3.9
Infectious and parasitic	13.1	41.6	62.5	1.0	4.1	7.3	3.3	15.6	0.6	2.8	3.3	10.0	15.3	0.5	4.0
HIV/AIDS	6.3	18.3	69.2	1.0	1.8	5.8	0.1	2.1	0.4	0.1	2.0	3.2	5.7	0.0	0.7
2. Non-communicable	1.1	1.2	1.3	1.0	1.2	0.9	1.2	1.3	0.9	1.2	1.4	1.1	1.2	0.7	1.0
Malignancies	2.5	1.2	1.4	1.0	0.9	0.7	0.9	0.9	1.1	1.2	1.2	0.9	0.8	1.0	1.3
Cardiovascular disease	1.5	1.4	1.4	1.0	1.2	0.6	2.1	2.2	0.9	2.2	2.4	1.4	2.1	0.6	1.1
3. Injuries	1.8	2.7	3.4	1.0	2.4	2.0	2.0	2.1	0.7	1.5	5.0	1.9	1.8	0.7	1.4
Intentional injuries	1.5	2.7	4.8	1.0	3.3	1.6	0.9	1.6	0.5	1.0	5.0	1.2	1.0	0.7	0.8
War and violence	2.1	5.1	9.3	1.0	6.3	2.9	1.2	2.5	0.2	1.1	5.6	1.7	0.7	0.1	0.7

* The reference region is AmrA.

Source: World Health Organization; 2002.

becomes a more important cause-of-disease burden in the noncommunicable disease cluster. However, in high mortality regions, infectious disease still imposes a greater share of disease burden.

Among the infectious and parasitic diseases, HIV/AIDS is now the fourth leading cause of mortality in the world. Currently 28 million (70%) of the 40 million people with HIV infection are concentrated in the AFRO region (AfrD and AfrE), but the epidemic is spreading rapidly elsewhere in the world. The development rate of new cases is highest in EurB and EurC subregions (23). In sub-Saharan Africa, life expectancy at birth is currently estimated at 47 years; without AIDS it is estimated that it would be around 62 years (24). The consequences of HIV/AIDS extend beyond mortality, as children are orphaned and entire economies can be affected in many countries. Therefore HIV/AIDS is considered to be one of the leading threats to human security, national security, and even economic growth because of its prolonged and large-scale effects on productive age groups (2, 25, 26).

Another immediate but often localized risk to human security includes intentional injuries such as those due to war and violence. The estimate of annual mortality figures for such entities is limited due to their dynamic and uncertain nature. Despite these difficulties, the GBD 2000 analysis on direct mortality suggests that there were approximately 0.7 million deaths due to war and violence, especially in AfrD, AfrE, AmrB, and EurC subregions, where nearly 65% of all deaths from war and violence took place. The estimated burden from war and violence seems relatively small (nearly 2% of total global burden of disease). However, only direct deaths and war-related disabilities have been taken into account in the present analysis, and there is great uncertainty in the magnitude of indirect deaths and other long-term sequelae. The future burden estimate of both direct and indirect consequences from the ongoing survey will provide a more accurate picture of the problem (5, 27). Given the greater weight attached to survival of the disadvantaged groups in the concept of human security, particular attention should be paid to the observed higher risks of mortality from communicable disease and injuries in developing regions.

DISEASE BURDEN ATTRIBUTABLE TO MAJOR RISKS

Comparative risk factor analysis suggests that there is a substantial variation in disease burden attributable to certain proximal risk factors. The selected major risk factors are responsible for a substantial proportion of the leading causes of death and disability as shown in Table 3.

The present analysis reveals the extraordinary concentration of risks in high mortality developing regions (15, 16). Not only are the rates of disease and injuries high, but also relatively few risk factors exert a major impact. For example, malnutrition and unsafe sex account for more than 25% of the entire disease burden in these countries. In contrast, the

Table 3.   Attributable disease burden in 2000, by region, sex, and
selected risk factors (% of total)

| Risk factor | Developing | | | | Developed | |
| | High mortality | | Low mortality | | | |
	Male	Female	Male	Female	Male	Female
Underweight	14.9	14.7	3.0	3.3	0.4	0.4
Unsafe sex	10.9	12.6	1.2	1.6	0.5	1.1
Unsafe water, sanitation, & hygiene	5.6	5.6	1.8	1.8	0.4	0.4
Indoor smoke from solid fuels	3.9	3.7	1.4	2.4	0.2	0.3
Zinc deficiency	3.3	3.3	0.3	0.3	0.1	0.1
Iron deficiency	2.8	3.5	1.5	2.2	0.5	1.0
Vitamin A deficiency	3.3	3.3	0.3	0.3	0.1	0.1
Blood pressure	2.6	2.4	4.9	5.2	11.3	10.7
Tobacco	3.3	0.6	6.7	1.3	17.3	6.3
Cholesterol	1.9	1.9	2.2	2.0	8.1	7.1

Source: World Health Organization; 2002.

leading risk factor in developed countries is tobacco, accounting for about
11% of burden.

It should be noted, however, that ranking the selected risk factors by
proportion of attributable burden might obscure the amount of burden
caused by risk factors in the large developing regions. Because such a large
proportion of the world's population lives in high mortality developing
countries, the absolute disease burden caused by a lower-ranked risk such
as hypertension would be almost as high as in the developed countries
(Table 4). These results clearly demonstrate an epidemiological transition
for risk factors. The comparative risk analysis also suggests the transition
in risk factors that determines the development of disease and injury patterns (16).

UNSAFE SEX AND HIV/AIDS

Particular attention is paid to unsafe sex since it is a major risk factor for
HIV/AIDS, one of the leading threats to human security as well as a potential risk to national security (2, 26). Sexual behaviors and characteristics vary greatly between countries and regions. Current estimates suggest
that unsafe sex accounts for more than 99% of the HIV infections prevalent in Africa. In the rest of the world, the estimated proportion of HIV/
AIDS deaths attributable to unsafe sex ranges from 13% in the WPRO
(WprA and WprB) region to 94% in the AMRO (AmrA, AmrB, and
AmrD) region (23).

Globally, about 2.8 million deaths (5% of total) and 94 million DALYs
(6.4% of all) are attributable to unsafe sex (15, 16). The vast majority of
this burden is due to HIV/AIDS in the AFRO region. In AfrD countries,

Table 4.   Attributable disease burden in 2000, by region, sex, and
selected risk factors (000s DALYs)

| Risk factor | Developing | | | | Developed | |
| | High mortality | | Low mortality | | | |
	Male	Female	Male	Female	Male	Female
Underweight	61,598	60,002	6,601	6,049	424	377
Unsafe sex	45,037	51,330	2,657	2,993	591	1,035
Unsafe water, sanitation & hygiene	23,332	23,049	4,042	3,371	429	396
Indoor smoke from solid fuels	16,023	15,203	3,149	4,349	254	295
Zinc deficiency	13,824	13,413	591	538	71	62
Iron deficiency	11,668	14,127	3,251	4,001	617	979
Vitamin A deficiency	13,824	13,413	591	538	71	62
Blood pressure	10,929	9,727	10,857	9,455	13,132	10,232
Tobacco	13,582	2,271	14,844	2,385	20,229	5,982
Cholesterol	7,768	7,833	4,892	3,716	9,463	6,764

Source: World Health Organization; 2002.

unsafe sex is responsible for about 12% of total disease burden, whereas
in AfrE countries it is responsible for about 27% of disease burden. In
addition, the African countries are unique in suffering more attributable
burden due to unsafe sex in women than in men.

DISTAL RISKS TO HEALTH: HEALTH AND POVERTY LINKAGES

As WHO's Director General Dr. Brundtland noted (28), "Poverty is the
most significant determinant of suffering and grief in today's world. We
must carry forward the fight against global poverty with all the energy we
can muster. We know that poor people are bound to remain poor if they
lack physical and human security. This means that freedom from terror,
violence, oppression, and disease are critical foundations for poverty reduction and a secure future for our world." The vast majority of threats
to health are commonly found in the disadvantaged sectors of society.
Risks tend to cluster and accumulate over time. An important component
of the strategy is first to assess how much more prevalent risks are among
the poor.

While this information is relevant to targeting interventions to the disadvantaged sectors of society, it should be noted that socioeconomic status is also a key determinant of health status. The current estimates shed
further light on the mechanisms through which poverty acts, by assessing
the distribution of risk factors by poverty levels (16). The WHO's analysis attempts to stratify selected global risks by levels of poverty (<U.S. $1,
U.S. $1-2, and >U.S. $2 per day), as well as by age, sex, and region. The
economically developed subregions (AmrA, EurA, and WprA) show neg-

ligible levels of absolute poverty and are excluded from all subsequent analyses. Available data are summarized on the links between poverty and certain risk factors (15).

Overall 20% of the world's population lives on less than U.S. $1 per day and nearly half live on less than U.S. $2 per day. The distribution of people living below the level of absolute poverty ranges from 17.6% living on less than U.S. $2 per day (3.0% living on less than U.S. $1 per day) for EurB, to 85.2% (42.4%) for SearD and 77.9% (55.5%) for AfrD. For all WHO regions there is a strong and monotonic correlation between increasing malnutrition and increasing absolute poverty, although the strength of the association varies considerably across regions. Unsafe water and sanitation and indoor air pollution are also strongly associated with absolute poverty. On the other hand, the associations of poverty with tobacco and unsafe sex are weak and variable in certain WHO regions, suggesting that such risks are not necessarily concentrated in the most disadvantaged sectors of society.

COST-EFFECTIVE INTERVENTIONS FOR HEALTHY LIFE YEARS

Given the results from comparative risk analysis, the effectiveness, costs, and cost-effectiveness of a series of interventions aimed at reducing specific risks to health were evaluated as well. The analysis allows decision makers with an interest in reducing the burden related to a specific cause — for example, the HIV/AIDS burden or child malnutrition — to assess what types of interventions would be cost-effective in that area, given available resources. One of the intrinsic goals of a health system is to improve population health; information about how best to achieve this goal with available resources is of vital importance (29). This requires deciding not only which combination of interventions is cost-effective in reducing the risks associated with unsafe sex, for example, but also which of the myriad health risks that could be targeted should be accorded priority (17).

For the purpose of illustration, some of the results of interventions against unsafe sex are presented here to show that feasible and cost-effective interventions can significantly extend healthy life years. To reduce the risk of HIV/AIDS transmission, the focus on a comprehensive approach to intervention is motivated in part by the success of such approaches as implemented in Uganda; it is also related to the uncertainty about the potential benefits of relying on any single intervention in settings that may differ widely from those reported. Estimates exist of the contributions and cost-effectiveness calculations for the range of interventions relating to HIV/AIDS, but also allow for comparisons with other health program interventions.

The interventions evaluated here include both prevention and treatment. A standard tool was used to translate age- and sex-specific changes in the risk of HIV/AIDS infections into changes in population health, quantified using DALYs. In this model, health effects are estimated by tracing what would happen to a given population over 100 years, with and without each intervention.

These interventions improve population health by reducing the incidence of HIV, which subsequently reduces mortality and morbidity. The exception is treatment with an antiretroviral regimen that reduces morbidity and mortality in those who are treated successfully. All the preventive interventions have a substantial impact on population health in the high mortality subregions. There is little difference between the preventive interventions in terms of their cost-effectiveness ratios in most settings; none of the preventive interventions considered here can be ruled out purely on cost-effectiveness grounds. Because of interactions between many of them, we conclude that the major preventive interventions are always cost-effective in high prevalence regions, and most are cost-effective everywhere. Offering antiretroviral treatment to people with clinical AIDS gains a substantial health benefit at the population level, although the gain is lower than for the preventive interventions. In these regions, preventive interventions gain each DALY at a cost of <$10 international.

Intervention-effectiveness can be translated into gains in healthy life expectancy (HALE), which is a measure of health gains. In AfrD, for example, a severe restriction of resources would result in attention to preventive interventions to reduce the impact of unsafe sexual behaviors. If the substantial increase in health resources for Africa that is now available allows all interventions costing less than three times GDP per capita to be funded (30), the optimal mix would include HIV prevention interventions combined with anti-retroviral treatment. Such intervention can extend health life expectancy up to 15 years compared to the null scenario in 2010 (Figure 4). Likewise, a similar analysis suggests that combining a relatively small number of feasible and cost-effective interventions for reducing health risks could significantly extend HALE (Figure 5).

DISCUSSION

TYPES OF RISKS TO HEALTH

The term security can be defined as "free from avoidable risks" and thus human security is a forward-looking concept in its own right (14). A number of individual preferences or characteristics influence how people translate their understanding of risks into health behavior. This includes one's level of aversion to health risks and how one values possible future health decrements compared to other competing life choices, such as wealth and lifestyle (31). Community and social value also play an important role in attitude and perception of risks to health (15).

Depending on the levels of aggregation (individual vs. population) as currently proposed by the WHO's Communicable Disease and Surveillance cluster, and the timing of risk incidence (ex ante vs. ex post), risk assessment of human security can be classified into four broad categories.

Figure 4.   Projected gains in healthy life expectancy assuming optimal mix of interventions*

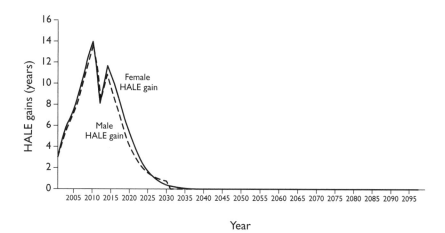

Year

* Interventions are assumed to have been implemented in 2000 and continued for 10 years.

Source: World Health Organization; 2002.

Figure 5.   Gains in healthy life expectancy from interventions* to reduce selected risk factors in AfrD and AmrB subregions in 2010

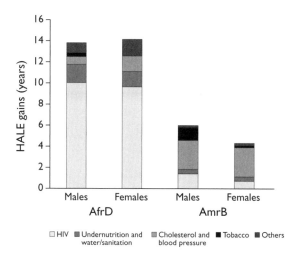

□ HIV   ■ Undernutrition and   ■ Cholesterol and   ■ Tobacco   ■ Others
water/sanitation   blood pressure

* Interventions are assumed to have been implemented in 2000 and continued for 10 years.

Source: World Health Organization; 2002.

A particular risk can be further classified by its magnitude (very small, small, moderate, or large), individual perception (perceived or objective), time-span (immediate, intermediate, or prolonged), and scale/space (subnational, national, regional, or global) (Figure 6).

Perceived risk is the subjective assessment of personal disease risk, based on an individual's interpretation of epidemiological and other types of data, while objective risk is the actual observed level of risk. There may be a difference between risk perception as an individual and cultural concepts of risk acceptability by society (31, 32, 33). Scale of the risks also matters since, for example, we may need to define both individual and population risks to health specifically among internally displaced populations that are often localized at the subnational level.

When it comes to health risks, individuals and societies sometimes exhibit positive time preference. The use of tobacco products and the consumption of alcohol, for instance, are perceived by some people as giving current pleasure despite running the risk of incurring future detrimental health effects; people give less weight to this possibility precisely because the effects will occur in the future. There seems to be considerable variation in the rate at which individuals discount adverse events that might happen in the future (34). Time preference is unlikely to be constant or stable across all groups in a society and for all conditions.

In economic literature, welfarists propose that assessment based on individual preferences under uncertainty for a societal perspective is a

Figure 6.   Classification of risks to health

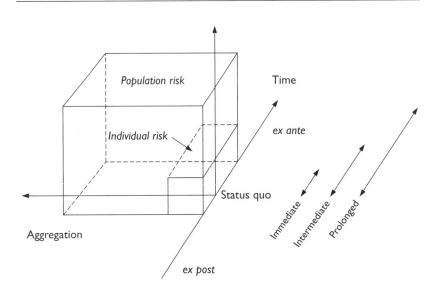

relevant concept (35). Likewise, one way of formalizing an individual risk to human security may be the form:

$$P_i^r(t \mid C)S_i^r(t)\sigma^t$$

where $P_i^r(t \mid C)$ is a risk to health in probability in time t conditional on the current status C of a person i in the region r, $S_i^r(t)$ is the survival probability of the same person, and δ is the discount rate if applicable. Population human security is an aggregation of individual humans' security, although there is a wide range of controversy when aggregating individual preferences (7). For simplicity, assume that the distribution of individual risk in a region is normal (for example, blood pressure and cholesterol levels, but not applicable to unsafe sex) and no distributional weights are considered. Then the regional risk is simply the mean of the individual risks of the form:

$$\frac{\sum_i P_i^r(t \mid C)S_i^r(t)\sigma^t}{N^r}$$

where N^r is the population in the region.

As in the case of conventional welfare economics, is only the ex ante subjective risk relevant to human security? Note that risk can be either subjective or objective and almost always is conditional on the current or past status. Given some difficulties in projecting future risks to health (in particular those risks with a small probability but a large consequence, including war and conflicts), what kind of risk assessment is feasible yet plausible with available information?

Economic analyses of choices made during periods of uncertainty generally assume that individuals exercise subjective probabilities over the occurrence of a set of exhaustive and mutually exclusive future states of the world. These probabilities are employed in the individual's calculation of his or her expected utility. This process is usually defined as an ex ante assessment. The economic literature on ex post welfare focuses on situations in which a social planner respects individuals' ex post preferences, but may not respect their subjective (ex ante) probabilities or their attitudes toward risks. Some economists have expressed the opinion that only ex post preferences should count (36, 37, 38).

The starting point for this literature is an article by Starr (39). He states, "The achievement of an Arrow (ex ante) optimum is a normative dead end. After all, we are not so much interested in expectations as in results." In other words, society may wish to achieve efficient allocations over realized rather than expected states of nature (40). In these cases, one is explicitly forced to adopt a social welfare function in which individuals' tastes count but their probability beliefs do not. Except in the case where all individuals have identical subjective probabilities over all states of nature and these probabilities coincide with social probabilities, an ex post optimum cannot be achieved without some form of government intervention.

The problem that ex ante subjective assessment is not always appropriate has implications for making welfare judgments as well as formulating risk assessment, as there may be a divergence between ex ante choice and ex post preference, and between perceived and objective risk. It is well known that a majority of people are generally concerned with immediate and large-scale risks with very low probability that have occurred in recent years (for example, natural disasters, bioterrorism, and air plane accidents; such risks are often overestimated through subjective judgments (32, 33, 41). On the other hand, people tend to underestimate the prolonged and localized risks (e.g., Afghanistan during the 1990s). Furthermore, subjective risk perception may be a function of the perception of others in society.

This situation raises the ethical question of whether someone should make decisions for ordinary people or force them to alter their beliefs, since they may not know what is best for them. Based on the questionnaire survey in Australia, Richardson and Nord suggest that the sample population did not accept the ethical basis of ex ante welfarism (42).

Although an individual's ex ante perceived risk plays an important role in formulating public opinions, many public policies are based on ex post objective assessment at the societal level rather than ex ante assessment at the individual level. In fact, many public policies are based on certain assessment, for example the number of deaths attributable to unsafe sex this year. This is simply because the probabilistic nature of assessment from an individual perspective turns out to be almost a sure thing from a social perspective, given a large enough number of people in society. Therefore, an approximate number of beneficiaries are known at population level through a health intervention such as an HIV/AIDS prevention program.

Furthermore, since future risks are most likely conditional on current risks, the ex post risk assessment of the current situation is still the basis for the future projection of risks. While human security emphasizes the importance of individual perspective, the balance between an individual's perceived and objective risks should be taken into account when operationalizing the concept into a concrete action agenda.

RISK ASSESSMENT AND FUTURE DIRECTIONS

A series of analyses presented in this chapter provides some evidence on the magnitude and distribution of current risks to health, and several implications for the health and human security linkage.

Firstly, the risk assessment shows a remarkable variation in disease burden and its distribution. It suggests the relative importance of immediate risks such as infectious disease and injuries in high mortality developing regions, as well as prolonged and large-scale health problems such as cardiovascular disease, cancers, and mental illness in low mortality developing and developed regions. The latter are most often 'present and clear.' On the other hand, the former are 'present' but not necessarily perceived as 'clear' or visible as risks to the public. It should be noted, however, that depending on the pace and scope of the spread of risks, both types — particularly the latter — are now observed in more parts of the world than expected.

Secondly, a further review of both proximal and distal determinants of health yields a slightly different picture. There are enormous gaps in distribution of major risks across regions, and high concentrations of risks in high mortality developing regions. Such risks may be closely correlated with root causes such as poverty. Understanding the magnitude of risks to health in the different strata of a society is essential to targeting and priority setting for protective interventions.

Thirdly, data on risk assessment is still incomplete, particularly in terms of epidemiological information for injuries and effectiveness of available interventions. Indirect and direct long-term consequences of war and violence have not been adequately quantified in health terms (5). There is a growing argument that health interventions could foster or support sustainable structures and processes that would strengthen the prospects for peaceful coexistence and decrease the likelihood of the outbreak, reoccurrence, or continuation of violent conflicts (43). Unfortunately this argument is still in early stages. There is little empirical evidence for the contention that health programs can mitigate conflict, nor are the mechanisms by which this process might function well articulated.

Fourthly, it is generally recognized that international collective actions can be justified when they aim to enhance public goods (for example, research and development) and deal with externalities through surveillance and control (such as disease outbreak) (44). Further supportive collective actions deal with problems that take place within individual countries, but may justify collective action at the international level owing to shortcomings in national health systems, such as technical cooperation and financing. The current analysis supports this view in bringing the health and human security agenda into action. In fact, interventions against some of the major risks to health, such as unsafe sex to prevent HIV/AIDS, are shown to be very cost-effective in many developing countries but additional funds are required for an individual country to make them feasible (15).

Finally, these observations suggest that priorities vary between countries and regions. Communities in disparate settings may differ in their ability and willingness to participate in specific risk reduction activities, and particular activities may be more difficult to incorporate into an existing health system infrastructure in some settings than others. The diverse priorities are not simply due to the differences in the levels and distributions of present risks. Most often, public concerns in the developed regions naturally focus on unanticipated and comparatively infrequent epidemics, including bioterrorism. On the other hand, people in developing regions are devastated by endemic infectious diseases in their daily life, which are potentially preventable with available interventions (11). It should be noted, however, that risks of unanticipated events also exist in developing regions, perhaps to a greater degree. As information prevails and people's perception changes, the double burden of both actual and perceived threats make priority setting more complicated among the most disadvantaged groups in the world.

It is clear that both perceived and objective risks are important in understanding and preventing risks to health. Perceived risks matter in the formulation of public opinions and even policies despite often being biased (34). Yet the evidence presented here, which is based on the ex post objective risk assessment, is one of the critical inputs required to inform the decision making process about efficient ways to reduce risks to health. The World Health Organization is in a unique position to focus on assessing global risk and enhancing international collective health actions in collaboration with its member states. In fact, one of the important roles of the government is to generate public confidence, reduce fear, and assure future security by facilitating informed communication and sharing the best available information with the public (5, 14).

Note

1. © Copyright World Health Organization 2003. All rights reserved. The World Health Organization has granted the publisher permission for the reproduction of this article.

References

1. Department of Foreign Affairs and International Trade. *Human security: safety for people in a changing world.* Ottawa: Department of Foreign Affairs and International Trade; 1999.

2. Ministry of Foreign Affairs of Japan. *Diplomatic bluebook 1999: Japan's diplomacy with leadership toward the new century.* Tokyo: Urban Connections Inc.; 1999.

3. United Nations Development Program. *Human development report 1994: new dimensions of human security.* New York: Oxford University Press; 1994.

4. Ogata S. *Globalization and human security.* New York: Weatherhead Policy Forum, Columbia University; 2002.

5. Murray CJL, King G, Lopez AD, et al. Armed conflict as a public health problem. *British Medical Journal* 2002;324:346–9.

6. Nef J. *Human security and mutual vulnerability: the global political economy of development and underdevelopment.* 2nd ed. Ottawa: International Development Center; 1999.

7. *Utilitarianism and beyond.* Cambridge: Cambridge University Press; 1982.

8. Goodin RE. Laundering preferences. In: Elster J, Hylland A, editors. *Foundations of social choice theory.* Cambridge: Cambridge University Press; 1986. p. 75–101.

9. Sen AK. *Inequality reexamined.* Cambridge (MA): Harvard University Press; 1992.

10. Anand S, Sen AK. *Concepts of human development and poverty: a multidimensional perspective.* Human Development Papers. New York: United Nations Development Programme; 1997.

11. Chen LC, Narasimhan V. *Human security: opportunities for global health.* Cambridge (MA): Kennedy School of Government, Harvard University; 2002.

12. MacLean, G. *The changing perceptions and human security: coordinating national and multilateral responses.* The United Nations and Security Agenda. Ottawa: United Nations Association in Canada; 1998.

13. Ul Haq M. *Reflections on human development.* Oxford: Oxford University Press; 1995.

14. King G, Murray CJL. Rethinking human security. *Political Science Quarterly* 2002;116:585–610.

15. World Health Organization. *World health report 2002.* Geneva: World Health Organization; 2002.

16. Ezzati M, Rodgers A, Lopez A, et al. *Comparative quantification of health risks: global and regional burden of disease due to selected major risk factors.* Geneva: World Health Organization; 2003.

17. Murray CJ, Evans DB, Acharya A, et al. Development of WHO guidelines on generalized cost-effectiveness analysis. *Health Economics* 2000;9:235–51.

18. Murray CJL, Lopez AD, Mathers CD, et al. *The global burden of disease 2000 project: aims, methods, and data sources.* Geneva: World Health Organization; 2001.

19. Lopez AD, Ahmad O, Guillot M, et al. Life tables for 191 countries for 2000: data, methods, results. GPE discussion paper No. 40. Geneva: World Health Organization; 2001.

20. Lopez AD, Ahmad O, Guillot M., et al. World mortality in 2000: life tables for 191 countries. Geneva: World Health Organization; 2002.

21. Salomon JA, Murray CJL. The epidemiological transition revisited: compositional models for causes of death by age and sex. *Population and Development Review* 2002;28:205–28.

22. Murray CJL, Lopez AD, editors. *The global burden of disease.* Cambridge (MA): Harvard University Press; 1996.

23. Joint United Nations Programme on HIV/AIDS (UNAIDS) and World Health Organization (WHO). *AIDS epidemic update — December 2001.* UNAIDS/01.74E - WHO/CDS/CSR/NCS/2001.2. Geneva: UNAIDS/WHO; 2001.

24. United Nations. *World population prospects — the 1998 revision*. Volume III: analytical report. New York: United Nations; 2000.

25. Bloom DE, Mahal AS. Does the AIDS epidemic threaten economic growth? *Journal of Econometrics* 1997;77:105–24.

26. United Nations Security Council. Security council holds debate on impact of AIDS on peace and security in Africa. Press release SC/6781; 2000.

27. Üstün TB, Chatterji S, Villanueva M, et al. WHO multi-country household survey study on health and responsiveness, 2000–2001. GPE discussion paper No. 37. Geneva: World Health Organization; 2001.

28. Brundtland GH. Speech to WHO regional committee for the eastern Mediterranean — 48th session. Riyadh, Saudi Arabia; 2001.

29. World Health Organization. *World health report 2000*. Geneva: World Health Organization; 2000.

30. World Health Organization. Macroeconomics and health: investing in health economic development. Report of the Commission on Macroeconomics and Health. Geneva: World Health Organization; 2001.

31. Viscusi KW. *Rational risk policy*. Oxford: Claredon Press; 1998.

32. Tversky A, Kahneman D. Judgement under uncertainty: heuristics and biases. *Science* 1974;185:1124–31.

33. Kahneman D, Tversky A. Choices, values, and frames. *American Psychologist* 1984;39:341–50.

34. Viscusi WK, Moore MJ. Rates of time preference and valuations of the duration of life. *Journal of Public Economics* 1989;38:297–317.

35. Johannesson M, Jonsson B, Karlsson G. Outcome measurement in economic evaluation. *Health Economics* 1996;5:279–96.

36. Drèze J. Market allocation under uncertainty. *European Economic Review* 1970;2:133–65.

37. Hammond P. Ex ante and ex post welfare optimality under uncertainty. *Economica* 1981;48:235–50.

38. Mirrlees J. Notes on welfare economics, information, and uncertainty. In: Balch M, McFadden D, Wu S, editors. *Essays on economic behavior under uncertainty*. Amsterdam: North-Holland; 1974. p. 243–58.

39. Starr R. Optimal production and allocation under uncertainty. *Quarterly Journal of Economics* 1973;87:81–95.

40. Harris R. Ex post efficiency and resource allocation under uncertainty. *Review of Economic Studies* 1978;45:427–36.

41. Zeckhauser RJ, Viscusi WK. Risk within reason. *Science* 1990;248:559–64.

42. Richardson J, Nord E. The importance of perspective in the measurement of quality-adjusted life years. *Medical Decision Making* 1997;17:33–41.

43. Editorial. Defining the limits of public health. *The Lancet* 2000;355:587.

44. Jamison DT, Frenk J, Knaul F. International collective action in health: objectives, functions, and rationale. *The Lancet* 1998;351(9101):514–7.

SECTION IV

POVERTY AND HEALTH ACTION

Human Security and Primary Health Care in Asia: Realities and Challenges

Mely Caballero-Anthony

Introduction

Human security has been a contested concept. It has evoked diverse views and generated a dizzying array of definitions — mostly predicated on where one is coming from. Yet, in spite of the differences on what and how human security should be, its value as a concept and as a viable framework for policy action still is not lost. In Asia, the discourse on human security has reached a threshold where action must take place to translate the goals and values of human security, otherwise it risks losing its relevance.

This chapter explores the potential of adopting a human security perspective to address health issues in Asia. Through an analysis of three case studies on primary health care in Cambodia, Indonesia, and the Philippines, the argument is put forth that unless health is 'securitized,' the threats to human survival can only rise and lead to more insecurities in the region. More importantly, a human security perspective also helps to identify gaps and opportunities, making possible closer multilateral cooperation and better cross-sectoral participation of both state and nonstate actors in addressing challenges to human security.

The chapter is divided into three parts. The first part provides a brief discussion on the conceptual development of human security and the extent to which this idea has been accepted and received in East Asia. It ends with a discussion on why human security can be a viable policy framework in the region. The second part attempts to locate health in the human security schema by drawing linkages between the issues and the conceptual framework. It then proceeds to discuss the findings of the case studies on the state of health and human security in East Asia. Finally, the third part provides a synthesis of some of the lessons learned from the case studies. It links back to the main concept to show that a human security approach can be a better way to respond to health and human security challenges in the region.

ADVANCING THE HUMAN SECURITY FRAMEWORK

WHY HUMAN SECURITY?

It has long been argued that a state-centric approach to security has been, at the very least, deficient. The post-Cold War international landscape and experiences of many conflict-ridden states point to several reasons why approaches to security should move beyond the state to individuals and communities. Among these reasons is that 90% of wars take place within rather than between states, and most of these wars are fought in the poorest of countries. A majority of victims caught in the vicious spiral of domestic conflicts are civilians, mostly women and children.

More importantly, there is the realization that security has been more than just the protection of state borders. In East Asia, for example, most of the pressing security issues that are prevalent in the region and pose real threats to the lives of individuals and communities are: pandemic diseases (such as AIDS, tuberculosis, and malaria that threaten to wipe out villages and entire communities), poverty and malnutrition, ethnic and communal conflicts, and environmental degradation, to name just a few. This list of security issues is certainly not exhaustive.

Against these developments, calls for policy shifts from national (state) security to human security became more resonant in the 1990s. This new security thinking was perhaps best articulated by Mahbub ul Haq in his seminal paper (1), *New Imperatives of Human Security*, which argued that the new concept of security must be based on the "security of individuals, not just security of the nations." According to Haq, fashioning a new concept of human security must be "reflected in the lives of our people, not in the weapons of our country." Haq, in effect, encapsulated the core human security concept: Security for whom? Whose security?

Haq's thinking extended to the United Nations Development Program (UNDP) when it introduced the Human Development Index (HDI) in the 1994 UNDP Human Development Report (2). The UNDP Report applied Haq's ideas to development planning, stressing that any formulation of development thinking and policies must take as its focus the welfare of individuals rather than simply the macroeconomy. Moreover, it expanded the concept of human security and defined it as having four essential characteristics:

1) it is a universal concern
2) the components are interdependent[1]
3) it is best ensured through early prevention than later intervention
4) it is people centered.

According to the UNDP Report, human security has two main aspects. "It means, firstly, safety from chronic threats such as hunger, disease, and repression. And secondly, it means protection from sudden and hurtful disruptions in the patterns of daily life — whether in homes, in jobs, or in communities." Essentially, the UNDP's definition of human security has been narrowed down to mean "freedom from fear and freedom from want." This definition subsequently became the point of reference of the many writings on human security.

Since the UNDP Report was launched, the literature on human security had expanded dramatically — reflecting the interests and contentions that this concept has generated. To date, there are at least 40 permutations to the meaning of human security, each differing in emphases and the values it promotes.[2] Indeed, as one author has noted, the conceptual journey of human security has been one of "dizzying complexity" (3).

TRENDS IN HUMAN SECURITY IN ASIA

In spite of the interest that this concept has generated, there has yet to be a major policy breakthrough on human security in Asia.[3] Among the reasons for this inaction are the following:

1) *The problem of conceptual ambiguity:* Human security has been critiqued for its lack of clarity. Although its definition has been narrowed to mean "freedom from fear and freedom from want," the main criticism has centered on the scope and possible parameters of the components of human security. What does it entail? How much does it cover? Although the UNDP's human security indicators have often been used by advocates and proponents of human security as policy guidelines for action, choosing a particular component or core value pertaining to either the "freedom from fear" or "freedom from want" categories has been controversial.

On the one hand, some governments have placed greater emphasis on the economic dimension of human security. From this perspective, human security can be attained if sustainable economic development is achieved. On the other hand, there are those who focus on the threats to individual security (i.e., personal safety and individual freedom) resulting from direct violence at either the domestic or international level. These threats could rise from various sources such as internal conflict, religious strife and ethnic discord, state repression, failed states, transnational crime, proliferation of weapons of mass destruction, and many others.[4] In the extreme, this approach calls for collective use of force as well as sanctions against the source(s) of direct violence.

From these two opposing trends, one can see that the lack of conceptual clarity and differences in emphases of human security threats present serious obstacles to moving ahead with the human security agenda.

2) *Economic development as a panacea:* The remarkable economic success over the past decades in East Asia — at least prior to the Asian financial crisis in 1997 — has led some Asian leaders to argue that most if not all the problems related to human security could be overcome as long as economic development continued. Thus in certain parts of East Asia, human security concerns were addressed in a 'sequential order' where political security (protection of political and human rights) was accorded lower priority in the pursuit of economic development. This approach has, to a large extent, hampered the effective implementation of human security goals.

3) *Noninterference principle:* The staunch adherence of most East Asian states to the principle of noninterference in internal affairs has also been a major stumbling block in the promotion of human security. In the ASEAN region for example, in cases where there have been urgent human security problems in member countries, traditional prudence has hampered any concrete and concerted action to address the problem.

4) *Absence of institutional framework:* The lacunae in institutional framework highlight the lack of resources and capacity in the region for collective action in coping with human security problems. For example, the Canadian policy for collective military action, involving intervention by peacekeeping forces in situations of gross human rights violations and violence, cannot have much support in a region such as Asia, where financial, institutional, and human resources are extremely limited.

Juxtaposed against these constraints, however, is the emergence of a nonending list of human security challenges that confront the region today. Perhaps the most vivid illustration of the extent of human security problems in the region is the picture that emerged in the aftermath of the Asian financial crisis.

The Asian financial crisis

There have been several accounts of the effects of the Asian financial crisis on human security.[5] In Southeast Asia, the effects were not only devastating but came in rapid succession. The sharp economic downturn that resulted wiped out many of the economic gains that these countries had made, particularly in poverty eradication and unemployment reduction. In a span of twelve months, depreciation in regional currencies against the US dollar ranged from 39% in Malaysia to as high as 84% in Indonesia. With the onslaught of the crisis, a host of problems ensued in a short period of time. These included massive private sector debt, a credit crunch, decline in economic production, decline in consumption, falling investments, high unemployment, inflation, labor migration, rising social problems, and political unrest (4). As these countries geared up for economic recession, it soon became clear that they were up against not merely a financial crisis, but — particularly for badly hit countries like Indonesia and Thailand — also a social and political crisis.

The Indonesian story mirrored the gravity of the Asian crisis. As a result of the recession, the country's economy was in shambles and prices of basic commodities such as food more than doubled. Unemployment rates ballooned from the precrisis level of 10% to 24% of the working population (5), meaning that at the height of the crisis, about 15 million people in Indonesia were unemployed. Poverty rates increased and the International Labour Organisation estimated that in mid-1998, about 37% of the population, or 75 million people, were expected to be living below the poverty line (defined as U.S. $1 per person per day).[6] It should be noted that up until 1997, Indonesia was cited by the World Bank as the only country in the world that had remarkably improved its Human Development Index (HDI), having started from a very low base in 1975.[7]

More distressing was the spiraling of these problems into ethnic riots in Indonesia's capital, Jakarta, and religious conflicts in the provinces of Aceh, Ambon, Sambas, and the Malukus. The impact of the crisis on the country was so severe that escalating political tensions eventually led to the collapse of the 35-year regime of President Suharto. Such was the extent of the problem in Indonesia at the height of the crisis that the major fear was the disintegration of the country. Indonesia is the biggest country in Southeast Asia and has the largest Muslim population in the world. Its implosion would have had tremendous impact on the region. More importantly, for years the country had provided leadership and a sense of stability in the Southeast Asian neighborhood.

Other countries in the region that were badly affected by the Asian crisis — like Thailand and Malaysia — experienced similar human security problems. But the situation was, to a certain extent, less grave than what Indonesia had suffered. These countries were spared the ethnic and religious conflict that followed. Nonetheless, the period during and after the crisis brought a host of human security problems to the region, including widespread poverty, pandemic diseases, illegal migration, trafficking of illegal drugs and small arms, and terrorism. In spite of the varying degrees of economic recovery that has taken place in some countries, serious problems persist domestically and transnationally.

The region's experience with the Asian crisis has therefore been instructive. One of the major lessons learned is that it is not enough for governments to promote economic development at the expense of other vital human concerns. The Asian crisis has shown that economic development devoid of a human face is simply inadequate. Governments and leaders in Asia have been criticized for neglecting issues such as good governance and accountability as they became singularly preoccupied with the goal of economic development. On the other hand, individuals and communities who found themselves coping with social and economic dislocations as a consequence of economic development have had to grapple also with the current forces of globalization that have engulfed many parts of the world today. The World Bank's study on *Voices of the Poor* provides valuable insights into the types of insecurities faced by the poor. To those in the study, insecurity meant poor health and sanitation, fear of disability or chronic illness, domestic violence, unemployment, and inflation (6). Paradoxically, as their problems became more complex, their voices became less audible. This has been the experience in Asia.

Thus, in crafting new policies and mechanisms to address many of these problems, strong arguments emerge to reexamine the orthodox approaches used to address these threats and to consider the merits of adopting a human security perspective.

Human security as a viable policy framework in Asia

Each of the security problems cited above demands urgent attention. To be sure, these problems will not subside in the short to medium term, and they all pose serious security threats to individuals and communities in the region. The task of confronting these challenges is daunting, and certainly beyond the capabilities of states acting on their own.

Consider the problems posed by terrorism, for example. The September 11, 2001 terrorist attack on the United States shocked the entire global community, as the tragedy unfolded on national television screens worldwide — in real time. Notwithstanding the need for a rapid military response to the perpetrators of acts of terrorism, many analyses on this subject have pointed to the need to examine the multidimensional root causes of the problem. This makes terrorism a much more complex phenomenon than is currently perceived. The United States' response to terrorism has been criticized for its shallowness and lack of cognizance of the fundamental root causes of terrorism and violent conflicts. These causes include such issues as distributive justice arising from economic and political marginalization, ethnic and religious isolation, and questions of identity, among others. As the dust of the September 11 terrorist attack began to settle in the U.S., the rest of the world has had to grapple with terrorist attacks in their own regions, as was the case in Southeast Asia with the October 2002 bombing attack in Bali, Indonesia. Many voices are appealing for a more integrated and comprehensive strategy to address the problems of terrorism.[8] In fact, many have argued that the campaign against terrorism is more than just a battle of might, but rather a battle of the hearts and minds. In this regard, a human security approach that answers the question — Security for whom? — may offer an alternative approach to dealing with many of the problems facing us today.

Beyond the arguments cited above for a reassessment of development and security policies, the imperative of treating many of these security threats as common human security threats is also compelling. This is part and parcel of the human security approach that allows for initiation of much needed collective and cooperative actions. More importantly, joint approaches help address not only the symptoms but also the root causes of problems, and generate more comprehensive and effective strategies to prevent conflict and crisis situations.

Recently, Madame Sadako Ogata, cochair of the Commission on Human Security, made this remark that reflects more succinctly the need to adopt a human security approach to security concerns. She stated:

> "The concept of 'human security' presents a useful entry point to the central security issue of the day; i.e., the security of the people. It represents a paradigm shift from the traditional resort to state as the provider of security. First of all, by focusing on the people who are victims of today's security threats, you come closer to identifying their protective needs. Secondly, by examining the people with their diverging interests and relations with each other, you uncover the social, economic, and political factors that promote or endanger their security..." (7).

Bringing people in and listening to security concerns from their perspective is one of the major facets of the human security approach. In doing so, this process engenders a more transparent and accountable system, since participation in policy formulation must be representative. Such processes therefore help create an environment conducive to working toward human security and human development. In sum, these processes quintessentially embody the human security approach.

Health and Human Security in Asia: Operationalizing the Human Security Approach

Regardless of the numerous criticisms of the vagueness of the human security concept, coherence can emerge once attempts are made to identify the specific areas that can be subsumed under human security. This section applies the human security concept and approach to an urgent human security problem in Asia — health. Specifically, it examines the challenges posed to primary health care since this speaks to the basic right of human survival. However, before addressing the challenges and operations of the human security concept, it is useful to first draw the interlinkages of health and human security.

Why health and human security?

Health and human security is not in the common lexicon in Asia, unlike in the more developed countries in the West, such as the United States. One of the reasons is that health has not been *securitized* in this region. To securitize an issue is to frame or present it as being susceptible to threats. More importantly, an issue is said to be securitized when it is able to find an audience or, for those who are securitizing it, persuade others that this referent object or issue is threatened and requires priority over and above other referent issues.[9] When something is securitized, exceptional measures are taken to secure the issue that faces existential threats.

However, the process of securitization is not merely an act of speech. It requires appropriate actions and policies to protect that which is threatened. Hence, securitizing demands both the discursive (i.e., the speech act and shared understanding) and the nondiscursive (i.e., policy implementation and action) dimensions. In this regard, securitizing health requires not only the use of language, but also the building of political constellations and policy implementation.

One could argue that the securitization of health need not be a difficult task in the Asian context since human security is not an alien concept in the region. In fact, if one were to locate the human security concept within the existing regional security frameworks, one would see that it fits in well with the Asian concept of comprehensive security. As argued by one Asian security expert, the human security concept is complementary to the notion of comprehensive security, in that it reviews security in a multidimensional manner, beyond the confines of state security. Comprehensive security includes, among others, political security, economic security, and environmental security. Hence, human security has homegrown roots in Asia (8). Moreover, comprehensive security reflects the kinds of individual and community threats and insecurities that require more than a state-centric approach, and instead emphasizes a more holistic and comprehensive approach to security threats. Comprehensive security also underscores the need for a more cooperative approach among actors, such as states, to address security issues. In this regard, the concept of comprehensive security and its modalities can be found in the human security paradigm. They are complementary.

Therefore, as far as health and human security are concerned, adopting a more comprehensive approach to security through the human security paradigm allows health to be included in the core values to be secured. In the process, health becomes no longer solely a medical issue but also a security issue. Within this framework, health is then securitized and not merely *medicalized*.

Why primary health care?

The argument for the securitization of health becomes more pertinent if one examines the state of health care within the Asian context. In a rapidly developing global environment, access to primary health care is considered a basic feature of a modernized world. Yet, the sad reality is that health care — like most basic human needs such as food and shelter — is still unavailable to many. The lack of access to, and deprivation of, health care are vivid examples of human insecurities. These insecurities, if not addressed, pose fundamental threats to the survival and well being of individuals. Moreover, they debase human dignity and deprive human beings of their freedoms.

When a core human need like health care becomes a scarce resource, the situation becomes a breeding ground for discontent and conflict among those individuals and communities that are affected. More importantly, it also causes the spread and cross-infection of complex diseases, and worst of all — death. As many of us know, pandemic diseases like AIDS have become more devastating than wars. Five years ago, it was estimated that 16,000 people were infected with HIV — 11 people per minute.[10] As noted in the most recent report of the joint UN-AIDS and WHO commission, nearly 500,000 people with the HIV virus died in the Asia-Pacific in 2001, and it is estimated that 11 million more people may contract AIDS by the end of the decade (9). Moreover, in East Asia, there is the stark reality that about 1,000 people die of tuberculosis (TB) every day — a figure much higher than victims of terrorism (10).

The effects of such diseases seriously undermine the social, economic, and political structures of states, not to mention the tremendous toll they take on human lives. It is worth noting that in many parts of the globe, including Asia, the impact of health issues on human security is magnified by a complex combination of factors ranging from limited resources, poor infrastructure, and endemic corruption, to a lack of commitment and understanding of the havoc health issues can wreak on individuals and communities. This situation underscores the importance of primary health care.

The cases of China and India are instructive here. China's Head of the Department of Disease Control of the Ministry of Health has announced that the country has about one million people infected with the HIV virus. He warned that if the AIDS epidemic is not dealt with efficiently, there could be more than 10 million HIV or AIDS patients in China by the year 2010 (11). In India, despite reports of a low HIV prevalence rate of 1%, this estimate translates to about four million Indians with the virus, the second highest figure in the world after South Africa (9). The problem is that reports of low prevalence of HIV cases in the world's most populous countries like China and India blur the extent of a major catastrophe that is already underway. Thus, inadequate attention is given to health care, such as preventive measures. But in proportion to the large population of both countries, the actual numbers of HIV-AIDS cases are already quite alarming. The extent of the problem has been described by an official at the U.N. Office for Drug Control and Prevention when he said, "In the past when making reference to the Asia-Pacific we talked of a low prevalence rate that could become terrible....I think it is now appropriate to say the disaster has already started" (9). For developing countries with low-quality health care, the impact of this pandemic disaster is magnified.

In Cambodia, HIV/AIDS is now reported to be the country's 'killing field.' Reports quoting a senior Cambodian health official state that by 2010, more than half a million of the country's 11.5 million population will suffer or die from AIDS (12). In Indonesia, there was a 50% increase in 2001 in injecting drug users who could be HIV positive, compared with a 0% increase in 1998. Similar stories are found in Malaysia, Myanmar, Nepal, and Thailand.

Thus, health issues no longer can be viewed solely within the purview of development and underdevelopment. The importance of primary health care — the first line of defense aside from prevention — is brought to the fore. Experience has shown that epidemics can reach crisis proportions beyond the capabilities of states to manage. The devastating effects brought about by neglect not only drain the resources of states, they can also reverse gains from economic growth and development. When health issues are ignored or sacrificed for other types of issues, the social and economic consequences can destabilize societies and threaten political stability. In worst-case scenarios, such crises could have devastating consequences, such as complex emergencies and failed states.

If we adopt the working definition of the Commission on Human Security that "the objective of human security is to *protect the vital core of all human lives from critical and pervasive threats, in a way that is consistent with long-term fulfillment,*" then a study on health, specifically access to primary health care in Asia, would give us a good idea of the extent to which this vital core — health — is secured or threatened in the region.

There is another reason why the concept of human security is a viable framework for addressing health issues. As mentioned in the first section of this paper, the division over which dimensions of human security must be emphasized has hampered the development of a human security agenda. Consequently, these contentions have prevented a meaningful application of this concept to state policies. It can be argued that using a human security perspective to understand health issues would help cut across the current conceptual impasse that has prevented a more effective deployment of this concept. Choosing health issues like access to primary health care, and highlighting the grave threats that a lack or absence of health care brings to the welfare and security of individuals in their personal surroundings, community, and environment, will leave little room for ideological differences or policy preferences.

Having argued the merits of the human security approach, the questions at this point are: What can these case studies on provision of health care contribute to the ongoing discourse on human security? In other words, what added value can a human security perspective bring to problems of primary health care? More importantly, how does this perspective move the human security concept beyond discourse to action?

PRIMARY HEALTH CARE IN EAST ASIA: A SNAPSHOT OF REALITIES AND CHALLENGES[11]

The human security approach behooves us to answer the questions: Security for whom? Whose security? The concept of human security gains more coherence when it specifies whom it is protecting. Thus, if we reiterate the working definition of human security by the Commission on Human Security, that is, *"to protect the vital core of all human lives from critical pervasive threats, in a way that is consistent with long-term fulfillment,"* then a study of primary health care goes to the very heart of what we are trying to secure. At the risk of sounding pedantic, the objective here is to actualize the freedom to survive, or freedom from preventable death. Hence, provision of primary health care ensures human survival that forms the core and ultimate goals of any human security agenda.

While primary health care is one of the basic entitlements people expect in today's modern, networked, and globalized world, the stories from Cambodia, Indonesia and the Philippines present a starkly different reality. In the interest of space, the following section provides a snapshot of the trends in primary health care that result from the case studies of these three countries. Common themes emerge from these trends and are relevant to one particular element of human security that this study examines, i.e., freedom from premature preventable death.

The three case studies focused their analyses on primary health care for the poor. The following are some highlights of their findings:

1) *Health-seeking behavior of the poor:* A typical 'health-seeking behavior' among the poor in these countries is either nontreatment or self-treatment in case of illness. Such behaviors are not surprising considering that the financing of health care for the poor comes mostly from their own pockets. It is often the case that a traditional method of cure is sought first and more often than not, referrals to tertiary health facilities are made at very late stages, as in the majority of cases in Cambodia.

In the Philippines, statistics from the Department of Health reveal that six out of 10 recorded deaths owing to nonviolent causes received no medical attention during the illness period prior to death. In the project on Health Care in Indonesia conducted by Naruo Uehara,[12] which examines health-seeking behavior of the poor communities in the district of Ancol, Jakarta, studies reveal that up to 80% of the cases on mortality in poor areas were intrinsically preventable. If these deaths were indeed preventable, the question is, What process in the system was critical in this event (i.e., death)?

Other consequences of health-seeking behavior are the irrational use of drugs and medicines, use of untested home remedies and cures, and neglect of preventive, promotive, and primary care services.

2) *Financing from out-of-pocket spending:* Most of the poor in these countries do not have access to health care, thus the spending pattern would be from their own pockets. In fact, as the Philippines case study shows, only those with the capacity to pay are able to access health care but do so under the following circumstances: i) by reducing current and future consumption, ii) by reducing future income, and iii) by tapping into existing social networks. The sad consequences of these methods are that the burden of paying for health care is passed on to future generations in the form of reduced investments in human capital and reduced future health and well-being.

However, the story for the poor is different since there is "almost no consumption to reduce, no future income to leverage, and they have very weak social institutions to depend on (13)." Yet, if they can, as Uehara's research findings reveal, the poor will sell all they can and borrow from all those they know just to save the lives of their family members.

This trend supports the findings of a recent WHO study on basic patterns in national health expenditure among low-income countries. The findings reject the assumption that the poorer a person is, the lower the threshold for catastrophic expenses, meaning that out-of-pocket spending ought to be lower. Instead, exactly the opposite occurs: in low-income countries, the average out-of-pocket spending is high, averaging from 20% to 80% of all health spending. Moreover, the study supports the catastrophic impact of out-of-pocket spending patterns on the poor. Even if consumers were willing to pay more for better quality services, it was not possible for the poor to pay much more. In addition, their expectation of lower or discounted charges required preferential treatment.[13] It is noteworthy that the poor, in spite of their obvious limitations, do in fact prioritize health — they are willing to pay all that they have for good health. Unfortunately, the political process does not accord them the same priority.

3) *Inaccessibility of health facilities:* While governments do provide services for the poor, in most instances the poor do not know that these services exist or how to access them. Consider the case of Indonesia when the Asian financial crisis struck. The government provided free social safety net programs for the poor,[14] but people in remote areas were unaware of these services. Even if they knew about the services, they did not understand the procedures on how to access them. Moreover, the poor in the remote villages were less likely to travel to health facilities.

In Cambodia, only 55% of the total population has geographical access to primary health care and these facilities can be accessed through a 10-km or two-hour walk. Furthermore, only 73% of these accessible health centers is able to provide minimum health services, and only around one-third of the population has physical access to the centers.

The common factor cited in the lack or inaccessibility of health care is the dire shortage of human resources. But studies reveal that it is not only the lack of doctors and medical personnel that affects access; there is also a lack of incentives for doctors and nurses to work in poorer communities. While these findings were reinforced in Uehara's research, another factor cited is the lack of recognition given to medical health workers by their own community for their oftentimes thankless jobs. This situation leads to lack of motivation and poor morale among health workers.

Sometimes it is not the lack of human or material resources that prevents access to health care. Countries like the Philippines have various types of health financing available from community-based schemes, charity, national and local budgets, and social health insurance. The findings reflect that it is not how much is being spent, but how existing resources are being spent on health. Some of the problems cited with regard to health financing programs are limited population coverage (particularly among the poorest populations), poor targeting, and crowding out by more affluent patients. In many instances, government subsidies are not accessible in the poorest regions. As a consequence, what happens over the long term is that an inefficient and inequitable health care system actually becomes a threat to health and human security, more serious than the threat from the resurgence of diseases like TB, polio, malaria, and schistosomiasis.

4) *Poor quality of health care:* Closely related to accessibility problems is the poor quality of health services and facilities. In the Philippines, health facilities operated by national and local governments tend to deliver poor quality services (e.g., lack of appropriate diagnostic facilities for surgeries, overprescription of antibiotics, poor health outcomes such as post operative infections and death in the case of pneumonia). The problem has become even more acute with the devolution of power to local government units. The performance of decentralized provincial and district hospitals is generally considered inadequate, and local governments have been blamed for their unwillingness and inability to maintain predevolution expenditure levels. This is one obvious risk in the process of devolution, as can be seen in the case of Indonesia: Provincial and district medical centers

are not ready to deal with the responsibility that used to be within the purview of the state or central government.

5)   *Lack of political will:* In spite of the limitations of primary health care in these countries, there are current programs to reform and improve the health services. Yet the reforms either never began or could not be sustained. A common theme that emerged from the three cases was the lack of political will among policymakers to sustain these reforms. This is because health is not considered as critical as jobs, prices, and issues of peace and order. Health spending is considered a luxury.[15] In Indonesia, for example, most regional governments do not consider health an investment. In the Philippines, commitment and support for health would not generate more votes. Moreover, bureaucrats at national levels who make decisions on budget allocations would not have to face elections.

6)   *Problems with external assistance:* In a country like Cambodia that is rebuilding after years of war and has only embarked on nationwide health service programs in recent years, external assistance from multilateral donor agencies has been crucial. In fact, external funding from donors, including both official development aid (ODA) and direct NGO funding, still exceeds government funding (i.e., 70% of health funds come from donor agencies).

While not underestimating the importance of external funding, there have however been coordination problems between donor agencies and the national government. Donor agencies are perceived to act independently from national agencies in planning health reforms, resulting in inconsistencies and ineffectiveness of training. There are also challenges in fitting program outputs to beneficiaries' needs. Similarly, there have been problems of poor targeting. The intended beneficiaries — the poor — either find themselves shut off from enjoying the benefits, or find that the health programs are inadequate and do not address the health problems of poor families.

MAJOR CHALLENGES IN HEALTH CARE

Against these trends, there are clearly major challenges in the delivery of primary health care in the region, including consistency in the delivery of primary health care to the poor. Even for countries like Indonesia with long experience providing highly subsidized primary health care, there have been serious limitations in this arena. Ideally, providing health care for the poor should be part of the comprehensive sociocultural and economic programs designed to reduce poverty in the country. Moreover, spending on health for the poor is not just a matter of public expenditure but also should be considered a good investment in poverty reduction.

The interrelatedness of poverty, malnutrition, and infectious diseases bears reiterating here. These three factors are 'silent killers' whose effects are often insidious. The number of deaths associated with poverty-linked infectious diseases and malnutrition is much higher than the deaths resulting from conflicts and violence. In this regard, primary health care must be seen as a public good. Unless this mindset is adopted, the incidence of health bipolarization between those who have the resources and those without, particularly the poorest, most vulnerable sectors of the society, can only worsen.

Another major challenge is widening the political space for nongovernmental actors to participate in the planning of health care programs. In local villages, community participation plays an important role in increasing access to basic health services and in making sure that information about health services and outreach programs reach the poor. More significantly, since poor families obviously have limited or no resources, they rely on the pooling of community resources, charities, and central and local government funds in order to access health services. Hence, people's participation in these programs must be included since as recipients or security referents, it is their health needs that must be addressed. It is the individuals and communities in need who are best able to define their health concerns.

There is also the challenge of how to generate political constituency in order to make 'good health, good politics.' The idea is to have the reforms in health services be consistent with political interests. To do this, one must be able to establish a clear linkage between health and human security, and the values that appeal to power holders. Since they are interested in issues of political stability and legitimacy, power holders must be sensitized to the idea that health and human security are integral to these issues.

Last but not least is the challenge to build a sound democracy to open up more political space for the marginalized sectors of society. The incongruity of the willingness of the poor to spend their life savings just to have good health, juxtaposed against a political process that does not give them the same priority, must be changed. There is clearly a dissonance when the suffering poor fails to gain acceptance into the political process. In a democratic system the poor — marginalized as they are — will at least have the power to vote and work to correct the imbalances in the system.

HEALTH AND THE HUMAN SECURITY APPROACH: SECURING PROTECTION FROM HUMAN INSECURITIES

How can human security be an alternative or a better policy framework to address health care issues? A human security perspective is essentially about protection. It recognizes that people and communities can be fatally threatened by events beyond their control: a natural disaster, a financial crisis leading to national policies cutting public and private investments in health care, a terrorist attack, and so on. The human security paradigm encourages institutions to respond by offering protection "which is constant — not episodic, nor static; and anticipatory rather than reactive, so that people will manage downturn with security" (14). Thus a human security approach that speaks of early prevention and people-centeredness will at least minimize if not prevent such events from occurring.

The foregoing discussion on the trends and challenges of health care woefully reflects the state of health care in the three country case studies. To be sure, health is human security! As is the case with most security concerns, these countries require urgent responses, such as allocating more resources to primary health care. But in many countries in Asia, access to primary health care has become more a privilege than an entitlement. In fact, health care services have been so inadequate that situations occur where six out of 10 recorded deaths owing to nonviolent causes are due to the absence of medical care. What about those deaths that were not recorded? Could the story be more dismal?

The trends cited above on primary health care in Cambodia, Indonesia, and the Philippines offer just a glimpse into the many untold stories of suffering, misery, and neglect that many poor people experience in this region. This need not be a permanent feature. The reason for this gloomy picture is that primary health care is not considered to be as critical as jobs or prices or military security. In Southeast Asia, defense expenditures and budgets far exceed those of health (Table 1 and Table 2). Some governments in the region have no qualms about spending U.S. $40 million to buy an F-16 plane, yet they cannot even provide basic health care to their own people. (For further examples of government allocation trends toward public health expenditures, see Table 3, Table 4, Table 5, and Table 6).

It is noteworthy that during the economic boom years in East Asia, public expenditure on health varied between 0.7and 2.7% of GDP (15). Moreover, with the low priority given to health care, there were also no provisions for times of crisis. It comes as no surprise then that at the height of the Asian financial crisis, one hears of tragic stories such as this: in 1998, half of the 130 health clinics in the Indonesian town of Bekasi, east of Jakarta, stopped providing services due to lack of medicines. Supplies in hospitals and public health centers elsewhere also were depleted (16). In this instance, health policies did not ensure early prevention. A major challenge then is how to insulate health care from the effects of economic catastrophe.

An important question at this point is: Who is responsible for providing primary health care to the poor? The obvious response would be the state. While human security shifts the security referent from the state to the individual, it does not obviate the state's responsibility to provide security for its citizens. Governments have the resources and instruments at their disposal to provide security for their people. In this context, a human security approach urges health officials and policymakers to be more accountable and responsive to the health needs of the people, and more importantly, to think of policies and programs from the perspective

Table 1.   Health expenditures in 1995 in selected ASEAN countries

	Total (% of GDP)	Public Sector (% of GDP)	Public Sector (% of Total)
Brunei	—	2.2	—
Cambodia	7.2	0.7	10.0
Indonesia	1.8	0.6	37.0
Malaysia	2.5	1.5	60.0
Philippines	2.4	1.3	56.0
Singapore	3.5	1.3	37.0
Thailand	5.3	1.4	26.0
Vietnam	5.2	1.1	22.0

Source: World Health Report 1999.

Table 2.   Government health and defense expenditure in 1995 in selected ASEAN countries

	Health (% of GDP)	Defense (% of GDP)
Brunei	2.2	5.5
Cambodia	0.7	5.9
Indonesia	0.6	1.3
Malaysia	1.5	2.7
Philippines	1.3	1.4
Singapore	1.3	4.7
Thailand	1.4	2.2
Vietnam	1.1	7.2

Source for Defense Budget: Based on data from *The Military Balance 1995/1996*. London: International Institute for Strategic Studies (IISS); 1995.

Table 3.   Total expenditure on health as % of GDP

	1995	1997	1998
Brunei	—	5.4	5.7
Cambodia	7.2	7.2	7.2
Indonesia	1.8	2.4	2.7
Malaysia	2.5	2.3	2.5
Philippines	2.4	3.6	3.6
Singapore	3.5	3.3	3.6
Thailand	5.3	3.7	3.9
Vietnam	5.2	4.5	5.2

Source: World Health Report 1999 and 2001.

Table 4.   Public expenditure on health as % of total expenditure on health

	1995	1997	1998
Brunei	—	40.6	43.5
Cambodia	10.0	9.4	8.4
Indonesia	37.0	23.8	25.5
Malaysia	60.0	57.6	57.7
Philippines	56.0	43.4	42.4
Singapore	37.0	34.4	35.4
Thailand	26.0	57.2	61.4
Vietnam	22.0	20.3	23.9

Source: World Health Report 1999 and 2001.

Table 5.   Private expenditure on health as % of total expenditure on health

	1995	1997	1998
Brunei	—	59.4	56.5
Cambodia	—	90.6	91.6
Indonesia	—	76.2	74.5
Malaysia	—	42.4	42.3
Philippines	—	56.6	57.6
Singapore	—	65.6	64.6
Thailand	—	42.8	38.6
Vietnam	—	79.7	76.1

Source: World Health Report 1999 and 2001.

Table 6.   Government expenditure on defense in year 2000

	% of GDP
Brunei	6.7
Cambodia	6.1
Indonesia	0.9
Malaysia	1.8
Philippines	1.8
Singapore	4.9
Thailand	2.0
Vietnam	3.1

Source for Defense Budget: Based on data from *The Military Balance 2000/2001*. London: International Institute for Strategic Studies (IISS); 2000.

of the beneficiaries. The cases of health financing not reaching the poorest citizens, as in the Philippines, ideally should not occur if there is awareness of the problems of inaccessibility and inability to access services. Yet in a typical top-down policy approach, directives and policies on health services generally come from Ministries of Health with little or no participation from nongovernment individuals and communities. But health is too important to be left in the hands of the medical professional and bureaucrats. One could argue that human security makes health everybody's business. This concept is an important part of the human securitization process.

Moreover, while the state is regarded as the main provider for security, we must recognize that the state's capabilities are limited. Political capabilities have become inadequate as governments respond to the ever-growing list of security issues confronting us today. Because of these shortcomings, human security allows nongovernmental actors or international agencies to provide help and carry out certain responsibilities to provide security. Effective participation from a diverse group of actors other than the state becomes inevitable, and multi-sectoral participation and cooperation become relevant. Hence within the context of human security, the importance of processes — governance, participation, transparency, capacity building, and institution building — must be emphasized.

Finally, a human security approach to health care also brings into focus the inter-relatedness of health issues with problems such as poverty, famine, illiteracy, environmental degradation, and others. Each of these issues feeds into the others. This characteristic of the human security framework allows for a more comprehensive approach to a core human security concern — health care. Human security recognizes the intrinsic value of weaving the other human security concerns into its analyses of health care.

In summary, one recalls the following phrase that succinctly captures the value of adopting a human security approach. "In the final analysis, human security is a child who did not die, a disease that did not spread, a job that was not cut, an ethnic tension that did not explode in violence, a dissident who was not silenced" (17).

CONCLUSION

Human security is at the juncture where it must be translated from the confines of conceptual discourse to action. Health is one area where a human security perspective can be a framework for this translation. Health — particularly the provision of primary health care — begs for an approach that comprehensively addresses the major challenges that confront it. This chapter has highlighted the seriousness of the failure to provide primary health care in Asia, particularly to the most vulnerable in societies — the poor. Common problems have been identified, including lack of resources, inefficient allocation of resources, inadequacy of governance, and institutional problems.

The challenge now is to move forward on the health and human security agenda. One of the significant themes of this paper is the question, How do we make good health, good politics? As the findings have shown, policymakers care less about health than they do about jobs and inflation. Obviously, primary health care is not considered a priority. Yet, good health is at the core of human survival. It ought to be a priority. Thus, unless we make good health equal good politics, the task of sensitizing the policy community to the primacy of health as a human security concern will be an uphill task.

In times of crisis, many governments in the region seem to resort to 'pump priming' their economies in response to the global economic slump. However, there are limitations to what fiscal stimuli can do to jump-start the domestic economy since the slow-down is externally driven. More importantly, there is a concern of expanding fiscal deficits (Figure 1).

Current developments like these pose vexing dilemmas to the policy community. Most often the challenge is how to prioritize certain core issues over others. What political process is involved in allocating resources to one issue instead of another? How does one avoid the inevitable tensions that arise in the midst of competing interests?

In the ladder of options available, the human security approach ideally can provide guidance in addressing these dilemmas. More importantly, the human security approach gives clarity; it brings into focus the vital issues of concern for the well being of individuals and communities. In an environment of competing interests, dialogue, sharing information, and learning from the experiences of others eases policy dilemmas. Moreover, by opening up the political space, new ideas and expertise can emerge to help address issues and prioritize competing interests. Finally, allowing more dialogue also provides windows for international cooperation to take place, as institutions are able to respond appropriately. The human security framework therefore allows for possibilities of multilateral and multisectoral approaches to realizing human security.

ACKNOWLEDGMENT

The author wishes to acknowledge the valuable contribution of Dr. Fujita Noriko, Dr. Purnawan Junadi, and Dr. Orville Solon who shared their case studies on Primary Health Care in Cambodia, Indonesia, and the Philippines, respectively. The case studies were commissioned by the Japan Center for International Exchange (JCIE) as part of its project on Health and Human Security in Asia, for which the author was Project Director. In this regard, the author is grateful to Mr. Tadashi Yamamoto, President

Figure 1. Budget balance in ASEAN-5 countries (2000 and 2001)

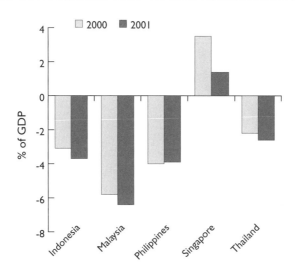

Source: Official sources, EIU.

of JCIE, and Mr. Makita Noda, Project Officer of JCIE, for supporting the project.

Notes

1   In the UNDP report, the following components are the core values or dimensions of human security: economic security, food security, health security, environmental security, personal security, community security, and political security.

2   See for example, CERTI, "Human Security: A Framework for Assessment in Conflict and Transition," 2000; Gary King and Christopher Murray, "Rethinking Human Security," working manuscript, 2000.

3   The geographical term Asia is used here for convenience. But the scope of this paper covers only southeast Asia as the case studies cited are from ASEAN countries.

4   See "Freedom From Fear: Canada's Foreign Policy for Human Security." Available at: URL: security/" http://www.dfait-maeci.gc.ca/foreignp/human security/ Human Security Booklet-e.asp.

5   See for example, Mely Caballero-Anthony, "Challenges to Southeast Asian Security Cooperation" and Rizal Sukma, "Security Implications of the Economic Crisis in Southeast Asia," in *An Asia-Pacific Security Crisis? New Challenges to Regional Stability*, Guy Wilson-Roberts, editor, New Zealand:

Centre for Strategic Studies, 1999, pp. 51-65 and pp. 39-51, respectively; *The Asian Crisis and Human Security*, Tokyo: Japan Centre for International Exchange, 1999; and *The Quest for Human Security*, Pranee Thiparat, editor, Bangkok: Institute of Strategic and International Studies, 2001.

6   See *The Asian Crisis and Human Security*, op. cit., pp. 56-57.

7   See United Nations Development Program (UNDP) Human Development Report, 1999.

8   On 12 October 2002, Bali, Indonesia experienced two simultaneous bombing attacks that claimed at least 190 lives of local residents and foreign tourists. Several injuries were also reported. Investigations point to terrorist attacks by Islamic militant groups called Jemaah Islamiyah (JI), allegedly linked to the Al-Qaeda terrorist network.

9   See Barry Buzan, "Human security in international perspective," *The Asia Pacific in the New Millennium: Political and Security Challenges*, Mely C. Anthony and Mohamed Jawhar Hassan, editors, Kuala Lumpur: Institute of Strategic and International Studies, 2001, pp. 583-589. For a more comprehensive discussion on "securitization," see Barry Buzan, Ole Waever, and Jaap de Wilde, *Security: A New Framework for Analysis*, Boulder, CO: Lynne Rienner, 1998.

10 See Mary Caron, "The Politics of Life and Death," *World Watch*, May/June 1999. Available at: URL: http://www.worldwatch.org/titles/titlesp.html.

11 This section draws extensively from the information provided in the country papers on Cambodia, Indonesia, and the Philippines as part of the JCIE project on Health and Human Security (referred to in the Acknowledgments). Available at: URL: http://www.jcie.or.jp.

12 Transcribed text of Naruo Uehara's report on "Health Care in Indonesia," presented at the Health and Human Security Workshop, Kisarazu, Japan, March 2002 (hereinafter referred to as Uehara's Report).

13 See Philip Musgrove, Riadh Zeramdini and Guy Carrin, "Basic Patterns in National Health Expenditure," *Bulletin of the World Health Organization 2002*, 80(02), pp. 134-142.

14 These health services include, among others, basic health care, basic maternity care, immunization and treatment of TB and malaria, and referral services to hospital.

15 This was supported in the WHO study (see Reference 8).

REFERENCES

1.   Haq M. New imperatives of human security. RGICS Paper No. 7. New Delhi: Rajiv Gandhi Institute for Contemporary Studies (RGICS); 1994.

2.   United Nations Development Program. *Human development report 1994*. New York: Oxford University Press; 1994. (Hereinafter referred to as the UNDP Report.)

3. Alkire S. Conceptual framework for the Commission on Human Security. Working manuscript 2001 Dec 6.

4. Caballero-Anthony M. Challenges to Southeast Asian security cooperation. In Wilson-Roberts G, editor. *An Asia-Pacific security crisis? New challenges to regional stability.* New Zealand: Centre for Strategic Studies; 1999. p. 51–65.

5. Steer A. Presentation to USINDO. In: USINDO economic briefing series. Washington; 2002 Oct 2.

6. Narayan D, Chambers R, Shah MK, and Petesch P. *Voices of the poor: crying out for change.* Published for the World Bank. New York: Oxford University Press; 2000.

7. Ogata S. State security — human security. The Fridtjof Nansen Memorial Lecture. Tokyo, Japan; 2001 Dec 12.

8. Acharya A. Human security: what kind for the Asia-Pacific? In: Dickens D, editor. *The human face of security: Asia Pacific perspectives.* Canberra: Strategic and Defence Studies Centre, Australian National University; 2002. p. 5–17.

9. UN says vast population masks Asian AIDS crisis. Reuters News Agency 2002 Nov 26.

10. Healthcare reforms, growth-stifling diseases. *Philippine Star.* Available from: URL: http://www.philstar.com/philstar/NEWS_FLASH090520021_1.htm.

11. China on verge of AIDS epidemic. *The Straits Times Interactive* 2002 Sep 6. Available from: URL: http://straitstimes.asia1.com.sg.

12. Rising health care costs alarm WHO. *The Straits Times Interactive* 2002 Sep 30. Available from: URL: http://straitstimes.asia1.com.sg.

13. Uehara N. Health care in Indonesia. Report presented at the Health and Human Security workshop; 2002 Mar; Kisarazu, Japan.

14. Sen A. Why human security? In: Alkire S. *Conceptual framework for the Commission on Human Security.* Working manuscript 2001 Dec 6.

15. The state in a changing world. *World development report 1997.* Published for the World Bank. New York: Oxford University Press; 1977.

16. *The Jakarta Post* 1998 March 8.

17. UNDP report 1994. p. 22.

CHAPTER 14

HARNESSING SOCIAL CAPITAL FOR
HEALTH, SECURITY, AND DEVELOPMENT
IN BANGLADESH

ALAYNE M. ADAMS AND MUSHTAQUE CHOWDHURY

INTRODUCTION

The nine-month war of independence in 1971 left Bangladesh in ruins. The economy was shattered, the infrastructure was destroyed, and the very fabric of society was under threat. Insecurities abounded and multiplied, particularly among those who were already poor and vulnerable. Disruptions in food production and distribution systems and loss of employment provoked widespread food and economic insecurity. The health situation deteriorated due to the collapse of any rudimentary services that existed before the war, while the ruthless slaughter of many students and teachers by the occupation army left the education system in similar disarray. With the liberation of the country, the acute or immediate threats to life due to civil unrest may have been averted, but persistent insecurities related to lack of income, employment, health care, or education prevailed or worsened.[1]

Thirty years later, Bangladesh has witnessed one of the most rapid health transitions in the developing world. Under-five mortality has decreased from 239 deaths per 1,000 live births in 1970, to 94 deaths in the late 1990s, and the fertility rate has dropped from 6.3 births per woman to 3.3 births in 2000 (1, 2). The gender gap in life expectancy favoring males, and biases in nutritional status and educational opportunity, have also diminished substantially (Table 1). Theories regarding the impetus behind these changes abound, although the most persuasive point to the success of nongovernmental organizations (NGOs) in addressing the multiple insecurities that afflict the poor (3).

In this chapter we explore the programmatic experience of BRAC, a large multisectoral NGO in Bangladesh whose origins coincide with the founding of the nation. In particular, we use the lens of social capital to interpret the evolution of BRAC's rural development approach. Key to this

Table I.   Changes in health and educational outcomes over the last 30 years

Indicator	1970	2000
Total fertility rate	6.3	3.3
Life expectancy at birth, total (years)	44.2	59.4
Female	43.5	59.5
Male	45.0	59.4
Infant mortality rate (per 1,000 live births)	140.0	66.3
Under-five mortality rate (per 1,000 live births)	239.0	94.0
Adult literacy rate, age 15+, total (%)	24	41
Female	11	30
Male	35	52
Gross enrollment rate, primary level (%)	49.8	100
Female	33.3	100
Male	65.7	100

Sources: World Bank HNP Stats; UNDP Human Development Report, 2002; BDHS 2001.

approach is BRAC's emphasis on building material and relational resources that support the health and security of the poor and excluded. Underscored by the Voices of the Poor study (4) and long recognized by BRAC, is that poverty is not merely a state of material deprivation, but a condition where multiple social and economic insecurities intersect to negatively impact health or exacerbate vulnerability to environmental, political, and other exogenous shocks. Indeed, for many of the poor, the psychological stress of chronic insecurity is no less supportable than the experience of acute deprivation. A critical resource in dealing with chronic insecurity is investment in relational resources that work to pool risk and provide assistance in times of need. As this chapter demonstrates, central to BRAC's success is its holistic approach to poverty alleviation in which multiple insecurities are addressed simultaneously, and social capital is forged deliberately and incrementally to enable the poor to help themselves.

The chapter begins with a brief orientation to key concepts from the social capital literature, followed by a description of the current health and human security situation in Bangladesh, and the nature of state and NGO-led responses over the past two decades. The example of BRAC is then discussed, focusing on how its health and poverty alleviation strategies have evolved in response to self-evaluation and increased understanding about the complex material and relational determinants of poverty and deprivation.

SOCIAL CAPITAL AND THE DEVELOPMENT PROCESS

Social capital is generally defined as resources that inhere in social relationships (5, 6, 7, 8, 9). These resources, including networks, and the norms of reciprocity and trust on which they are based, assist the group or community as a whole by facilitating cooperation for mutual benefit. Thus conceptualized, the construct of social capital is somewhat analogous to notions of social integration, social support (10, 11), community capacity (12, 13), and community participation (14, 15) that have influenced health and development approaches over the last several decades, but with a specific emphasis on the structure and role of social relationships in achieving individual and collective security and well-being.

Advocates of the concept refer to a growing literature that documents associations between social capital, variously measured and defined, and a host of beneficial outcomes including political participation, increased income, and macroeconomic performance (8). The putative health benefits of social capital are also extolled, although empirical evidence of their association is limited to the aggregation and extrapolation of individual level data (16, 17). Despite criticisms regarding problems of measurement and lack of conceptual specificity, the concept has captured the attention of a wide range of policymakers and practitioners concerned with the health and development of the poor and excluded. How can social capital be created, enhanced, and harnessed to promote the health equity and security of the most vulnerable in society?

Four distinct dimensions of social capital have been identified in the sociological literature that operationalize the concept in ways useful to action. These are notions of integration and linkage at the micro level, and organizational integrity and synergy at the macro level (18). Sometimes referred to as 'bonding' social capital (17), *integration* denotes relationships among relatively homogenous groups such as the family, ethnic, or fraternal organizations. Characterized by a high degree of density and closure, these embedded relationships facilitate informal exchange and support among the group. On the downside, in addition to excluding those who do not meet the criteria for inclusion, high degrees of integration may impose constraints on more successful members of these communities as they attempt to transition to membership in larger exchange networks coordinated by formal institutions and the rule of law (18). The *linkage* dimension of social capital consists of relationships — with more distant associates, noncommunity members, or larger organizations — that tend to be weaker and more diverse. The concept of linkage comes from Simmel (19), who recognized that poor communities needed to generate 'centrifugal' social ties extending beyond the primordial group if long-term developmental outcomes were to be achieved. Akin to Granovetter's (20) notion of weak ties and Putnam's concept of 'bridging' social capital, these microlevel relationships are particularly potent in creating opportunities for advancement by enabling groups to leverage resources, ideas, and information from beyond the community.

At the macro level, the first dimension of social capital of pertinence to development and human security is *organizational integrity*, or the competence, coherence, and capacity of institutions to organize individual interests towards collective well-being. This dimension has its origins in Weber (21), who argued that economic development is associated with the emergence of "routines of administration" that provide a secure and predictable basis from which individual interests and abilities can be channeled into the attainment of larger collective enterprise.[2] Extending the Weberian thesis, the internal structures that establish and perpetuate capacity and credibility, and external ties to clients and constituents, are critical to successful development by the state or any large organization (22). The fourth and final dimension of social capital proposed by Woolcock (18) is *synergy*, which refers to macro-level relationships that connect representatives of formal organizations. In its most ideal form, synergy is achieved when social ties between state and society permit the pursuit of a coherent development framework, and when institutionalized mechanisms exist for the negotiation and renegotiation of goals and policies (22).

We argue in this chapter that efforts to address human insecurity through social action must harness and develop social capital in each of these dimensions. We also argue that this process should be dynamic, as development will alter the nature of baseline social relationships. Given that each form of social capital may confer costs as well as benefits, the challenge for activists and policymakers alike is to nurture mechanisms that will create and sustain the types and combinations of social relationships that are conducive to a healthy, secure, and participatory society. Optimal developmental outcomes are attained when people are willing and able to draw on social ties from within and beyond their local communities, and when macro-level connections between civil society and both public and corporate institutions work to support sustainable, equitable, and participatory development (18).

HEALTH AND HUMAN INSECURITY IN BANGLADESH

Since independence in 1971, remarkable improvements in the health and security of Bangladeshis have occurred. Despite these positive trends, Bangladesh remains one of the poorest countries in South Asia.[3] It is estimated that half the population is poor, as indicated by the upper cost-of-basic-needs (CBN) poverty line, while 34% live in extreme poverty based on the lower CBN cutoff (23).[4] Rapid urbanization from 10% in 1975 to 25% in 2000 has also marked this 30-year period, prompted in large part by rural exodus due to the increasing scarcity of cultivable land (24). Although the incidence of poverty remains higher in rural areas (53%

vs. 37%), urban dwellers are experiencing new insecurities including the high cost of living, rising local terrorism (extortion by *mastans*/mafia), and lack of access to social safety nets (23, 25). A quarter of all urban households are located in slum neighborhoods often characterized by high population densities and the absence of sanitary latrines, electricity, and easily accessible water sources. Twelve percent of urban families are squatters or are homeless (26, 1, 27).

ENVIRONMENTAL INSECURITIES

A deltaic country formed by the confluence of the great river systems of the Ganges, the Brahmaputra, and the Meghna, Bangladesh is flooded by seasonal monsoon rains over much of its landmass. The country is also susceptible to tropical cyclones, drought, tidal bores and riverbank erosion, and associated water-borne epidemics. A tribute to the effectiveness of early warning systems, emergency shelters, and timely relief operations mounted by both the government and NGOs across the county, the most recent flood of 1998 (similar in scale to that of 1974), resulted in only a few deaths, none of which were attributed to food shortage or flood-related diseases such as diarrhea.

An emerging environmental hazard is the problem of arsenic contamination in water sources across Bangladesh. Ninety-seven percent of the population relies on shallow tube wells for drinking water. It is estimated that approximately 27% of the total tube wells installed in the country have an arsenic concentration above tolerable levels (28). Hundreds of arsenic-related deaths have already been reported, and without immediate attention, the problem may grow to epidemic proportions over the next several years.

HEALTH AND NUTRITIONAL INSECURITIES

Both infant and child mortality rates have declined substantially since the early 1970s. In the last 15 years alone, the infant mortality rate has dropped from 105 to 66 deaths per 1,000 live births. Similarly, the under-five mortality rate declined from 152 to 94 deaths per 1,000 live births during the same period (2). While the rural-urban differential in mortality rates is disappearing, differentials between advanced communities and infrastructurally backward areas persist (29). For example, infant and under-five mortality rates are lowest in Khulna with 64 and 79 deaths per 1,000 live births respectively, and highest in Sylhet with 127 and 162 deaths per 1,000 live births respectively (29). The maternal mortality rate in Bangladesh (4.5 deaths per 1,000 live births) is among the highest in the world (30); however, recent data estimate a reduction of about 20% over the last 15 years (31).[5]

While overall levels of malnutrition in Bangladesh have declined in recent years, they remain among the highest in the world and present a picture of chronic food insecurity. It is estimated that approximately one-third of the population in Bangladesh is undernourished (24). Forty-five percent of children are stunted or short for their age, and 18% are severely stunted. Forty-eight percent of children under age five are underweight, a measure that takes into account both acute and chronic malnutrition, while 13% of children are classified as severely underweight (2).

GENDER-RELATED INSECURITIES

Access to education and literacy rates has improved over the years, signifying an increase in capacity beneficial to human security. Although gender disparities in primary school enrollment have all but disappeared, with 80% of girls reportedly in school, only 64% of boys and 57% of girls who complete primary school achieve literacy (32, 33). On average, however, only 30% of adult women are literate, compared to 52% of adult men (24). Bangladesh is also one of the few countries in the world in which gender differentials in life expectancy contradict expected patterns that reflect women's biological advantage (34, 35, 36, 37, 38). While this gap has closed in the last 15 years, its persistence highlights the deep and pervasive nature of discrimination afflicting women in Bangladesh.

In addition to greater numbers of girls attending school, other societal changes affect the social and economic security of women in Bangladesh. For example, employment opportunities for young women in the rapidly expanding garment sector and the widespread availability of women's microcredit are challenging powerful gender-related sociocultural norms that limit women's full participation in the economy and society. Despite these positive changes, women remain highly vulnerable and powerless in their ability to participate in household decision-making or decide how best to care for themselves and their children. According to the national Demographic Health Survey, 46% of women in Bangladesh are not involved in decisions regarding their own health care, and 35% have no say in decisions regarding health care for their children (2). Limits on women's mobility also persist. In the same survey, only 14% of women report being able to leave the village alone, while 27% claim that they can travel to a hospital or health center unaccompanied (2).

ADDRESSING INSECURITIES

While the government of Bangladesh has adopted many proactive policies to target poverty and its manifestations, public sector programs alone have been inadequate in addressing the diverse insecurities that threaten the poor. The bureaucratic culture that defines the government system has impeded innovation and flexibility, characteristics that are valuable in the design and implementation of effective development programs at the local level.

Compared to other developing countries, Bangladesh has built a fairly extensive human and physical infrastructure for the delivery of health services, particularly in rural areas of the country (3). However, despite efforts to promote community participation and decentralization, the management of state-led health programs remains quite rigid. For example, thana-level managers have limited discretion in their work and must seek clearance from higher-level authorities on most decisions. The government system in general focuses on the "implementation of directives from the 'top' (often without recognition of varying local circumstances), on rules and regulations, on not overstepping authority, and on not making a mistake" (3). This type of institutional structure results in a fixed plan, a blueprint, rather than a dynamic approach to development.

These limitations of government programs have partly fueled the growth in Bangladesh of the NGO sector that focuses on localized, more holistic approaches to development. Central to the NGO model of development are the importance of creating social capital through institution-building among the marginalized, and the assumption that both social and economic development are necessary in addressing insecurities. Community influence and participation are also considered hallmarks of NGO activities (39). In addition, the organizational culture of NGOs offers staff more potential for initiative and ingenuity (3).

NGOs in Bangladesh, for example, are considered leaders in microcredit financing for the poor. Microcredit is assumed to reduce vulnerability through a number of mechanisms. Most obvious is the beneficial impact of an increase in income generation and assets, particularly among women who have largely been excluded from the formal economy. Of equal importance, however, are the social benefits associated with participation in group-based microlending programs. For women these include increased self-esteem, decreased dependency, and greater power and prestige within the household and community. These benefits accrue as women gain access to and control over resources, and develop confidence as group members (40, 41, 42).

Bangladesh's NGOs are unique in their impact and scale of activities. Through close ties to local communities, they have been better able to recognize the complexities of human insecurity and formulate multisectoral responses that attempt to target the core issues involved. The next section highlights the experience of one NGO, BRAC, and its approach to addressing poverty and insecurity in Bangladesh.

THE CASE OF BRAC

Since its inception in early 1972, BRAC's main mission has been to reduce the insecurities of the poor and marginalized. Since these insecurities are multiple and complex, BRAC's strategy has been to employ multipronged interventions for the best synergistic effect. These programs have evolved dramatically over time in response to changing development needs and greater understanding of the nature and determinants of poverty in Bangladesh.

THE FIRST PHASE: RELIEF AND REHABILITATION

BRAC was originally founded to provide relief to refugees returning from India following the birth of Bangladesh. In the words of its founder, Mr. F. H. Abed:

> "Right after the War of Liberation, 10 million refugees started trekking back home to Bangladesh from India. We followed a large party of them from Meghalaya in India to the Sulla region of Bangladesh and found village after village completely destroyed. Houses — with utensils, tools, and implements left behind in terror — had been burned to the ground, and livestock killed and eaten. We felt that the great suffering of the people of this region, because of its remoteness, would not attract very much relief assistance" (as quoted in 43).

The first year's goal was to organize relief and rehabilitation. Over 14,000 houses were built, tools were supplied, livestock bought, and food and medical services provided. However, it soon became apparent that relief measures that sufficed as short-term solutions could not be a basis for sustainable development. BRAC staff began a process of experimentation, and a series of development programs were planned and fielded. At first, many of these programs were adapted from other experiments or efforts in Bangladesh and elsewhere. However, as the inappropriateness of borrowed ideas became increasingly clear, a new set of programs was developed and tested, including functional education for men and women, village group formation for collective economic activities, agricultural programs through demonstration plots, and health and family planning. Underlying these programs was the belief that investment in human capabilities in the form of education, health, economic opportunity, and institution formation is fundamental to the development process (44).[6]

THE SECOND PHASE: INTEGRATION AND ORGANIZATIONAL INTEGRITY

Then came a major strategy shift. In the initial phase, BRAC had attempted to work with the entire village community, with a particular emphasis on the poor. However, the social realities of village life soon intruded on this community-wide approach. Critical analysis by program staff and ethnographic research undertaken by BRAC researchers revealed a multiplicity of social factions within the village based on economic status, class, tradition, occupation, and political affiliation. Bringing conflicting interest groups under one umbrella of a village cooperative proved virtually impossible, as were efforts to include the truly disadvantaged such as women, landless peasants, and fishermen.

Also emerging from this early phase was an appreciation of the importance of social integration and linkage as a means of coping with insecurity. Greater resilience was observed among households well positioned in the social hierarchy and in institutions of power. By contrast, social exclusion and lack of institutional representation typified households suffering chronic insecurity and poverty. These observations led BRAC in 1977 to adopt a 'target group' approach wherein the poor and disadvantaged became the focus of BRAC's development activities. Initial eligibility criteria limited BRAC membership to households with less than 0.5 acres of land and reliant on wage labor for at least 100 days per year.

Beginning in the early 1990s, membership criteria were further refined to specifically target poor women who figured among the most disadvantaged and powerless in Bangladeshi society.[7] Prior to the arrival of NGOs such as BRAC, women were largely confined to their homes and lacked formal opportunities to associate or organize. For many women members, participation in BRAC's Village Organization (VO) represented their first exposure to a social world beyond the household. The process of forming a VO, which involves 40 to 50 women, begins with a period of consciousness and awareness raising and compulsory savings. Women are made aware of the society around them, and analyze the reasons underlying their poverty and political marginalization, and how their situation might be ameliorated. A formal course on human rights and legal education (HRLE) — covering constitutional and citizens' rights, and family, inheritance, and land laws — is also provided to members.

More important, however, are the empowerment activities that are part of BRAC's regular rural development program, such as participation in weekly and monthly meetings and interactions with BRAC staff that take place on an almost daily basis. Weekly meetings deal mainly with the collection of savings and loan transactions, while monthly meetings are designed to discuss issues ranging from local menaces such as dowry and domestic violence, to health education on issues such as childhood immunization, oral rehydration therapy (ORT), hygiene and sanitation, and safe delivery. At the end of each meeting, VO members chart out action plans on how to deal with the particular problem they have discussed.

In addition to nurturing and harnessing social capital to address collective health and gender-related insecurities, the VO also serves as a place where the skills of individual members are developed and made available to the community. Members are trained by BRAC in a variety of trades including poultry rearing, health care, and veterinary work. These cadres fill a critical vacuum in the village and cater to the needs of both VO members and the community. By serving the collective, VO members gain important social and economic credibility that is a critical next step in redressing the social and structural barriers that have kept them poor.

During this second phase, BRAC also has been working to scale up its activities to the national level, beginning with the widely celebrated ORT program that reached every household in Bangladesh (43). The rapid expansion of the microfinance program throughout the country, the improvement of nonformal primary schools for children, and BRAC's innovative TB program (see descriptions below), have challenged BRAC to develop even more efficient systems of operation, while at the same time maintaining its integrity as an institution for the poor.

BRAC's increasing size and prominence as a national institutional actor has enabled the organization to leverage its influence to advocate for the poor at state and international levels. Strategic partnerships with the government of Bangladesh and various NGOs were initiated in this phase, in which BRAC played a major role in developing, training, and facilitating national programs in nutrition, family planning, and development activities for destitute women. In the latter instance, the government with the support of the World Food Program had been providing food rations to destitute women for a period of several years. On the advice of BRAC, the government introduced a training component whereby women also received instruction on poultry rearing, thus providing a potential source of income to reduce or even alleviate dependence on food aid. Implemented jointly by the government and BRAC, over 300,000 women currently receive training through this program.

Although BRAC's visibility and high public regard has made the VO a legitimate and enduring social institution for women and the poor, periods of fundamentalist backlash have taken place, the most recent occurring in the mid 1990s. During this period, several BRAC schools and offices were torched and the homes of VO members were attacked and damaged. BRAC dealt with this challenge to its organizational integrity by successfully mobilizing civil society to support BRAC's programs, and by using the media to expose the hollowness of the fundamentalist cause.

THE THIRD PHASE: LINKAGE

Emerging from the experience of the second phase were concerns that BRAC's rapid expansion had resulted in insufficient attention to the organizational development and autonomy of the VO, and a tendency to regard the VO as a means to channel services. In the third phase, attempts to reverse this trend are apparent through increased training in leadership and organizational management at the VO level. Greater attention to fostering linkages between VOs and higher-level institutions at the union and subdistrict levels also marks this period. In this respect, BRAC encourages the efforts of local VOs to organize supralevel institutions to increase their collective bargaining power and to effectively voice demands for their rightful share in local resource allocation, including health services. Evidence of the increasing salience and power of the VO was seen in recent local and national elections as VOs functioned as important 'vote banks' that were consulted and lobbied by local political candidates.

BRAC's CURRENT PROGRAMS

BRAC currently serves 3.5 million households throughout Bangladesh. BRAC's poverty alleviation program operates in 60,000 villages managed by field-based Area Offices staffed by over 60,000 full- and part-time staff (Table 2). Beyond its own programs, BRAC is also involved in synergistic development activities with the government and various NGOs in the areas of health and family planning.

ADDRESSING INCOME INSECURITY

BRAC uses microfinance as a means for VO members to increase their income and employment chances. Within a month of VO formation, members are encouraged to apply for BRAC loans that are provided for three main purposes: 1) traditional economic activities such as rural trading, transport (boat or rickshaw), and rice processing; 2) nontraditional activities such as rural grocery and restaurant management, or technology-based activity such as raising poultry, sericulture, or mechanized irrigation; and 3) housing loans. Interest on housing loans is 10%, while for other activities a 15% rate is applied. The high proportion of loans that are repaid (99%) is attributed to peer group pressure, careful monitoring, and BRAC staff supervision.

An important feature of income and employment generation activities supported by BRAC is the attempt to create backward and forward linkages. For example, in the case of poultry programs, BRAC starts by training VO members on how to rear high-yielding varieties of chicken. Loans are then granted to finance low-cost hatcheries that enable VO members to sell day-old chicks to other women in the village. These chicks are reared until they start laying eggs, after which time they are sold back to the

Table 2.   The scale of BRAC's activities (June 2002)

Full-time staff	27,000
Part-time staff	34,000
Participants in BRAC's microfinance programs	3.5 million households
Villages with BRAC microfinance programs	60,000
Districts with BRAC microfinance programs	64 (out of 64)
Field offices	1,200
Total loans disbursed to the poor	U.S. $1.64 billion
Percentage of loans repaid	99%
Total saved by VO members	U.S. $80.4 million
Nonformal primary schools run by BRAC	34,000
Total students enrolled	1.1 million (66% girls)
Mothers taught ORT for diarrhea	13 million
Total budget (annual)	U.S. $166 million

hatchery or on the open market. One of the major risks of poultry rearing is the high mortality of birds. While the government livestock department keeps stocks of vaccines, these have typically been underused. To overcome this inefficiency, an agreement was made with the government that VO members trained as poultry workers be supplied vaccines and provide inoculation services to their community for a small fee. The VO member thus increases her own income and averts the spread of disease.

Addressing educational needs

Until recently, the primary education system in Bangladesh was beset with many problems. Enrollment was low, dropout high, attendance poor, and the quality of education mediocre. In the mid-1980s, BRAC initiated a program to provide basic education to children of poor parents. Over the years this program has expanded and now caters to the primary educational needs of over a million children, almost 70% of whom are girls. The recent achievement of gender parity in primary schools is largely due to this affirmative action by BRAC in favor of girls' schooling. The success of the program in terms of achieving basic competencies has also spurred greater attention to the quality of education in the state system.

Addressing health insecurities

BRAC implements a variety of health programs, both preventive and curative, with a particular emphasis on the diseases that afflict the poor, women, and their children.

Increasing women's capacity to treat diarrhea at home

Diarrhea was once a major killer in Bangladesh, particularly of young children. During the decade from 1980 to 1990, BRAC carried out a nationwide program to teach every mother in Bangladesh how to treat diarrhea at home with salt and sugar. The dramatic fall in infant and child mortality in Bangladesh is attributed in part to this program (43).

Enhancing human resource capacity in health at the village level

Although Bangladesh has a large public sector health program with a high density of personnel, village-level services are lacking. In response to this paucity of local care, BRAC has trained a cadre of village women as health workers. Being female and part of the VO, they are especially well suited to serve the health needs of women and the poor. In addition to selling essential drugs and contraceptives for a small profit, village health workers are trained to treat common diseases, such as TB using Directly Observed Therapy (DOTS) and pneumonia using antibiotics.

Enhancing public sector capacities in health

To help support the delivery capacity of the large and often inefficient public health sector in Bangladesh, BRAC provides training and human resources to government personnel involved in national family planning and nutrition programs. BRAC has launched a social mobilization campaign around childhood immunization, and provides assistance with research and monitoring.

Meeting the health needs of the 'ultrapoor'

One of the greatest challenges that BRAC has encountered in the last several decades is how to reach the poorest of the poor (the ultrapoor). Acknowledging the inappropriateness of microcredit as a means of poverty alleviation for this group, BRAC recently initiated a new program called Targeting the Ultrapoor, Targeting the Social Constraints. This program has several components including asset transfer, food rationing, and skills training. Recognizing that sudden health shocks and associated costs due to treatment and income loss frequently provoke a free fall into ultrapoverty, BRAC also provides health services to this population.

Tuberculosis (TB)

BRAC also has developed an innovative TB program with the village health worker (VHW) responsible for case finding and treatment. Patients enrolled in the program are obliged to sign a deed and pay a bond (equivalent to five days' wages) in order to be offered treatment. This system has yielded remarkable results with a nearly 90% cure rate (45). The government has appointed 106 subdistricts (out of 460) to carry out BRAC's program with drugs supplied free by the state.

RESEARCH AND MONITORING

Key to BRAC's strategy is the role of research in monitoring program implementation and performance, documenting program learning, and developing new ideas and approaches. Unlike most other NGOs, BRAC has made substantial investments in research capacity development within the organization, and supports a Research and Evaluation Division consisting of nearly 100 staff members. Although the mandate of this division is to conduct research for the benefit of BRAC's programs, its activities extend beyond BRAC both in terms of collaborations with other institutions, and the range of public health and development issues it addresses.

Of particular note is a longitudinal study undertaken in collaboration with the Bangladesh-based ICDDR,B Centre for Health and Population, an international research center of high repute, and several North American universities. Initiated in 1992, this study explored the impact of participation in BRAC's programs on health and well-being in a sample of 60,000 households in Matlab (46). Among the various analyses conducted was the comparison of child survival rates among three groups of women: 1) women who joined BRAC (BRAC members), 2) poor eligible women who didn't join BRAC (poor nonmembers), and 3) nonpoor women not eligible to join BRAC (nonpoor nonmembers). Striking differences were

Figure 1.   Life table probability of survival of children belonging to households of BRAC members, poor nonmembers, and nonpoor nonmembers

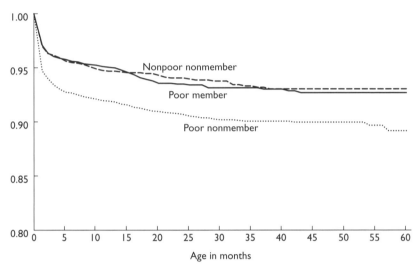

Source: Bhuiya et al., 2002.

observed. Figure 1 suggests that the survival rate of children belonging to BRAC households is higher than that of children from poor nonmember households, and remarkably similar to the survival rate of children from nonpoor households. Interestingly, further analysis indicates that the survival advantage associated with BRAC membership among the poor is largely due to mortality differences in the first few months of life, particularly in the neonatal period (47).

Using the same data set, a cross-sectional analysis of self-reported violence provides a glimpse into the degree to which gender-related insecurities have been affected by membership. Table 3 compares the incidence of reported physical violence against women in BRAC member and nonmember households. Surprisingly, it shows a higher incidence of violence among BRAC members than among nonmember households. However, when incidence figures are analyzed according to length and depth of membership, a different picture emerges. Results indicate a lower prevalence of reported violence with increasing membership length. Correspondingly, violence appears significantly greater among women who have only received credit, and tapers off with the addition of later inputs such as training. These results suggest that women's participation in economic and social life may provoke initial tension as their role in the household is redefined. As this new role is normalized, a decrease in levels of reported

Table 3. Occurrence of physical violence during last four months by BRAC membership, membership length, and membership depth, Matlab 1995

	Physical violence %
BRAC membership	
BRAC member (n=438)	8.9
Poor nonmember (n=1550)	5.8
X^2 significance	p<.05
Length of BRAC membership	
≤2 years (n=185)	10.8
2+ years (n=260)	7.3
X^2 significance	NS
Depth of BRAC membership	
Poor nonmember (n=1595)	5.6
Savings only (n=56)	5.4
Savings + credit (n=268)	11.2
Savings + credit + training (n=119)	3.4
X^2 significance	p<.01

Source: Khan et al., 1998.

violence is evident, although it is unclear whether these levels will eventually fall below community norms (48).

DISCUSSION

The case of Bangladesh illustrates the multidimensional and dynamic nature of human insecurity and its influence on equity in health outcomes and life opportunity. It also exemplifies the critical importance of relational resources in allowing individuals, households, and communities to cope with and become more resilient to these persistent insecurities.

At the micro level, BRAC has played a key role in developing individual and relational capabilities through the creation of viable social institutions that integrate the poor and excluded, and link them to the larger economy and society. Initially, given the fractured nature of civil society after the war of Liberation, a top-down approach was employed to reconstruct and develop social capital among the poor through institution-building and group-based lending. A pyramidal and multisectoral organizational structure has since evolved in response to the multidimensional nature of poverty and BRAC's desire to maximize contact with the grass roots.

At the field operations level, frontline workers in a particular sector (health, credit, training, education) report to a specialist supervisor, a group of whom report to the next level of specialist management, and so on. Due to this pyramidal structure, central management is very small in size relative to the total number of field-based staff. However, as the VO becomes a durable institution in society, BRAC is encouraging its transformation as a change agent and autonomous advocate for the poor.

At the macro level, organizational integrity has been a critical dimension of BRAC's social capital, and fundamental to its success in mobilizing government and civil society around issues of health, education, and the needs of women and the poor. Clear rules and expectations and their systematic enforcement has earned trust and respect from poor clients and the government alike. Another factor key to BRAC's organizational integrity is the emphasis placed on financial transparency through regular internal and external audits and careful attention to building a culture of honesty, commitment, and community service within the organization. BRAC's politically neutral stance as an advocate for the poor despite frequent changes in government has similarly earned the respect of the local communities in which it works, as well as of NGO partners and the donor community.

Although the impact of BRAC's overall programs on health, education, and gender relations has been marked and at times remarkable, it remains unclear to what extent this success is attributable to an emphasis on social capital creation and institution building. An important next step is the challenging task of measuring the specific impact of BRAC's relational investments on health and human security, such that these investments can be made even more effective.

Recognizing the uniqueness of the Bangladesh development experience over the last 30 years, a number of policy and programmatic lessons are apparent, relevant to settings in which human insecurity is unacceptably high. First is the importance of long-term investment in the development process that tackles poverty and related gender, social economic, and health insecurities in an integrated manner. Supporting this holistic approach is a commitment to ongoing monitoring and evaluation, and the willingness to innovate and respond to changing circumstances. Finally, the case study emphasizes the added value of investment in both material and relational resource development through institution and group formation and social capital creation at micro and macro levels. Efforts to organize the poor and create institutional linkages with the state and civil society will enhance access to resources and opportunities critical to greater health and human security.

ACKNOWLEDGMENT

Special thanks go to Caroline Min for her efficient research assistance, and to Timothy Evans for his valued editorial advice.

Notes

[1] Affecting 38 million people, the flood and subsequent famine of 1974 further eroded the health and livelihood security of Bangladeshis, resulting in a human toll of 28,700 lives (29).

[2] It was Weber's view, however, that having attained a certain measure of size and stature, large bureaucracies would become "iron cages," unable and unwilling to change to meet new circumstances.

[3] The GDP per capita in Bangladesh of U.S. $1,602 (purchasing power parity — ppp — U.S. $2,000) is markedly lower than both Pakistan (U.S. $1,928) and India (U.S. $2,358) (24).

[4] The cost-of-basic-needs poverty line represents the level of per capita expenditure needed for members of a household to meet their basic needs (including both food consumption to meet caloric requirements and nonfood consumption).

[5] By contrast, the maternal mortality rate is 3.4 in Pakistan, approximately 3.5 in India, and 2.4 in Sri Lanka (29).

[6] For Sen, the "overarching objective" of development is to maximize people's "capabilities" — their freedom to "lead the kind of lives they value, and have reason to value" (44).

[7] Also influential in this decision to target women in particular was their greater availability and interest in sustained participation, and their comparatively greater reliability as borrowers.

References

1. World Bank HNP Stats. Available from: URL: http://devdata.worldbandk.org/hnpstats, accessed on 2003 Mar 19.

2. Bangladesh Demographic and Health Survey. Mitra and Associates and ORC Macro. Calverton: National Institute of Population Research and Training; 2001.

3. Perry H. *Health for all in Bangladesh: lessons in primary health care for the twenty-first century.* Dhaka: The University Limited Press; 2000.

4. Narayan D, Patel R, Schafft K, Rademacher A, Koch-Schulte S. *Voices of the poor: can anyone hear us?* Published for the World Bank. New York: Oxford University Press; 2000.

5. Bourdieu P. The forms of capital. In: Baron S, Field J, Schuller T, editors. *Social capital: critical perspectives.* New York: Oxford University Press; 1986. p. 241–58.

6. Coleman JS. Social capital in the creation of human capital. *American Journal of Sociology* 1988;94(Suppl):S95–120.

7. Coleman JS. *Foundations of social theory.* Cambridge (MA): Harvard University Press; 1990.

8. Putnam RD. The prosperous community: social capital and public life. *The American Prospect* 1993;(Spring):35–42.

9. Putnam RD. Bowling alone: America's declining social capital. *Journal of Democracy* 1995;6(1):65–78.

10. House JS, Landis KR, Umberson D. Social relationships and health. *Science* 1998;241:540–5.

11. Heany CA, Israel BA. Social networks and social support in health education. In: Glanz K, Lewis FM, Rimer BK, editors. *Health behavior and health education: theory, research, and practice.* 2nd ed. San Francisco: Jossey-Bass; 1997. p. 179–205.

12. Parker EA, Eng E. Conceptualizing community problem-solving capacity: results of a grounded theory study. Unpublished paper. Ann Arbor: The University of Michigan; 1995.

13. Goodman RM, Speers MA, McLeroy K, Fawcett S, Kegler K, Parker E, et al. Identifying and defining the dimensions of community capacity to provide a basis for measurement. *Health Education and Health Behavior* 1998;25(3):258–78.

14. Rifkin SB. Paradigms lost: toward a new understanding of community participation in health programmes. *Acta Tropica* 1996;61(2):62–79.

15. Minkler M, Wallerstein N. Improving health through community organization and community building: a health education perspective. In: Minkler M, editor. *Community organizing and community building for health.* New Brunswick: Rutgers University Press; 1997. p. 30–52.

16. Kawachi I, Kennedy BP, Lochner K, Prothrow-Stith D. Social capital, income inequality, and mortality. *American Journal of Public Health* 1997;87:1491–8.

17. Putnam RD. *Bowling alone: the collapse and revival of American community.* New York: Simon & Schuster; 2000.

18. Woolcock M. Social capital and economic development: toward a theoretical synthesis and policy framework. *Theory and Society* 1998;27:151–208.

19. Simmel G. Group expansion and the development of individuality. In: Levine D, editor. *Georg Simmel: on individuality and social forms.* Chicago: University of Chicago Press; 1971[1908]. p. 253–255.

20. Granovetter M. The strength of weak ties. *American Journal of Sociology* 1973;78:1360–80.

21. Weber M. *General economic history.* Translated by Frank Knight. New Brunswick, NJ: Transaction Books; 1923[1981].

22. Evans P. Government action, social capital and development: reviewing the evidence on synergy. *World Development* 1995;24(6):1122.

23. World Bank. Bangladesh: progress in poverty reduction. Background Paper. Bangladesh Development Forum. Washington: World Bank; 2002.

24. United Nations Development Program. *Human development report 2002: deepening democracy in a fragmented world.* New York: Oxford University Press, Inc.; 2002.

25. Islam N, Huda N, Narayan FB, Rana PB, editors. *Addressing the urban poverty agenda in Bangladesh: critical issues and the 1995 survey findings.* Published for the Asian Development Bank. Dhaka: University Press Limited; 1997.

26. Asian Development Bank. *Project Administration Memorandum (PAM) for the loan to the People's Republic of Bangladesh for the Urban Primary Health Care Project.* Dhaka: Asian Development Bank; 1998.

27. World Bank and Bangladesh Centre for Advanced Studies. *Bangladesh 2020: a long-run perspective study.* Dhaka: University Press Limited; 1998.

28. Chowdhury AMR, Hossain Md Z, Nickson R, Rahman M, Jakariay Md, Shamimuddin Md. *Combating a deadly menace: early experiences with a community-based arsenic mitigation project in Bangladesh.* Research Monograph Series 16. Dhaka: BRAC; 2000.

29. Bangladesh Institute of Development Studies (BIDS). *Fighting human poverty: Bangladesh human development report 2000.* Dhaka: BIDS; 2001.

30. Ministry of Health and Family Welfare (MOHFW). Towards a safer motherhood for the women of Bangladesh: the power of partnership. Bangladesh Country Paper. Technical consultation on Safe Motherhood; 1997 October 19–23; Colombo. Dhaka: Government of the People's Republic of Bangladesh, MOHFW; 1997.

31. National Institute of Population Research and Training (NIPORT). The maternal mortality study. Draft report. Dhaka: NIPORT; 2002.

32. Chowdhury AMR, Nath SR, Choudhury RK. Enrolment at primary level: gender difference disappears in Bangladesh. *International Journal of Educational Development* 2002;22:191–203.

33. Watkins K. *Education now: break the cycle of poverty.* Oxford: OXFAM; 1999.

34. D'Souza S, and Chen LC. Sex differentials in mortality in rural Bangladesh. *Population and Development Review* 1980;6(2):257–70.

35. Bhuiya A, Zimicki S, and D'Souza S. Socioeconomic differentials in child nutrition and morbidity in a rural area of Bangladesh. *Journal of Tropical Pediatrics* 1986;32(1):17–23.

36. Koenig MA, D'Souza S. Sex differentials in childhood mortality in rural Bangladesh. *Social Science and Medicine* 1986;22(1):15–22.

37. Bhuiya A, Wojtyniak B, and Karim R. Malnutrition and child mortality: are socioeconomic factors important? *Journal of Biosocial Science* 1989;21(3):357–64.

38. Sen AK. More than 100 million women are missing. *The New York Review* 1990 Dec 20:61–6.

39. World Bank. Bangladesh: from counting the poor to making the poor count. World Bank Country Study. Washington: World Bank; 1999.

40. Hashemi SM, Schuler SR. Rural credit programs and women's empowerment in Bangladesh. *World Development* 1996;24(4):635–53.

41. Rahman A, et al., editors. *Early impact of Grameen.* Dhaka: Grameen Trust; 2002.

42. Chowdhury AMR. The impact of development interventions on health in Bangladesh. In: Rohde J, Wyon J, editors. *Community-based health care: lessons from Bangladesh to Boston.* Boston: Management Sciences for Health; 2002. p. 61–86.

43. Chowdhury AMR and Cash R. *A simple solution: teaching millions to treat diarrhoea at home.* Dhaka: University Press Ltd.; 1996.

44. Sen AK. *Development as freedom.* Oxford: Oxford University Press; 1999.

45. Chowdhury AMR. Success with the DOTS strategy. *The Lancet* 1999;353:1003–4.

46. Chowdhury M, Bhuiya A, Vaughan P, Adams A, Mahmud S. Effects of socioeconomic development on health status and human well-being: determining impact and exploring pathways of change. Proposals for phase II of the BRAC-ICDDR,B Matlab joint project 1996–2000. BRAC-ICDDR Working Paper No. 6. Dhaka: International Center for Diarrhea Disease Research; 1995.

47. Bhuiya A and Chowdhury AMR. Beneficial effects of a women-focused development programme on child survival: evidence from Bangladesh. *Social Science and Medicine* 55(9):1553–60. In press 2003.

48. Chowdhury AMR, Bhuiya A. Do poverty alleviation programmes reduce inequalities in health? The Bangladesh experience. In: Leon D, Walt G, editors. *Poverty, inequality and health: an international perspective.* Oxford: Oxford University Press; 2001. p. 312–31.

CHAPTER 15

LIVELIHOOD SECURITY THROUGH COMMUNITY-BASED HEALTH INSURANCE IN INDIA

MIRAI CHATTERJEE AND M. KENT RANSON

SUMMARY

For poor families, disease and illness are major risks that keep them in poverty. Rising medical costs are obstacles to their quest for health and human security. In this context, community-based health insurance (CBHI) is of special relevance to the poor.

SEWA Insurance, or Vimo SEWA, is one example of CBHI developed by the Self-Employed Women's Association (SEWA). SEWA is a labor union of 700,000 informal women workers based in Gujarat, India; all these women are economically active. SEWA is designed for and managed by women workers of the informal economy. The women are not covered by basic social protection measures, yet sickness is a major crisis and economic leakage. In the absence of state-sponsored or other social insurance, SEWA developed its own, and now reaches almost 103,000 insured persons. Operating for the last ten years, the SEWA plan is an integrated insurance package with health insurance as a major component.

One of the lessons learned is that insuring the poor can be financially viable. Sustainability is enhanced if insurance is built upon existing solidarity networks and tailored to local people's needs, but based on sound actuarial principles. Also contributing to the sustainability of Vimo SEWA are partnerships with and technical support from government insurance companies, as well as technical support from external partners.

Emerging concerns in Vimo SEWA include the continuing need for further education and awareness about both health and insurance, especially preventive and risk reduction measures, access to and quality of health care obtained (especially by poor women), prevention of adverse section (disproportionate inclusion in the scheme of those who know they are at risk of falling ill), and affordability for the poorest women and their families.

Another lesson learned from Vimo SEWA is that CBHI schemes need to be encouraged and promoted, bearing in mind access and affordability for the poorest families and women in particular. Governments, employers, donors, and others must join forces to create an environment that promotes and encourages CBHI schemes that can be developed and run by the poor themselves.

In summary, CBHI schemes offer an opportunity to increase access to health care for informal workers, especially women. They have the potential to protect workers from financial risk and from slipping further into the cycle of indebtedness, poverty, and illness. Thus, CBHI schemes can be an important economic support to the poor; however, they must be part of an integrated, holistic approach to address poverty. Only then will health and human security be possible for all, especially the poorest of workers — women workers in the informal economy.

Savitaben is a 47-year-old widow and mother to six children. She works as a traditional midwife for SEWA in Vichchiya village, the drought-prone desert district of Banaskantha. Over the years, she and her family members have suffered many episodes of illness, resulting in accumulated debts of 195,000 rupees. "Somehow in my family, whatever we earned through sheer hard labor was spent on sickness. A few months ago, I had acute appendicitis. I had to be admitted to a private hospital in Ahmedabad for an emergency operation. The whole episode cost me 8,000 rupees. Then each of my grandsons was very sick — one with meningitis and the other with pneumonia. We spent a total of 19,000 rupees on their medical expenses. The village people have been kind and understanding — they told us we could take time to pay off our debts. But we still have a long way to go" (1).

Shantaben is a 52-year-old resident of Bharoda village in Kheda district — the centre of Gujarat's dairy and tobacco industries. A member of Vimo SEWA for five years, Shantaben works for daily wages, either as an agricultural laborer or as an assistant with the midday meal program at the village school. Recently, while closing a high window at the school, she fell and injured her back. Initially, she tried to treat the injury at home by applying salt and turmeric, but the pain only worsened. She was taken by rickshaw to a nearby, nonprofit hospital, where she was admitted for ten days and treated with bed rest and medicines for her pain. The cost of hospitalization and transportation was around 1,800 rupees, which she was able to borrow from her nephew at the time of discharge. After only two weeks, Vimo SEWA reimbursed her. She has now paid back her nephew, and says that because of the health insurance, she has been able to continue saving money to replace her kuttcha house (built from bricks of sun-dried mud).

For more than ten years, Vimo SEWA has provided health, life, and assets insurance services to women working in India's informal sector, and today has almost 103,000 insured members (FY 2001–02). Based on

SEWA's experience and data, this chapter will: 1) describe Vimo SEWA's health insurance services and highlight some of the lessons learned in providing these services; 2) discuss whether (and if so, what kind of) support is required to strengthen, replicate, and scale-up CBHI schemes like Vimo SEWA's. The first section discusses the potential benefits of CBHI and the extent to which these benefits have been realized by existing schemes. The second section of the chapter documents Vimo SEWA's experience to date, including: a) a description of the scheme's technical design and management; b) an assessment of the scheme's impact; and c) a discussion of the factors that have contributed to the scheme's impact. The third and final section of the chapter discusses ways in which government, multinational organizations (like the ILO and WHO), and external donors can help to strengthen and support CBHI schemes.

BACKGROUND

For over two decades, there have been calls for communities in developing countries to participate in the planning, financing, organizing, and operating of health care services. The Declaration of Alma Ata (2) implied that community participation was integral to the achievement of health for all, and stated that "primary health care requires and promotes maximum community and individual self-reliance and participation…making fullest use of local, national, and other available resources." The Bamako Initiative aimed to make primary health care universally accessible through community financing and management (3). But questions remain as to whether, how, and how much poor people in poor countries can or should be expected to contribute toward the provision of health care.

The issue is of greatest importance to the poor themselves. Material wealth, health, and the ability to cope with adverse health events are intimately related. The World Bank defines poverty as "encompassing not only material deprivation but also low achievements in education and health…[and] vulnerability and exposure to risk." (4). An individual of low income may be unable to afford preventive care, or curative care in the event of illness, which may result in the worsening of his or her state of health. In the event of serious illness, the poor are particularly vulnerable to the financial burden resulting from lost income and out-of-pocket medical expenditures as they have low levels of the assets (physical, natural, and financial) necessary to cope. Disease or illness can cause an individual or household to enter a vicious downward spiral in which poor health results in the depletion of assets, and low levels of assets in turn lead to worsening health and the inability to cope with future illness episodes. In theory, government provision of health care should cover the poor, but in practice it often does not. Thus, there is a need to find ways to protect the poor from the costs of medical care.

The term *community-based health insurance* refers to schemes wherein individuals or households regularly pay a premium in exchange for coverage of the costs of future, unpredictable medical expenses. What distinguishes these community-based schemes from public or private-for-profit insurance is that the targeted community is involved in defining the contribution level and collecting mechanisms, defining the content of the benefit package, and allocating the scheme's financial resources (5).

Policymakers hope that CBHI will contribute to the health system goals of better health, fair financing, and responsiveness as proposed recently by the WHO (6). In many developing countries, the potential for expanding or improving the health sector through increased government funding is limited due to a narrow tax base (7). CBHI allows pooling — the joint contribution of resources to cover the future costs of illnesses that may afflict anyone in the group — in those settings where institutional capacity is weak to organize nationwide risk-pooling, which may allow a health sector starved for funds to tap resources that would otherwise not be available. A fundamental question is whether CBHI will be able to expand to cover sufficiently large populations to 1) put to use the pooling functions, and 2) be considered a serious alternative (to state-run social security and tax-financed public health services) for providing social protection to the poor.

Since the Alma Ata Declaration's call for resource mobilization, there have been a number of thorough reviews of CBHI or more general community financing (8, 9, 10, 5). Authors have generally bemoaned the lack of empirically derived data on the schemes, particularly regarding their impact on health status, utilization of services, and financial protection. All of the reviews have commented that CBHI schemes face many threats to long-term financial sustainability, often stemming from poor design and management. Nonetheless, the reviewers have generally been cautiously optimistic in their recommendations. For example, Working Group 3 of the Commission on Macroeconomics and Health recommended:

> "That out-of-pocket expenditures by poor communities should increasingly be channeled into 'community financing' schemes to help cover the costs of community-based health delivery.... Community-financing schemes are no panacea, and have often failed, but for many places they seem a promising and flexible mechanism that can often be harnessed to local needs" (11).

The Vimo SEWA experience

Figure 1 (adapted from 12) illustrates some of the elements of Vimo SEWA that will be described in this section, including the context in which the scheme operates, the design and management of the scheme (and the related nature of the interaction between the insured members, Vimo SEWA, health care providers, the government, and donors); and the economic and social impact of the scheme.

CONTEXT

The Self Employed Women's Association is a labor union of 700,000 women workers engaged in the informal economy, based in Ahmedabad, Gujarat, India. SEWA members have no fixed employer-employee relationship, nor are they covered by protective labor legislation. SEWA's membership can be categorized by four main occupation groups: 1) manual laborers and service providers such as agricultural workers, construction workers, and cleaners; 2) street vendors; 3) home-based workers, for example, incense stick rollers and embroiderers; and 4) small-scale producers such as gum collectors and craft workers. These women work long, hard hours, and because of the nature of their employment and the absence of laws covering them, they do not obtain even basic social protection such as health insurance, maternity benefits, and sick leave.

It was in this context that SEWA began to organize women for their economic rights in 1972. The goals are full employment and self-reliance — both economic and in terms of decision-making and control. Full employment includes security of work and income, food security, and social security, which in SEWA's experience must include at least health care, child care, insurance, and shelter.

Figure 1. Vimo SEWA: context, design, and outcomes

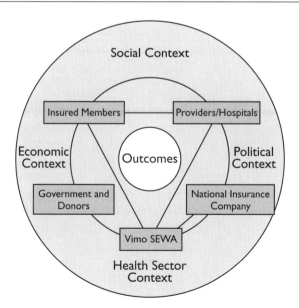

Source: Adapted from Bogg L, Hengjin D, et al. The cost of coverage: rural health insurance in China. *Health Policy and Planning* 1996;11(3):238–52.

One of SEWA's first initiatives was to address women's needs for financial services — savings and credit. These needs were filled through the women's own microfinance cooperative, SEWA Bank. A study in 1977 of women who were not repaying their loans regularly revealed that the major cause was sickness of the woman or her family members. We regularly witness women selling or mortgaging assets and utilizing their hard-earned savings during illness episodes. These experiences resulted in the establishment of a community-based primary health care program at SEWA in 1984.

Being the poorest of workers, and often living in environments without basic water and sanitation, SEWA members and their families are frequently sick. The high cost of health care usually prevents an informal sector worker from seeking treatment, which may result in the worsening of her state of health. The poorest quintile of Indians is 2.6 times more likely than the richest to forego medical treatment when ill, and despite higher rates of illness, is only one-sixth as likely to undergo hospitalization (13). Poor health, when it results in lost wages or health care expenditures, leads to indebtedness, loss of assets, and further poverty. According to an analysis by Peters, et al. (13), at least 24% of all people hospitalized in India in a single year fell below the poverty line because they were hospitalized. In theory, government provision of health care should cover the poor, but in practice it often does not.

Social insurance and private health insurance (outside of Vimo SEWA) are largely unavailable to SEWA members and other workers of the informal economy. Social insurance in India is provided through the Central Government Health Scheme (CGHS) and the Employee State Insurance Scheme (ESIS). Introduced in 1954, CHGS is a contributory health scheme that provides comprehensive medical care to central government employees and their dependents. Some 4.4 million beneficiaries were covered under the scheme in 1996 (13). The Government of India (GOI) heavily subsidizes the CGHS. The ESIS, which became operational in 1952, is an insurance system providing both care and medical benefits to poor factory workers and dependents. As of 1998, 35.4 million people were covered (13). Employers contribute to the ESIS an amount equal to 4.75% of the wages payable to employees, while employees contribute 2.25% of their wages. State governments contribute a minimum of 12.5% of the total ESIS expenditure on medical care in their respective states (14).

Private insurance coverage in India is very limited. Four national insurance companies (falling under the control of the semiautonomous General Insurance Company, or GIC), along with a few new private insurers, offer a full range of non-life insurance types with health as a very small share of their total. As of the end of calendar year 1995, there were 1.8 million people covered by Mediclaim, the main health insurance policy sold by the GIC. Premiums are generally paid directly by households, and in 1996 ranged from 175 to 5,770 rupees per year (for coverage from

15,000 to 300,000 rupees per year (14). Individuals are eligible for a rebate on income tax up to a sum of 10,000 rupees per year. While the government's insurance companies have designed a voluntary policy — *Jan Arogya Bima* — targeted at poorer populations, most people are not familiar with it or do not have access to an agent who could sell them this insurance. Besides, premiums offered are generally unaffordable to most poor families.

SCHEME DESIGN AND MANAGEMENT

Given the need for protection from sickness and other frequent risks, SEWA Insurance or Vimo SEWA was established in 1992 to complement the primary health care work. This scheme provides life insurance, health (hospitalization) insurance, and asset insurance. This section deals exclusively with the health insurance component.

The scheme is targeted at members of the SEWA Union across eleven districts in Gujarat state, their spouses, and — as of this year — their children. In order to join, adults must be between 18 and 58 years of age. Under Vimo SEWA's most popular policy, those who pay the annual premium of 85 rupees (22.5 rupees of which is earmarked for medical insurance) are covered to a maximum of 2,000 rupees per year in case of hospitalization (Table 1). Women also have the option of becoming lifetime members of the Social Security scheme by making a fixed deposit of 1,000 rupees; interest on this amount is used to pay the annual premium and the deposit is returned to the woman when she reaches age 58.[1] Exempted from coverage under SEWA's health insurance are certain preexisting diseases (for example, chronic tuberculosis, certain cancers, diabetes, hypertension, piles) and disease caused by addiction.

The choice of health care provider is left to the discretion of the SEWA member. Members are eligible for reimbursement whether they use private-for-profit, private-nonprofit, or public facilities. After discharge, the

Table I.   Premiums* and benefits for Vimo SEWA's health insurance

	Policy I	Policy II	Policy III
Premiums for package inclusive of health, life, and assets insurance:			
Female annual premium	85	200	400
Female fixed deposit	1,000	2,400	4,800
Male (spouse) annual premium	55	150	325
Male (spouse) fixed deposit	650	1,800	4,000
Amount (from above premiums) earmarked for health insurance	42	56	218
Hospital benefit	2,000	5,500	10,000

* Note that these premiums are for the health, life, and assets components combined.

member is required to submit the following documents within a three-month period: a doctor's certificate stating the reason for hospitalization and the dates of admission and discharge, doctors' prescriptions and bills for medicines purchased, and reports of laboratory tests done during the hospital stay. After submission of these documents, a SEWA employee usually visits the member to verify the authenticity of the claim. A consultant physician reviews all documentation, and a final decision on the claim is then made by an insurance committee, most of whom are self-employed workers. Finally, the insured member is notified of the committee decision, and when applicable, is paid by check.

Vimo SEWA is run by local women leaders called *aagewans* and supported by a team of full-time staff. The latter help the aagewans become managers of the insurance program. A team of experienced professionals, including insurance, public health, and medical experts, help in capacity building, maintaining technical competence, and quality control.

The design and management of SEWA's health insurance have evolved considerably since 1992. Initially the plan was administered jointly by SEWA and the United India Insurance Company (UIIC, a subsidiary of the government's general insurance companies). SEWA negotiated with the UIIC to develop a special package to cover members. At that time, coverage included only allopathic, inpatient care, and did not include gynecologic illnesses. The maximum amount of reimbursement was 1,000 rupees per year.

The collaboration with the insurance company proved to be a mixed experience. Difficulties arose in part due to the nature of the risks covered, and also because these companies had very little experience in insuring the poor. Consequently, systems and procedures were slow and not suited to the reality of women workers. When we began facing bureaucratic delays and procedural problems, we first tried to change the policies of the insurance company. Finally, in 1994, we decided to run the health insurance component of Vimo SEWA ourselves. It proved to be less complicated and risky than we had imagined. By taking over the management of the health insurance scheme, we learned that we could run health insurance for poor women in a sustainable way (retaining any profit for the benefit of our members). By improving the quality of our insurance services, we could also increase our membership markedly.

In 1995, coverage was expanded to include treatment from traditional bonesetters, occupational diseases, obstetric and gynecologic problems, and in exceptional cases, traditional homeopathic or ayurvedic medical care (still to a maximum of 1,000 rupees per year). In 1998, the maximum coverage was increased to 1,200 rupees per year. In 2001, Vimo SEWA began offering health insurance to men, and implemented three different insurance policies for adult men and women. Since then, Vimo SEWA has again started purchasing medical insurance from a government general insurance company, this time the National Insurance Company (NIC).

However, Vimo SEWA remains fully responsible for enrollment of members, and for approval and processing of claims. The NIC receives premiums from Vimo SEWA once per year, and pays Vimo SEWA a lump sum on a monthly basis for all claims reimbursed.

IMPACT OF VIMO SEWA'S MEDICAL INSURANCE FUND

Currently, SEWA Insurance has 102,897 members in Gujarat in both urban and rural areas (Figure 2). This number represents about 20% of SEWA Union's total membership in Gujarat state (535,674 members).

As one would expect, given the increasing membership, the number of claims has steadily increased with time (Figure 3). However, rates of utilization of the scheme have remained relatively stable at around 18 to 20 claims per 1,000 members per year. This rate is low in comparison to rates of hospitalization among Gujarati women, generally in the range of 48 to 78 per 1,000 per year (15, 16).

Among the 1,930 claims submitted over a six-year period from July 1, 1994 to June 30, 2000, claimants had a mean age of 41.0 years (median = 40 years). The leading causes of hospitalization (N = 1,914) were accidents and injuries (14%), malaria (10%), acute gastroenteritis (10%), and hysterectomy (9%); the mean duration of hospitalization was 6.1 days (N = 1,929; median = 4 days). Care was given in private-for-profit (63.9% of claims), government (28.6%), and private-nonprofit (7.5%) hospitals.

Vimo SEWA recognizes the need for improvements in the quality of health care availed of its members. An in-depth study of hysterectomy cases

Figure 2.   Membership in Vimo SEWA by year

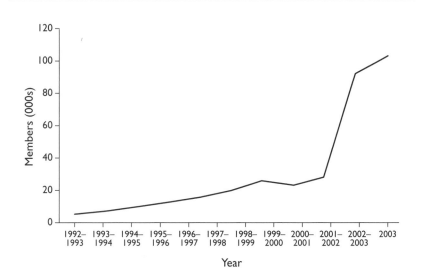

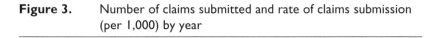

Figure 3.   Number of claims submitted and rate of claims submission
(per 1,000) by year

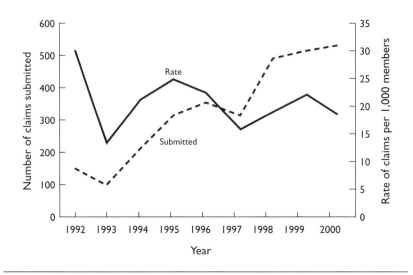

among Vimo SEWA members in the Kheda district found that quality
varies tremendously, from potentially dangerous to excellent (17).

Among those who have submitted medical claims to SEWA, the degree
of financial protection appears to have been substantial (18). The average rate of rejection over the last eight years has been only 11%. Among
the claims that were reimbursed, the mean rate of reimbursement varied
from an average of 50% (in recent years) to 85% (in 1995 to 1996) of total
reported hospital costs. In recent years, the delay between hospital discharge and reimbursement of the insured was just over three months, with
more than half of this delay occurring between discharge from hospital
and submission of the insurance claim to Vimo SEWA. Women who submitted medical claims to Vimo SEWA experienced difficulties in compiling the necessary receipts and certificates. The difficulty seems to result
from a lack of information regarding the documentation required, problems finding time to collect documentation, and attempts by doctors to
make things difficult or extract money from the insured. Decentralization
of the claims process has been piloted in one district (Kheda) with reduced
delays in the submission and processing of claims.

Since the health insurance scheme's inception, the premiums paid by
annual members plus the interest received from the fixed deposits of lifetime members have always exceeded medical claim payments (Figure 4
shows that the claims/premiums ratio is consistently less than 100%).

However, administrative costs of the scheme have been quite high. It
is difficult to estimate the costs of the health insurance component, as many

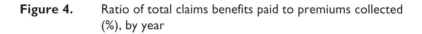

Figure 4.   Ratio of total claims benefits paid to premiums collected (%), by year

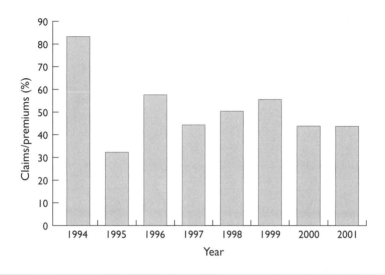

of the administrative functions are shared with the life and asset insurance components as well as with other activities of SEWA. A recent study by the International Labour Office (ILO) found that basic administration costs accounted for 10.2% to 22.9% of SEWA's Integrated Social Security Scheme expenses annually (19).

Data on the maternity benefits provided under Vimo SEWA have been less thoroughly investigated. Preliminary analyses suggest that most recipients deliver in a public hospital; however, it is also common to deliver in a private hospital or at home with the assistance of a *dai* (traditional midwife). On average, the 300 rupees maternity benefit seems to cover a significant portion of the cost of delivery services, but represents only a fraction of the total costs of pregnancy and delivery (including indirect costs such as transportation and antenatal care). Costs were higher among urban than rural women, and were far higher among those who had experienced complications at delivery or had undergone cesarean section. Most respondents received their Vimo SEWA benefits only after delivery (usually around three months afterwards).

FACTORS THAT HAVE CONTRIBUTED TO THE GROWTH OF VIMO SEWA'S HEALTH INSURANCE

There is no established framework for reviewing the success or effectiveness of CBHI schemes. Figure 5, adapted from Ranson and Bennett (20), is a simple conceptual map of the associations between overall health system goals, obstacles to promoting these goals through CBHI schemes,

Figure 5.   Social goals for CBHIs, obstacles to achieving them, and corrective mechanisms

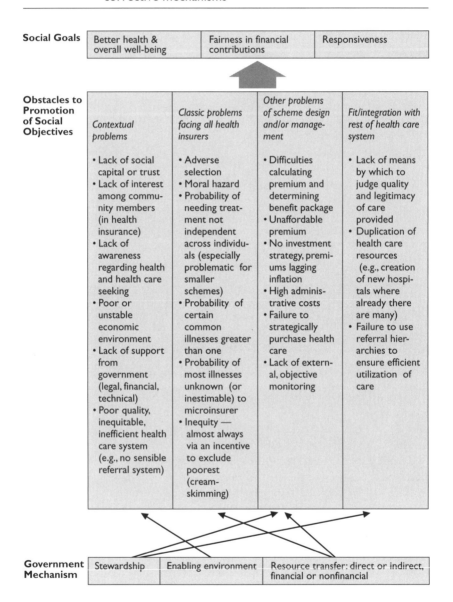

Source: Adapted from Ranson and Bennett (20).

and the categories of external interventions that can be used to overcome these obstacles. This map provides a useful framework for exploring the factors that may act as obstacles to the successful operation of CBHI schemes and their contribution toward social objectives.

Contextual (environmental) problems refer to the economic, political, social, or cultural context in which the scheme operates. People in a poor or unstable economic setting, for example, may be unable or unwilling to participate in a CBHI scheme. The classic problems facing all insurers include adverse selection, moral hazard, covariant risks (affecting groups of households, communities, regions, or nations), and unknown probability of illness (21). Schemes may also fail to meet social objectives due to problems of design and management, such as failing to increase premiums to keep pace with inflation and rising health care costs. Finally, CBHI schemes may fail to contribute to social goals if they are not well integrated with the rest of the health care system. For example, a hospital-based insurance scheme may adequately cover the risks of a high-cost hospital admission, but in the absence of a network of preventive, primary, and referral services, it may function inefficiently or fail to attract the people who need it most.

Here we address two questions. First, to what extent has Vimo SEWA been subject to the problems in Figure 5? Second, what aspects of the context, scheme design, and management have helped or hindered Vimo SEWA in addressing these problems?

Table 2 again lists the problems that may prevent CBHI schemes from operating successfully and contributing toward social objectives (as per Figure 5). It then indicates the importance of each problem to Vimo SEWA and characteristics of the scheme that have helped either to prevent or to overcome the problem. Through highlighting, this table showcases Vimo SEWA's strengths and identifies problems that still impede the scheme's ability to achieve social goals.

Four factors have contributed to the growth of Vimo SEWA: 1) the nesting of Vimo SEWA within a larger, membership-based organization; 2) rational, data-based setting of premiums and benefits packages, owing in part to the (on-off-on) partnership with the Government Insurance Company; 3) technical and (small but reliable) financial support from external partners and donors; and 4) dynamic management that has not hesitated to make changes to the scheme in response to members' needs.

Vimo SEWA's close association with SEWA Union and other sister organizations (SEWA Bank, SEWA Health, and SEWA Academy in particular), has helped to prevent and overcome a variety of problems. SEWA Union is the workers' own organization, based on the principles of solidarity, trust, and unity among workers, and organized for their overall economic rights and basic security. As a result of decades of repeated, successful, collective activities carried out by SEWA Union, members are more willing to participate in Vimo SEWA. The literacy training provided

Table 2.   Potential problems, their importance/relevance for Vimo
              SEWA, and characteristics of Vimo SEWA that have helped
              to prevent or overcome them

Potential problems	Problem for Vimo SEWA?	Characteristics of Vimo SEWA
Contextual problems		
Lack of solidarity (sense of community) or trust in leadership	No	Nesting of Vimo SEWA within SEWA Union, whose members avail of various development-oriented services.
Lack of interest among community members in health insurance	No	Vimo SEWA evolved out of a demand for insurance services, voiced by SEWA's members. As well, SEWA members are provided with periodic, recurrent education regarding the benefits of insurance.
Lack of knowledge/ awareness among community members in health and health care seeking	Yes	Literacy training provided by SEWA Academy and health education provided by SEWA Health have helped. But many members, particularly women, remain unaware of health care problems and how/ where to seek treatment.
Poor or unstable economic environment	Yes	While the savings, credit, and income-generating services offered by SEWA have helped to provide a stable economic environment, poorer SEWA members still cannot afford the premium.
Lack of support from government (legal, financial, technical)	Yes	External donors have stepped in to provide financial and technical support (particularly GTZ and ILO).
Poor quality, inequitable, inefficient health care system	Yes	Vimo SEWA has begun to forge relationships directly with the providers, but poor quality of care remains a significant problem.
Classic problems facing health insurers		
Adverse selection	Yes	Preexisting diseases are excluded from coverage, and there is a minimum 30-day waiting period between enrollment and eligibility for benefits. As well, people are encouraged to enroll the whole family, rather than just the old or infirm. Nonetheless, the old and infirm are more likely to join.
Moral hazard	No	Vimo SEWA covers only the direct costs of hospitalization (so in effect, all claimants face a 'co-payment' in the form of indirect costs) and the scheme covers to a maximum of 2,000 rupees. But as mentioned below, there is a financial incentive to use inpatient versus outpatient facilities.
Covariant risks (probability of needing treatment not independent across individuals)	No	Large and steadily increasing population covered.

Potential problems	Problem for Vimo SEWA?	Characteristics of Vimo SEWA
Probability of certain common illnesses greater than one	No	The scheme only covers inpatient (presumably infrequent) illnesses. It excludes maternity benefits, which are covered under a special bonus for fixed deposit members.
Probability of most illnesses unknown	No	Vimo SEWA originally partnered with the Government Insurance Company, which has the best available illness statistics.
Preferential inclusion of the wealthy/healthy (cream-skimming)	No	One of the primary goals of Vimo SEWA is to include the very poor (which has probably contributed to the problem of adverse selection). Nonetheless, the cost of joining prevents some, particularly the poorest, from joining.

Other problems of scheme design and/or management

Difficulties calculating premium and determining benefit package	No	Vimo SEWA has been able to set rational (actuarially sound) premiums and benefits packages through its partnership with the GIC.
Unaffordable premium	No	Vimo SEWA has attempted to set an affordable premium, and sells the insurance at the time of harvest. As well, it offers payment options (annual versus fixed deposit). Nonetheless, some of the very poorest SEWA members cannot afford.
Problems of financial management: no investment strategy, premiums that do not keep pace with inflation	No	Since Vimo SEWA's inception, there has been support from SEWA Bank and from external donors (GTZ, ILO, CGAP).
High administrative costs	Yes	The costs of providing, educating, promoting, and selling insurance among a scattered, largely rural and illiterate population are high. Financial assistance from external donors has helped to offset these costs.
Failure to strategically purchase health care	Yes	Vimo SEWA has initiated dialogue with health care providers, but strategic purchasing is hindered by lack of any financial relationship between Vimo SEWA and providers, which is made difficult in turn because the providers are many and scattered.
Lack of internal monitoring and evaluation	No	Since Vimo SEWA's inception there has been a paper-based MIS, regularly analyzed to provide information to administrators. This system has now been computerized.
Lack of external, objective monitoring	No	Regular external accounts audits. Numerous external researchers have studied the scheme.

Continued on next page

Table 2.   Potential problems, their importance/relevance for Vimo
SEWA, and characteristics of Vimo SEWA that have helped
to prevent or overcome them *(continued)*

Potential problems	Problem for Vimo SEWA?	Characteristics of Vimo SEWA
Fit/integration with rest of health care system		
Lack of means by which to judge quality and legitimacy of care provided	Yes	As per GIC guidelines, Vimo SEWA encourages its members to use facilities that are registered with local authorities or have at least 15 inpatient beds. In reality, this does little to assure quality of care.
Duplication of health care resources (e.g., creation of new hospitals where already there are many)	No	Not an issue, given that Vimo SEWA members use existing hospitals that are not run by SEWA.
Failure to use referral hierarchies to ensure efficient utilization of care	Yes	There is a 'perverse incentive' for Vimo SEWA members to seek inpatient rather than outpatient care. Aside from providing health education to Vimo SEWA members, this matter has not yet been addressed.

by SEWA Academy and the health awareness and education provided by
SEWA Health have increased demand for health care services among the
members of Vimo SEWA (and thus increased their demand for insurance
services). The financial services offered by SEWA Bank (savings and
credit), along with income-generation and marketing activities carried out
by SEWA — through its Trade Facilitation Center, *Mahila Gram Haat*
(Rural Women's Market), and the Federation of Cooperatives it has promoted — help to provide members with a sense of economic security, and
so facilitate payment of the insurance premium. Finally, Vimo SEWA
draws on the infrastructure and human resources of its sister organizations,
particularly at the time of the annual membership drive.

Vimo SEWA's partnership with the government's insurance companies
— and particularly its early partnership with the United India Insurance
Company — has contributed to its long-term financial viability. By collaborating with the UIIC, Vimo SEWA was able to draw on: 1) the wealth
of information regarding disease frequency and cost of health care seeking that the UIIC (and GIC) had accumulated during its decades of operation in India (since 1946); and 2) the technical skills and experience of its
staff, including the actuarial skills required in setting Vimo SEWA's origi-
nal premium and benefits package. While the premiums and benefits have
changed gradually over the last ten years, their levels at the time of the
scheme's inception have doubtless been important to its success.

Technical and financial support provided by partner and donor organizations have also helped Vimo SEWA achieve what otherwise would have been impossible. Technical support has been particularly useful in making year-to-year adjustments in the premium and benefits package, and external financial support has covered some of the costs of capacity building, marketing, and promotion. The costs of marketing the scheme among its scattered, largely rural and illiterate population are high. Education and promotion must be provided face-to-face, which involves significant labor and transportation costs.

Vimo SEWA's management has used the data collected through its paper/computer-based monitoring system and during periodic studies to make adjustments over the years to the premium and benefits package. Management's willingness to change and experiment with scheme design has surely contributed to members' sense of consumer satisfaction and to increased membership. Being open to external evaluation (for example, audits and research) has also helped to make evidence-based changes to the insurance scheme.

Sidebar 1.   Lessons learned from the Vimo SEWA experience

---

1. Insurance is an essential economic support to women during crises. In ten years, 18,000 women have received 20 million rupees or US $400,000 by way of claims.

2. People's own insurance programs — those run by the poor, for the poor — can be viable.

3. Health insurance creates demand for government health services.

4. To maintain affordability, a panel of providers can be developed.

5. Linkage with health programs focused on prevention and promotion enhances the viability of health insurance.

6. Linking insurance to other financial services (such as savings and credit) promotes long-term insurance coverage.

7. Women begin future planning through insurance.

8. Insurance promotion can be a source of employment.

9. Education about insurance accelerates membership.

10. Insurance by and for poor women encourages them to organize and contributes to their economic empowerment.

11. Promotional, marketing, and claim-servicing costs are high when insuring the poor.

12. Expanding the number of insured members helps spread costs.

13. The increase in premiums must be gradual.

14. Both government and private equity are required for overall sustainability.

15. Worker, government, and private contributions should be one-third each.

16. Investing in the poor, especially women, through social insurance is viable.

Sidebar 1 lists a number of other lessons learned from the Vimo SEWA experience.

Vimo SEWA has encountered a number of obstacles that have been particularly difficult to address (Table 2):

1. Owing largely to a lack of awareness regarding their own health and the availability of different health care treatments, many people (particularly women) fail to recognize illness and present for medical treatment in a timely manner. Thus, even Vimo SEWA members may succumb to treatable illnesses such as malaria, typhoid, or acute gastroenteritis, when they could be cured with medical (perhaps inpatient) treatment. Addressing this problem requires gender-specific education and literacy training that are provided repeatedly from an early age.

2. Improving people's access to health care is a mixed blessing in a setting where quality of care is variable, and at worst, dangerous. Poor quality is an issue both with private and (perhaps to a lesser degree) public inpatient facilities. To date, the government has done nothing to monitor or regulate the quality of health care (in part due to resistance from national, state, and local medical associations). In the absence of any national quality guidelines, it has been difficult for Vimo SEWA to work for better quality of care. While it is possible to assemble a list of preferred providers (inpatient facilities that offer an acceptable standard of care), this would mean limiting the choice of providers available to Vimo SEWA's members, and potentially reducing geographic accessibility for those who live in more remote areas.

3. Despite its efforts to prevent adverse selection (upper age limit of 58 years, exclusion of preexisting disease, and minimum waiting period of 30 days between enrollment and eligibility for benefits), Vimo SEWA (more in some geographic areas than others) has attracted a membership that is older and more likely to experience illness than the general population. It is only logical that households with limited resources will preferentially enroll those who are most likely to fall sick (or to die, given that the insurance package also includes life insurance). Vimo SEWA encourages all SEWA members (age 18 to 58) and their spouses and children to join the scheme. But by allowing individual as opposed to family (or household) membership, it is inevitable that even in households that can afford the insurance, some of the young and healthy will opt out.

4. Despite Vimo SEWA's best efforts to design an insurance package that is affordable to the poor, some very poor households find the premiums unaffordable. Failure to include the very poor limits the overall equity impact of the scheme.

5. SEWA's health insurance covers only the cost of inpatient care; however, there is no referral mechanism (or 'gatekeeper') to ensure that only the more serious cases proceed to hospital. Thus in some cases the insured have a financial incentive to be treated as an inpatient rather than as an outpatient (as the cost to them after reimbursement will be less). This calls for Vimo SEWA to rely more heavily upon its sister organization, SEWA Health, to set up a referral network that will prevent unnecessary hospitalization.

In the following section, we discuss how these and other problems might be addressed with the assistance of government, the private sector, and other NGOs and international agencies.

DEVELOPING, STRENGTHENING, AND UPSCALING CBHIS: USING THE LESSONS FROM VIMO SEWA

Certain external interventions may lessen or overcome obstacles to the success of CBHI schemes and their promotion of social objectives (Figure 4). The mechanisms used can be categorized as stewardship, creation of an enabling environment, and transfer of resources, both financial and nonfinancial. Stewardship includes developing a policy framework; implementing relevant legislation; mandating or obliging the performance of certain activities; monitoring and regulating the quantity, quality, and price of CBHI and health care; and generating and disseminating information on disease prevalence and treatment costs. The creation of an enabling environment is a broader concept that includes ensuring economic and political stability; providing literacy training and health education; and preventing corruption in the legal, health care, and banking systems (these mechanisms generally fall outside the realm of the Ministry of Health). The transfer of resources to CBHIs may occur directly, from government to insurer, or indirectly, from government to health care provider (usually government-owned) or the insured. Resources (financial or otherwise) may be transferred routinely or only when the scheme faces bankruptcy. Nonfinancial transfers include targeted technical or managerial support or provision of a reinsurance function, wherein groups of CBHIs create a solidarity fund for protection against covariant risks.

The Vimo SEWA experience suggests that the following interventions would be particularly useful:

CREATION OF AN ENABLING ENVIRONMENT

- Encouraging people's organizations (POs) and NGOs that are already providing broad, development-oriented interventions, to implement CBHI schemes

■ Creating interventions aimed at improving literacy and awareness of health care problems and their treatment (particularly among girls and women)

■ Ensuring that adequate quality of inpatient care is available at a fair price

FINANCIAL SUPPORT

■ Direct transfer of resources to the CBHI scheme, perhaps earmarked for administrative costs or marketing and promoting the scheme among the poor

■ Development of special loans either to the CBHI scheme or to households, so that even the poorest households are able to join

TECHNICAL SUPPORT

■ Both private and public insurers could custom-design health insurance schemes for poorer populations, and partner with POs and NGOs in marketing these schemes

■ Technical support for the setting of premiums and design of benefits packages

■ External evaluations and audits

■ Support in establishing a referral network that emphasizes cost-effective preventive and primary health interventions, and limits unnecessary hospitalizations

These external interventions may come from a variety of different sources, either alone or in combination:

1. *The health care sector (both private and public).* It is hoped that, as has happened in many developed countries, doctors (and perhaps other health care providers) will unite to establish certain quality guidelines, and will self-monitor for adherence to these guidelines.

2. *Private sector industry.* Many informal sector workers, including many of SEWA's self-employed laborers, work either directly (for daily wages) or indirectly for large, private-sector companies. These employers should be required to make some financial contribution toward CBHI schemes, in the same way that they contribute toward insurance for their salaried (formal sector) employees. In fact, all employers should be required to contribute toward a Social Security Fund for informal workers that will be used to develop CBHI schemes to be implemented by POs and NGOs.

3. *Other people's organizations and nongovernmental organizations.* In Africa, and South and Southeast Asia, there are increasing num-

bers of CBHI schemes. While they are generally unlikely to be a source of financial resources for one another, they comprise a rich source of skill and experience. Vimo SEWA, for example, is often called upon to document its experience and provide technical expertise to new schemes being developed in India. Friends of Women's World Banking's (FWWB's) Insurance Promotion Program has developed out of a partnership between SEWA and the German Technical Cooperation (GTZ), and functions as an 'apex NGO' providing technical and limited financial support to microfinance institutions interested in starting CBHI schemes. Similarly, an international network of cooperatives is committed to providing insurance — the International Cooperatives and Mutual Insurance Federation (ICMIF).

4. *Government*. The role of government in furthering social goals through CBHI schemes is particularly controversial. Some argue that the strength of CBHI is due to the community-driven nature of the schemes, which must be responsive and accountable to their target populations or they risk going out of business. As such, they tend to be far more dynamic and innovative than government health financing initiatives. Any intervention by government should not counteract these strengths.

In their study of the role that central governments can play in facilitating CBHI schemes, Ranson and Bennett concluded that (20):

■ Broad policy statements by government are helpful, particularly in creating an environment conducive to building confidence in CBHI schemes (otherwise people may worry that schemes will be shut down).

■ Regulation of CBHI schemes should be embarked upon only with caution in developing countries, given capacity constraints and the frequent perversion of regulation to serve private interests. Tighter government control over schemes may stifle innovation and limit their variety, another reason not to encourage regulation. Any regulation used should be simple and easy to understand.

■ Mandating scheme membership, for example at the level of local or village government, is an interesting idea, but there is limited evidence on how it works and how feasible it is to implement in the contexts where CBHI schemes can make the biggest contribution.

■ Environment is important, but we have little understanding of the impact of government measures on environment (how frequently does government succeed at uniting disparate groups?). Nor do we fully understand the effects of the environment upon the scheme (for example, how important is trust among members, or between members and the insurer or provider, to the success of a scheme?).

■ Technical assistance of adequate quality is desirable and not very controversial.

■ Financial support is critical but it is not clear how this should be delivered. Is it best to provide financial support on a regular and sustained basis, or only when schemes are financially strained (for example, due to poor investment strategy, or because premiums were set too low), or only when schemes are financially strained due to covariant risks? If governments provide support in the first two scenarios, they risk fostering inefficiently managed schemes. However, this type of support may be required if governments wish to encourage coverage of populations that are poor and at high risk of illness. CBHI schemes may require reinsurance against covariant risks, but the question is whether, to what extent, and how reinsurance should be coupled with other forms of financial or technical support.

5. *International organizations and donors.* International organizations (such as the World Bank, ILO, and WHO) can do much to facilitate beneficial mechanisms between government and microinsurers (a macrostewardship role). They can help shape policy, encourage governments to promote CBHIs, and build capacity. In addition, they can recommend suitable mechanisms to be implemented by government, encourage research on the relative impact of mechanisms, and help disseminate the lessons learned.

International donors can make financial transfers directly to CBHI schemes as equity. Among other possibilities, this money can be earmarked for administrative costs, targeting the scheme to particularly poor or hard-to-reach populations, or supporting experimentation in CBHIs, accompanied by sound monitoring and evaluation. International organizations are also well positioned to facilitate the sharing of experience and technical support between countries and regions.

CONCLUSIONS

In summary, CBHI schemes present a number of possibilities to increase the accessibility of appropriate and timely health care to workers in the informal sector, and protect them from financial risk and slipping further into indebtedness, poverty, and illness.

Our experience at Vimo SEWA shows that health insurance is not only a growing need and demand of workers in the informal sector — the bulk of the working poor — but also a significant economic support. Time and again, our SEWA sisters have said that this support prevented their slipping back into poverty from which they had struggled to emerge.

However, our experience also points to the need for setting CBHIs in the wider context of organizing the poor, especially women, for their economic rights. It is not simply a matter of implementing a single intervention — health insurance — but rather developing a holistic and integrated approach to address the many facets of poverty. An integrated approach will ultimately lead to health and human security for all, especially the poorest of workers — women workers of the informal economy.

NOTE

[1] The fixed deposit, which can be paid at any time of the year, must be paid in cash into the member's account in SEWA Bank, where it remains. The annual interest, ranging from 11% to 13% up to 1999 — but now only 9.5% — is used to pay the annual premium.

REFERENCES

1. Self-Employed Women's Association. *'Tana Vana': warp and weft of life.* Ahmedabad: Self-Employed Women's Association; 2002.

2. International Conference on Primary Health Care. Declaration of Alma-Ata. *The Lancet* 1978 Nov 11;2:1040–1.

3. McPake B, Hanson K, et al. *Implementing the Bamako initiative in Africa.* Health Economics and Financing Programme, Health Policy Unit. London: Department of Public Health and Policy; 1992.

4. World Bank. *World development report 2000/2001: attacking poverty.* Oxford: Oxford University Press; 2001.

5. International Labour Organization, Universitas Programme. *Extending social protection in health through community based health organizations: evidence and challenges.* Geneva: International Labour Organization; 2002. p. 79.

6. World Health Organization. *The world health report 2000.* Health systems: improving performance. Geneva: World Health Organization; 2000.

7. Mills A. Economic aspects of health insurance. In: Lee K, Mills A. *The economics of health in developing countries.* Oxford: Oxford University Press; 1983. p. 64–88.

8. Stinson W. Community financing of primary health care. *Primary Health Care Issues* 1982;1(4):90 pages.

9. Bennett S, Creese A, et al. *Health insurance schemes for people outside formal sector employment.* Division of Analysis, Research, and Assessment, World Health Organization (WHO). Geneva: WHO; 1998.

10. Working Group 3 of the Commission on Macroeconomics and Health. Mobilisation of domestic resources for health. Draft report. Geneva: World Health Organization; 2001. 130 pages.

11. World Health Organization. *Macroeconomics and health: investing in health for economic development.* Geneva: World Health Organization; 2002.

12. Bogg L, Hengjin D, et al. The cost of coverage: rural health insurance in China. *Health Policy and Planning* 1996;11(3):238–52.

13. Peters D, Yazbeck A, et al. *Raising the sights: better health systems for India's poor.* Health, Nutrition, Population Sector Unit. Delhi: The World Bank; 2001. p. 173.

14. Naylor CD, Jha P, et al. *A fine balance: some options for private and public health care in urban India.* Human Development Network. Washington: The World Bank; 1999.

15. Sundar R. Household survey of health care utilisation and expenditure. New Delhi: National Council of Applied Economic Research; 1995. p. 95.

16. Gumber A, Kulkarni V. Health insurance for informal sector: case study of Gujarat. *Economic and Political Weekly* 2000 Sep 30:3607–13.

17. Ranson MK, John KR. Quality of hysterectomy care in rural Gujarat: the role of community-based health insurance. *Health Policy and Planning* 2001;16(4):395–403.

18. Ranson MK. Reduction of catastrophic health care expenditures by a community-based health insurance scheme in Gujarat, India: current experiences and challenges. *Bulletin of the World Health Organization* 2002;80(8):613–21.

19. International Labour Organization and STEP. *Women organizing for social protection: the Self-employed Women's Association's integrated insurance scheme, India.* Geneva: International Labour Organization and STEP; 2001.

20. Ranson MK, Bennett S. Role of central governments in furthering social goals through microinsurance units. In: Dror DM, Preker AS. *Social reinsurance: a new approach to sustain community health financing.* Washington: The World Bank and the International Labor Organization; 2002.

21. Barr N. *The economics of the welfare state.* Oxford: Oxford University Press; 1998.

INDEX

A
Aagewans, 284
Abington, 12, 119
Abstinence, 155
Abuse of women, 165
Acceptable standard of care, 294
Accessible health centers, 245
Accordion effect, 134
Adams AM, vii, xxiii, 257, 276
Adolescent girls, 190
Adolescent men, 189
Adolescent sexual health agendas, 204
Adult AIDS, 147
Adult HIV, 128
Adult life expectancy, 127–128, 147
Aedes aegypti, 62, 98, 107
Affirmative action, 268
Affordable access, 76
Affordable medicines, 154
Afghanistan, 5, 11, 18–19, 29, 115,
    226
Africa, vii, ix–xii, xiv, xvii, xx–xxi, 8–
    9, 18, 28, 38, 40–41, 58, 62–63, 68,
    80, 87–88, 93–96, 101–103, 106–
    109, 111, 119–120, 125–130, 132–
    134, 136–139, 141–144, 146–154,
    156–158, 166–167, 169, 179, 187,
    190–191, 201, 203, 213, 218–219,
    222, 230, 241, 296, 299
Ahmedabad, 278, 281, 299
AIDS, vii, ix–xii, xiv–xv, xvii–xviii,
    xx–xxii, 8–9, 27, 62–63, 67, 72, 75,
    78–82, 88, 96, 100, 103, 105–106,
    108–112, 117–118, 120–121, 123,
    125–139, 141–158, 167, 178, 182–
    183, 185–192, 197, 199, 201–204,
    207, 213, 216–219, 221–222, 226–
    227, 229–230, 234, 241–242, 255
AIDS activists, 148–149
AIDS care, 133
AIDS epidemic, xii, xxi, 80, 108, 120,
    125–127, 129–131, 133–134, 142–
    143, 145, 155–157, 187, 191, 202–
    203, 229–230, 241, 255
Alcohol abuse, 197

Alkire S, 12, 255
Al-Qaeda, 254
Anarchy, 28, 109, 175
Angola, 150
Annan K, 201
Anthrax, xx, 4, 8, 105, 112, 115–117
Antimicrobial, 88, 93, 101, 120
Antiretroviral regimen, 222
Antivirals, 105, 110
Anxiety, xiv, 94, 197
Apartheid, 147
Argentina, 48
Arie S, vii, 13, 28, 82
Armed conflict, 6, 17, 23, 30, 143,
    157, 170, 174, 192, 196, 228
ASEAN, 249, 253
Asian crisis, 237, 254
Asian Development Bank, vii, 177, 275
Asian financial crisis, 4, 9, 236, 244,
    248
Australia, 41, 194, 204, 207, 226

B
Bacteria, 8, 71, 90–91, 97, 101
Bali, 238, 254
Balkans, 174
Bangladesh, vii, ix, xxiii, 6, 65, 74, 95,
    115, 127–128, 169, 194–195, 205,
    257–258, 260–264, 266–268, 271–
    276
Banking systems, 295
Barrier protections, 95
Benin, 186, 202
Berlinguer G, vii, xix, 12, 53, 65, 83,
    101
Besir Center, 206
Bettcher DW, vii, xxi, 161, 178, 180
Biodiversity, 102
Bioethics, vii, xix, 30, 53, 55–56, 64–
    65, 139
Bioterrorism, xx, 4, 8–9, 67, 94, 105,
    111–113, 115–117, 121–122, 226,
    228
Bolivia, 92
Bosnia-Herzegovina, 5, 18, 17, 196

Botswana, xi–xii, 88, 127–128, 142, 144, 146–147, 150, 153–154, 184
BRAC, vii, ix, xxiii, 74, 257–258, 263–272, 275
Brazil, vii, 55, 63, 92, 127–128, 168, 170, 178, 191, 195, 205
Breakdown of social mores, 144
Breastfeeding, 98
Britain, xiii, xix, 32–33, 37, 40, 47, 49–52, 69
Bruderlein C, viii, 13, 28–29, 82
Brundtland, GH, xiii, 149, 156
Brunei, 249–250
Brussels, 7, 156
Bubonic plague, 141, 147
Burden of AIDS, 144
Burden of disease, xxii, 70, 73, 83, 171, 199, 202, 209–213, 218, 229
Burkina Faso, 115
Bush G, 49
Bushmeat, 93, 103

C
Caballero-Anthony M, viii, xxii, 64, 233, 253, 255
Caloric requirements, 273
Cambodia, 18, 188, 233, 242–243, 245–246, 248–250, 252, 254
Cameroon, vii, 93, 188
Capital accumulation, 33, 41
Capital formation, 40
Cardiovascular disease, 215–217, 226
Caribbean, 41, 143, 179
Catastrophic illness, 4, 10–11
Centers for Disease Control (CDC), x, xiii, 8, 102, 120, 206
Central America, 168
Central Asia, 143
Central government, 69, 246, 282
Chatterjee M, viii, xxiii, 277
Chechnya, 18, 29
Chemical weapons, 122
Chen LC, ix, xviii, xix, 3, 12, 65, 67, 207, 229, 275
Child abuse, 165
Child care, 134, 281
Child deaths, 101, 147
Child health, xi
Child labor, 58, 69
Child malnutrition, 135, 221
Child marriage, 193
Child mortality, 127, 131, 134, 147, 213, 261, 268, 275

Child nutrition, 275
Child soldiers, 151, 157
Child survival, 147, 269, 276
Childhood immunization, 110, 112, 265, 269
Childhood mortality, 275
Chile, 168, 188, 194, 205–206, 208
Chloroquine, 100, 103
Cholera, 8, 59, 69, 94, 106, 115, 119, 180
Chowdhury M, ix, xxiii, 257, 276
Civil rights, 39
Civil society, xix, 22, 27, 41, 54, 69–70, 78, 133–134, 138, 149, 152, 155, 260, 266, 271–272
Civil war, 17, 25, 170, 173, 178–180
Clinical AIDS, 222
Clinton W, 62
Collective enterprise, 14, 260
Colombia, 92, 100, 170, 194, 205
Commission on Human Security (CHS), ix, xv, 3–4, 154, 166, 239, 242–243, 255
Communal violence, 19
Communicable disease, 101, 122, 167, 175, 212, 214, 218, 222
Concept of 'human security,' xviii, 3, 11, 24, 55, 165–166, 218, 234, 239, 242–243
Condom, 144, 146, 188–190, 197, 203
Conflict, viii, xi, xv, xviii–xix, xxi, 4–6, 10–11, 13–23, 26–30, 37, 48, 58, 67, 82, 109, 121, 138, 143, 149, 151–152, 157, 166, 168, 170, 172–174, 177–180, 184–185, 192–193, 196, 210, 227–228, 235, 237, 239, 241, 253
Congo, 17, 28, 151
Congo-Rwanda border, 6
Containment response, 115
Contraception, 188
Control of infectious diseases, 88
Coping capacities, 130
Coping strategies, 16, 26
Core values, 175, 240, 253
Cost of health care, 282, 292
Cost of hospitalization, 278
Cost of inpatient care, 295
Costa Rica, 188
Cost-effective interventions, xii, xxii, 211, 221–222
Côte d'Ivoire, 107, 115

Criminal assault, 192
Criminal, 23, 71, 163–164, 180, 192
Cuba, 92, 112
Czech Republic, 196

D
Dai, 287
de Waal A, ix, xx, 125, 138–139
Debt burdens, 27
Decision-making, 152, 185, 262, 281
Demographic, xiii, xx, 33, 40, 58, 70,
    87–88, 95, 106, 121, 125, 127,
    132, 134–137, 145, 147–148, 156,
    186, 205–206, 214, 262, 273
Dengue fever, 4, 8, 92
Denmark, 205
Directly Observed Therapy (DOTS),
    74, 83, 268, 276
Disability-adjusted life years (DALYs),
    87, 213, 222
Disease burden, xii, 96, 118, 217–220,
    226
Disease, ix–xiii, xv, xviii–xx, xxii, 4,
    7–8, 24, 33, 35, 50, 52, 55–56, 58,
    62, 68–70, 73, 75, 78, 82–83, 87,
    92–96, 98–103, 105–108, 110–122,
    126, 138, 141, 144, 149–152, 162,
    167, 171, 174–175, 181–182, 186,
    191, 199, 202, 206, 209–220, 222,
    224, 226–227, 229, 235, 241, 251,
    268, 276–277, 279, 283, 292, 294–
    295
Displaced persons, 22, 178
Domestic violence, ix, xxi, 6, 197,
    205–208, 238, 265
Dominican Republic, 92
Donor agencies, 246
Donor community, 272
Drèze J, 15, 28, 230
Drought-prone, 278
Drug trade, 174
Drug–resistant viruses, 97

E
Ebola, x, 8, 94–95, 106, 112, 114
Economic constraints, 95
Economic crises, 143
Economic development, xxi–xxii, 10,
    38, 42, 51–52, 60, 77–78, 81, 84,
    111, 120, 125, 130, 133, 136, 144,
    147, 170, 230, 235–238, 260, 263,
    274, 300

Egypt, 94, 99, 103, 115, 194, 198, 205
El Salvador, 92, 168
Emergency preparedness, 107, 116
England, xiii, 32, 38, 41, 51, 101, 104
Environment, ix, xix, 4, 12, 35–36, 39,
    54–55, 58, 60, 62, 92, 162–163,
    184, 193, 198, 213, 239–240, 242,
    252, 278, 290, 295, 297
Epidemic, xii, xvii, xx–xxi, 19, 24, 64,
    67, 71, 75, 80, 98, 104, 107–108,
    110, 112, 115, 119–120, 122, 125–
    127, 129–131, 133–134, 137, 142–
    143, 145, 147, 151, 153, 155–157,
    169–170, 178–179, 182, 187, 191,
    202–203, 218, 229–230, 241, 255,
    261
Epidemiology, xii, xxi, 31, 102–103,
    106, 119, 157, 173, 202–203, 205
Ethics, xi, xvii–xviii, 1, 12, 22, 48, 55,
    61, 65, 82–83
Ethiopia, 115, 137, 194, 205
Ethnic cleansing, 168
Euphoria-induced amnesia, 36
European Union, 47, 72–73

F
Faith-based groups, 78
Family planning, 186, 205, 264, 266–
    267, 269
Famine, ix, 38, 131, 134–136, 138–
    139, 165, 251, 273
Fecal contamination, 118
Female condoms, 144, 153, 189
Female genital mutilation, 193
Food insecurity, 133, 137, 139, 261
Food rationing, 269
Freedom from fear, 5, 17, 181, 195,
    235, 253
Freedom of expression, 152

G
García-Moreno C, ix, xxi, 181, 201,
    204, 207
Gastrointestinal pathogens, 91
Gaza Strip, 194
Gender bias, xxi
Gender disparities, 262
Gender-based violence, 182–183, 191–
    193, 195, 197–199
General Agreement on Trade in
    Services (GATS) 63, 76
Genocide, 6, 24, 30, 149, 157, 165,
    167–168

Germany, x, 47, 69, 78
Ghafele R, x, xxi, 52, 161
Global burden of disease, 70, 73, 83, 171, 209–210, 212, 218, 229
Global Equity Initiative, ix, xi, xiii, xv–xvi, 52, 64, 82–83, 207
Global Fund for AIDS, Tuberculosis, and Malaria (Global Fund), 9, 63, 72, 80, 111, 118, 123, 148–149, 155
Global health crises, 80
Global health security, 117–118, 122
Globalization, viii, x, xix, 4, 10, 34, 50, 52, 57, 59, 65, 68, 75, 82–83, 87–88, 110, 132, 170, 172–174, 176, 180, 228, 238
Gore A, 157
Great Britain, 51
Gross domestic product (GDP), 10, 27, 33, 111, 130–131, 147, 150, 170, 222, 248–250, 273
Guatemala, 6, 92
Guinea worm disease, 118
Guinea, 118, 146, 185, 188, 194, 198, 202, 206

H
Haiti, 143–144, 146
Hajj, 98, 101, 103
Hantavirus, 106, 112
Health Canada, 114, 122
Health care, ix, xxii, 10, 26, 59–60, 64, 69, 78, 81, 94, 107, 109, 122, 130–131, 149, 151, 155, 167, 182, 184, 186, 194, 198–200, 233, 239–248, 251–252, 254–255, 257, 262, 265, 273, 275–279, 281–283, 285, 289–292, 294–296, 298–300
Health equity, ix, xix, 12, 62, 65, 73–74, 83, 259
Health infrastructure, xix–xx, 9, 82, 96, 116, 154
Health insurance, xxiii, 245, 277–284, 286–287, 290, 293, 295–296, 298–300
Health intervention, 226
Health life expectancy, 27, 222
Health outcomes, 163, 165, 167, 182, 213, 245, 271
Health promotion, vii
Health security, viii, 5, 11, 56–57, 62, 68, 80–82, 105, 116–118, 121–122, 165, 175, 178, 181, 212, 253, 257

Health threats, xxii, 9, 11, 33, 36, 67, 70–71, 82–83, 210
Healthy life expectancy (HALE), 185, 200, 222–223
Hepatitis B, 8, 90, 94–95
Hepatitis C, 94–95, 99, 103
Heymann DL, xvi, xx, 105, 119–120, 122
HIV
    HIV incidence, 135
    HIV infection, 126, 132, 143, 145, 150, 153, 188–189, 197, 207, 218
    HIV–infected, 97
    HIV–positive, 8
    Transmission of HIV, 89, 135, 152–153, 200
    Spread of, 90, 144, 153
Holleufer G, x, 13, 29, 82
Honduras, 92
Hong Kong, 98, 100, 115
Human Development Index (HDI), 27
Human Rights and Legal Education (HRLE), 265
Human Rights Watch, ix, 207
Human rights, ix, xi, 5–7, 21–24, 26, 29–30, 53, 55, 72, 133, 180–181, 192, 196, 204, 207, 236, 265
Human Sciences Research Council (HSRC), xii, xiv, 146
Human security, viii–ix, xii, xv–xxiii, 3–6, 8–18, 20–25, 27–28, 32–35, 37, 39, 42–49, 52–57, 61, 64–65, 67, 71, 76–78, 80–83, 117–118, 125–126, 136, 141–142, 145, 154, 157, 161–162, 164–166, 168, 170, 173, 175–179, 181–182, 185, 187, 190–193, 195–196, 198–201, 203, 207, 209–210, 218–220, 222, 225–229, 233–243, 245, 247–248, 251–255, 258, 260, 262, 272, 277–278, 299
Humanitarian principles, 22
Humanitarian workers, 20, 25

I
Immigrants, 90, 93
Immunization, xiii, 107–108, 110, 112, 254, 265, 269
Income insecurity, 4, 267
Indebtedness, 278, 282, 298
Indonesia, 48, 95, 233, 236–238, 242–246, 248–250, 252, 254–255

Industrial capital accumulation, 41
Inequality, 9, 15, 26, 36, 44, 71, 131, 136, 138, 179, 181–182, 184, 186, 188, 190–193, 198, 200–202, 210, 229, 274, 276
Infectious disease, xiii, xviii, 8, 82, 87, 94, 100, 105–106, 108, 111–113, 115–119, 121–122, 138, 162, 174, 215, 218, 226
Insect vectors of human diseases, 102
Insecurities of daily life, 4, 9
Institution-building, 263, 271
Insurance promotion, 293, 297
Inter-American Development Bank, 197, 205–206, 208
Internal conflict, 19, 149, 235
International AIDS Vaccine Initiative, 79
International Centre for Diarrhoeal Disease Research (ICDDR), 269
International Committee of the Red Cross (ICRC), x–xi, 18, 25, 28–29
International donors, 298
International Labour Organization (ILO), 47, 201, 279, 287, 290–291, 298–300
International Monetary Fund (IMF), 36, 60, 63
International Rescue Committee (IRC), 28
Interventions, xii, xxi–xxii, 7, 25, 77, 92, 94, 97, 153, 199–200, 211, 214, 220–223, 227–228, 263, 276, 289, 295–296
Iraq, 29
Ireland, 38
Irrigation, 267
Islam, 129, 275
Italy, vii, 59, 65, 207

J
Japan, xvi, 12, 47, 69, 78, 127–128, 146, 195, 228, 252, 254–255
Johnson S, x, xxi, 181, 207

K
Kampala, 206
Karachi, 96, 179
Kenya, 153, 191, 194, 204–205
Key competencies, 27
Killing of women, 201
Korea, 194, 205
Kosovo, 5, 17–18, 115

L
Labor markets, 41
Labor migration, 237
Latin America, ix, 8, 38, 40–41, 70, 94, 96, 107, 110, 143, 178–179, 197
Latvia, 173
Leaning J, xi, 13, 28–30, 52, 64, 82–83, 207
Legal status, 190
Lesotho, 88, 142, 148, 150
Lethal infection, 90
Liberia, 102
Life expectancy, 27, 68, 88, 111, 127–129, 133, 137, 147, 184–185, 200, 218, 222–223, 257–258, 262
Life insurance, 130, 283, 294
Life tables, 128, 138, 184, 202, 229, 270
Life years, 87, 167, 213, 215, 221, 230
Local government, 37–38, 42, 45, 54, 69, 138, 245, 247
Local health care workers, 94
Local initiative, 24
Local interventions, 97

M
Macroeconomic, 4, 9, 39, 83, 130, 259
Malaria, xi, 8–9, 36, 58, 63, 72, 78–80, 87–88, 95, 100, 104, 107, 110–112, 118, 123, 148–149, 155, 163–164, 185–186, 234, 245, 254, 285, 294
Malawi, 127–128, 133, 148, 150, 190
Malaysia, 236–237, 242, 249–250
Maldives, 184
Male condoms, 189
Male dominance, 193, 206
Male sex workers, 189
Mali, vii, 128
Malignancies, 216–217
Malnutrition, 10, 70, 78, 135, 167, 174, 186, 210, 218, 221, 234, 246–247, 261–262, 275
Marginalized people, 152
Market economy, 37
Marriage, xiii, 189–190, 193, 201, 204, 206
Mass migration, 109, 175
Meddings DR, xi, xxi, 52, 161, 178, 180
Médecins Sans Frontières, 149

Medical ethics, xi
Medical insurance, 283–285
Mental health, xiv, 207
Mental illness, 71, 215, 226
Merck, 79
Merck-Gates Initiative, xi
Mexico, 92, 112, 116, 146, 194, 196
Microbe, 58, 95
Microbial contamination, 91
Microcredit, 262–263, 269
Microfinance cooperative, 282
Middle East, 53, 143, 187
Migrant labor, 143
Millennium Development Goal, 130
Morbidity, xviii, xxi–xxii, 10, 68, 102, 131, 134, 164, 167, 212, 222, 275
Mortality, xiii, xviii, xx–xxii, 10–11, 27–28, 37–38, 50–51, 64, 68, 70, 73, 78, 83, 87, 100, 102, 108, 117, 126–131, 134–135, 147–148, 164, 166–167, 169, 178–179, 185, 200, 210, 212–216, 218–220, 222, 226–227, 229, 243, 257–258, 261, 268, 270, 273–275
Mother-to-child transmission, 131, 135, 139, 157
Movement of people, 4, 89, 92
Mozambique, 148, 150, 154
Multilateral donor agencies, 246
Myanmar, 242

N
Namibia, 88, 142, 148, 150, 184, 195, 203–204
Narasimhan V, xi, xvi, xviii, 3, 52, 64–65, 82–84, 103, 207, 229
National security, xvii, 3–4, 9, 32, 49–50, 62, 105–106, 108–109, 111, 117, 120–121, 133, 141, 145, 151, 209, 218–219
Natural disaster, 247
Nepal, 184, 204, 242
Netherlands, 29, 194, 205
New Zealand, 253, 255
Nicaragua, 92, 178, 194, 205–206, 208
Nigeria, 95, 137, 194, 206
Nongovernmental organization (NGO), 246, 257, 263, 272, 297
Noncombatant distinctions, 27
Noncommunicable disease, 212, 214–215, 218

North Africa, 143, 187
Norway, xiii, 78, 194
Nuclear arms race, 109
Null scenario, 222

O
Ogata S, xv, 3, 177, 239, 228, 255
Oman, 74, 83
Operational efficiency, 109
Oral rehydration therapy, 74, 265
Organization for Economic Cooperation and Development (OECD), 73, 78
Orphaned diseases, 8, 73, 79
Oslo, xiii
OXFAM, 30, 275

P
Pakistan, 95, 273
Pan American Health Organization, 69, 168, 178
Panama, 92
Pandemic diseases, 234, 237, 241
Papua New Guinea, 146, 185, 188, 198, 202, 206
Paraguay, 194, 206
Paralysis of government, 8
Partner violence, 193, 197, 207
Partners In Health, xiii
Pathogen, 90, 104, 108, 115–116, 122
Perinatal death, 197
Peru, xiii, 8, 40, 74, 146, 194–195, 207
Pervasive threat, 125, 166, 168
Pharmaceutical companies, 78–79, 148–149, 151, 153–155
Philippines, 188, 194, 233, 243–246, 248–252, 254
Physical abuse, 206
Plague, 8–9, 91, 94, 103, 108, 112–113, 141, 145, 147
Plutocratic system, 49
Polio, 245
Political marginalization, 53, 238, 265
Political repression, 165
Political security, 165, 181, 236, 240, 253
Political stability, 148, 242, 247, 295
Political structures, 148, 241
Population growth, 96, 147–148
Population health, 6, 50, 211, 214, 221–222

Portugal, 104, 146
Post-conflict, xviii, 20–22, 24–26
Poverty alleviation, ix, 77, 258, 267, 269, 276
Poverty eradication, 236
Poverty reduction, vii, 220, 246, 274
Poverty, vii, ix, xvii–xviii, xxi–xxii, 5, 9–10, 27, 44, 53, 62, 64, 68, 77–78, 88, 101, 112, 130–132, 143, 152, 155, 165, 182, 186, 190–191, 193, 195, 199, 206, 210, 220–221, 227, 229, 231, 234, 236–237, 246, 251, 258, 260, 262–265, 267, 269, 271–279, 282, 298–299
Premarital relationships, 189
Premature death, xvii, 78, 147, 197, 213
Preventable death, 243
Prevention programs, 142, 144–145, 154, 188
Prevention strategies, viii, 27, 119, 155, 199
Preventive action, xviii
Preventive care, 279
Primary care, 207, 244
Protection of civilian human rights, 23
Providing, 17, 25, 32, 78, 148, 162, 184, 246, 248, 266, 279–280, 282, 291–292, 295, 297
Psalm, 125
Psychological abuse, 192, 198
Psychological harm, 161, 192
Public health infrastructure, 9, 96, 116
Public opinion, 36, 54, 62, 211
Puerto Rico, 194, 206

Q
Quality of health care, 245, 277, 285, 294
Quality of life, 127, 154, 191

R
Racism, 53
Racist ideology, 41
Random violence, 164, 174
Ranson MK, xi, xxiii, 277, 287–288, 297, 300
Rape, xxi, 6, 144, 151, 163, 169, 174–175, 196, 201, 206
Rapid response, 113
Rate of infection, 150
Reemerging infectious diseases, 111

Refugee, 17, 25, 174
Relief agencies, 25
Relief convoys, 18
Relief efforts, 7
Relief operations, 28, 261
Religious conflict, 237
Religious strife, 235
Reproduction, xxi, 119, 133–136, 177, 200, 228
Reproductive health, ix, 64, 167, 197, 205–206
Reproductive ill health, 186
Resource allocation, 214, 230, 266
Resource mobilization, 280
Rethinking human security, 12, 229, 253
Rift Valley fever, 93, 107
Risk assessment, 207, 210, 222, 225–228
Risk factor, 182, 210, 213, 218–220
Rural credit, 276
Russia, 120, 137, 143, 196
Rwanda, 5, 17, 23–24, 30, 197

S
Safe sex, 189–190
Salmonella, 93
San Salvador, 168
Sanitary diseases, 34, 37
SARS, xvii, xx, 67, 71, 75, 80–81, 100, 106, 108, 110, 115
Saudi Arabia, 230
Satcher D, 145, 156
Scarlet fever, 58
Schistosomiasis, 94, 99, 245
Securitization of health, 240
Securitization, 240, 251, 254
Security challenges, viii, 166, 176, 234, 236, 254
Security paradigm, 176, 240, 247
Security policies, xxii–xxiii, 239
Security threat, 9, 72, 87, 106, 109, 111, 116, 141, 157, 162, 168
Sen A, xv, 3, 12, 15, 28, 33, 38, 50, 62, 65, 184, 202, 255
Senegal, 107, 119, 153
September 11, 4–5, 11, 32, 53, 105, 238
Serial partners, 153
SEWA, viii, xi–xii, xxiii, 277–287, 289–299
Sex industry, 190, 196

Sex selection, 185, 202
Sex workers, 135, 144, 151, 189
Sexual activity, 98, 201
Sexual assault, 195
Sexual behavior, 71, 144, 188–189
Sexual violence, 17, 25, 164, 193,
    195–198, 205, 207
Sexually transmitted disease (STD),
    156
Shibuya K, xii, xxii, 209
Shisana O, xii, xxi, 82, 141
Shisana W, xii, xxi, 82, 141
Sierra Leone, 115, 127–128, 196, 207
Simian immunodeficiency viruses, 93,
    103
Slum neighborhoods, 261
Smallpox, 8, 42, 58–59, 105, 112, 116,
    141
Social anthropology, ix
Social capital, xiii, 35, 38–39, 42, 45–
    47, 50, 52, 257–260, 263, 265,
    271–274
Social development, ix, 135, 164
Social justice, 68
Social mores, 89, 144
Social reproduction, xxi, 133–136
Social services, 39, 76
Social values, 75, 211
Social violence, 174
Sociocultural, 153, 246, 262
Socioeconomic, 4, 77, 88, 93, 135,
    137, 152, 164, 168, 173, 182, 187,
    193, 201, 206, 210, 213–215, 220,
    275–276
Sociological literature, 259
Solidarity networks, 277
Somalia, 18, 29, 130
South Africa, xii, xiv, 18, 63, 88, 111,
    120, 126–128, 130, 132, 137–138,
    142, 144, 146–150, 152–154, 157–
    158, 169, 179, 190, 241
South Asia, xxii, 51, 260
Southeast Asia, xxii, 40, 100, 106,
    142, 185, 236–238, 248, 253, 296
Southeast Asian Security Cooperation,
    253, 255
Southern Africa Development Commu-
    nity (SADC), 139, 142, 144–145,
    148
Spain, 156–157, 178
Spread of AIDS, 62
Spread of infectious diseases, xx, 89,
    96, 113, 122

Sri Lanka, 273
State security, 11, 62, 108, 234, 240,
    255
State sovereignty, 110, 168, 175–176
State stability, 109–110
Strategic partnerships, 266
Street vendors, 281
Streptococcus pneumoniae, 90, 95, 97,
    104
Støre JG, xiii, xix, 67
Sub-Saharan Africa, x, xvii, xx, 9, 68,
    87–88, 106–109, 111, 125, 129,
    136, 141–143, 148, 153, 156, 166,
    187, 191, 213, 218
Sudan, 11, 115, 146
Suez Canal, 49
Sustainability, 80–81, 277, 280, 293
Sustainable basis, 151
Sustainable development, xviii, 12, 77,
    264
Swaziland, 88, 142, 148, 150
Sweatshop labor, 196
Sweden, 78, 205
Switzerland, xv, 29, 83, 194, 201, 203,
    206
Szreter S, xiii, xix, 31, 50–52, 83

T
Tanzania, 185, 195, 202
Target populations, 297
Terror, xviii, 17, 87, 102, 105, 112,
    115, 220, 264
Terrorism, 4, 26, 53, 62, 122, 165,
    174, 178, 237–238, 241, 261
Thailand, 189, 194–196, 207, 237,
    242, 249–250
Theories of human welfare, 209
Thompson T, 148
Threat assessment, 15
Tobacco, viii, xxi–xxii, 76, 84, 110,
    210, 219–221, 224, 278
Trafficking, xxii, 169, 193, 195–196,
    207, 237
Transitional states, 173
Transmission mechanisms, 41
Transmission of blood, 103
Transmission of infections, 95
Transmission of virus, 99
Transnational contagion, 121
Transnational problems, 176
Tuberculosis, xi, xiii, xv, 8–9, 36, 63,
    72, 74, 79–80, 87, 90, 95, 97–98,
    100, 107, 110–111, 118, 123, 134–

135, 148–149, 155, 186, 230, 234, 241, 254, 266, 268–269, 283
Tularemia, 91–92
Turkey, 184, 194, 206
Types of violence, 161, 192
Typhoid fever, 58

U
Uganda, 115, 142, 146, 151, 153, 157–158, 178, 184, 186, 194, 204, 206, 221
Ukraine, 196
UN Human Security Trust Fund, xvi
UN indices, 15
UN Security Council, 9, 72, 111, 121, 138
UNAIDS, 80, 120, 128, 143, 146, 148, 150, 155–157, 187–188, 191, 202–204, 229
Unarmed refugees, 24
Unavoidable health crises, 6
Undernourished, 262
Underreported, 195, 198
Unilateral approach, 79
United Nations, viii, xvi, 3, 9, 12, 28–30, 64, 83, 103, 114, 123, 137, 141, 144, 154, 156, 164, 177, 180, 192, 202–204, 207, 228–230, 234, 254, 275
United Nations Children's Fund (UNICEF), 78, 157, 187, 207
United Nations Development Program (UNDP), xvi, 9, 12, 28, 74, 78, 156, 164–165, 181, 201, 203, 234–235, 253–255, 258, 275
United Nations General Assembly Special Session on HIV/AIDS (UNGASS), 192
United Nations High Commission for Refugees (UNHCR), 144, 156, 174, 180
United Nations Population Fund (UNFPA), 207
United Nations Security Council, 30, 141, 154, 230
United States, xi, xiii, xvii, xix, 91, 102, 119, 121–122, 128, 138, 169, 194, 196, 206–207, 238–239
United States Indonesia Society (USINDO), 255
Urban slum, 169
Urban violence, 168, 178–179

Urban yellow fever, 107, 112
U.S. global leadership, 121

V
Vaccination, 103, 110, 167
Vaccine
    Vaccine delivery, 99
    Vaccine development, 153
    Vaccine initiatives, 79
    Vaccine price, 119
    Vaccine shortages, 112
    Vaccine stocks, 107
Vector-borne infections, 92, 97, 120
Victimization, 178, 207
Victims of terrorism, 241
Victims of violence, 168–169
Vietnam, 115, 196, 249–250
Vimo SEWA, xi–xii, 277–287, 289–295, 297–298
Violence prevention, xi, 179
Violence, ix–xi, xv, xvii–xviii, xxi, 4–6, 9–10, 12, 14, 16–20, 23, 25, 27, 29, 36, 46, 52, 54, 59–60, 71, 127, 144, 159, 161–179, 181–183, 186, 189–200, 202, 204–209, 216–218, 220, 227, 235–236, 238, 247, 251, 265, 270–271
Violent conflicts, 227, 238
Violent death, 164, 176
Violent relationships, 184
Viral pathogens, 92
Virus, 8–9, 67, 90–92, 94, 98–100, 102–103, 105–108, 112, 115, 120, 137–138, 143, 150, 203, 241
Voices of children, 157
Voices of the Poor, 10, 12, 238, 255, 258, 273

W
War-related disabilities, 218
Warring factions, 196
Warring parties, 13, 18, 22–23
Weapon of terror, xviii
Welch J, xiii, xix, 67
Welfare economics, 225, 230
Welfare expenditures, 172
Welfare state, 32, 37, 43–44, 55, 300
West Nile virus, 91, 99–100, 102, 107, 112, 120
Wife-beating, 205–206
Wilson ME, xiii, xx, 82, 87
Women's empowerment, ix, 200, 203, 276

Women's fear, 184
Women's insecurity, 181
Women's productivity, 197
Women's reproductive health, 197
Women's vulnerability, 193
World Bank, vii, 10, 12, 47, 60, 63, 78, 137, 147, 150, 179, 202, 237–238, 255, 258, 273–276, 279, 298–300
World disasters, 29
World Health Assembly, 71, 83–84, 113, 119, 122
World Health Organization (WHO), viii–xiii, xv, xx, 10, 12, 57, 59, 64, 68, 83–84, 101, 103–104, 113, 119–120, 122, 138, 143, 161, 164, 177–179, 194–195, 200, 202–204, 207, 211–213, 215–217, 219–220, 223, 228–230, 254, 299–300

World Health Report, 12, 74, 84, 101, 166, 178, 184, 202, 229–230, 249–250, 299

Y
Yellow fever, 58, 62, 107, 112, 115, 119
Yemen, 115
Youth violence, 179

Z
Zaire, 24, 29, 204
Zambia, 88, 128, 150, 154
Zero tolerance attitude, 200
Zone of protection, 21
Zungu-Dirwayi N, xiv, xxi, 82, 141